FIFTH EDITION

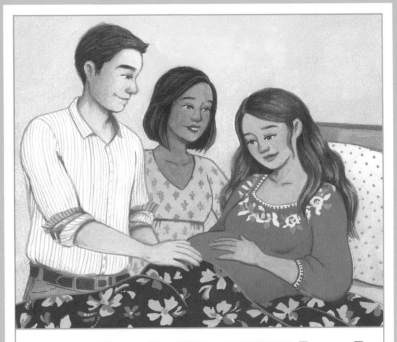

THE **BIRTH PARTNER**

A COMPLETE GUIDE TO CHILDBIRTH FOR DADS,
DOULAS, AND OTHER LABOR COMPANIONS

PENNY SIMKIN, P.T.
WITH KATIE ROHS

HARVARD
COMMON
PRESS

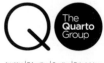

The
Quarto
Group

Inspiring | Educating | Creating | Entertaining

Brimming with creative inspiration, how-to projects, and useful information to enrich your everyday life, quarto.com is a favorite destination for those pursuing their interests and passions.

Copyright © 2018 by Penny Simkin
Cover illustration © 2018 by Lola and Bek
This edition first published in 2018 by The Harvard Common Press,
an imprint of The Quarto Group,
100 Cummings Center, Suite 265-D, Beverly, MA 01915, USA.
T (978) 282-9590 F (978) 283-2742 Quarto.com

The Harvard Common Press titles are also available at discount for retail, wholesale, promotional, and bulk purchase. For details, contact the Special Sales Manager by email at specialsales@quarto.com or by mail at The Quarto Group, Attn: Special Sales Manager, 100 Cummings Center, Suite 265-D, Beverly, MA 01915, USA.

22 10

ISBN: 978-1-55832-910-2

Digital edition published in 2018
eISBN: 978-1-55832-911-9

Originally found under the following Library of Congress Cataloging-in-Publication Data
Simkin, Penny with Katie Rohs
The birth partner : a complete guide to childbirth for dads, doulas, and all other labor companions / Penny Simkin
pages cm
ISBN 978-1-55832-819-8 (pbk.)
1. Pregnancy. 2. Natural childbirth--Coaching. 3. Labor (Obstetrics)—Complications. 4. Childbirth. I. Title.
RG525.S5829 2013
618.2—dc23
2013007371

Photographs by Shutterstock (pages 19 and 60) and Patti Ramos (pages 236 and 363)
Cover illustration by Susie So
Drawings by Gayle Isabelle Ford; except pages 115, 174 (top left), 176, 177 (middle), 194, 249 (left), 252, 259, 350, and 378 by Dolly Sundstrom
Cover and text design by Laura H. Couallier, Laura Herrmann Design
Page layout by Tabula Rasa

Printed in China

Dedication

Contents

PREFACE   8

ACKNOWLEDGMENTS   13

HOW TO USE THIS BOOK   16

A NOTE TO DOULAS   18

PART ONE Before the Birth   19

1. The Last Weeks of Pregnancy   20

What Kind of Birth Partner Will You Be   21
Getting Ready for Labor   23
Preparing for Life with the Baby   51
On to the Next Step . . .   59

PART TWO Labor and Birth   60

2. Getting into Labor   62

The Difference Between Prelabor and Labor   63
How Long Will Labor Last?   66
Signs of Labor   67
If the Bag of Waters Breaks Before Labor Begins   71
"False" Labor, or Prelabor   72
Labor Progresses in Six Ways   74
Timing Contractions   77

3. Moving Through the Stages of Labor   81

Compare Labor to Running a Marathon   82
Prelabor   85
The Dilation, First, Stage   90
Early Labor   92
Getting into Active Labor (3 to 5 Centimeters Dilation)   99
Active Labor   102
Transition   109

The Birthing, Second, Stage   116

The Resting Phase   117

The Descent Phase   121

The Crowning and Birth Phase   127

The Placental, Third, Stage   131

The Recovery and Bonding, Fourth, Stage   135

Normal Labor—in a Nutshell   138

4. Comfort Measures for Labor   143

Pain versus Suffering   144

The Three Rs: Relaxation, Rhythm, and Ritual   147

Self-Help Comfort Measures   153

Comfort Aids and Devices   176

Comforting Techniques   187

Taking Care of Yourself   197

Checklist of Comfort Measures for Labor   198

5. Strategies for Challenging Variations in Normal Labor   201

The Take-Charge Routine   202

On-the-Spot Coaching (When You Have Had No
    Childbirth Classes)   206

The Very Rapid Labor   207

The Emergency Delivery   209

When Labor Must Start (Labor-Stimulating Measures)   212

The Slow-to-Start Labor   216

Slow Progress in Active Labor and the Birthing Stage—
    with or without Back Pain   221

When the Birthing Person Must Labor in Bed   224

A Breech Baby   226

A Previous Disappointing or Traumatic Birth Experience   231

Incompatibility with the Nurse or Caregiver   233

PART THREE The Medical Side of Childbirth   236

Key Questions for Informed Decision-Making   237

6. Tests, Technologies, Interventions, and Procedures   239

Late-Pregnancy Tests   240

Essential Observations During Labor   243

Conditions Influencing the Use of Intervention
During Labor   245

Common Obstetric Interventions   246

7. Complications in Late Pregnancy, Labor, or Afterward   270

Complications for the Pregnant Person   272

Complications with Labor Progress   285

Complications with the Fetus   290

Complications in the Placental Stage   295

Complications with the Newborn   297

After It Is All Over   303

8. Medications for Pain During Labor   304

Management of Normal Labor without Pain Medications   305

What You Both Need to Know About Pain Medications   307

Know How the Birthing Person Feels About Using
Pain Medications   326

9. Cesarean Birth and Vaginal Birth After Cesarean   340

Know the Nonmedical Reasons for Cesarean Birth
and Factors to Consider   341

Know the Medical Reasons for Cesarean Birth   343

Know What to Expect During Cesarean Birth   346

Your Role During and After a Cesarean Birth   353

Vaginal Birth After Cesarean (VBAC) and
Trial of Labor after Cesarean (TOLAC)   356

PART FOUR After the Birth   363

10. The First Days Postpartum   364

The First Few Hours   364
The First Few Days for the Baby   376
The First Few Days for the Birthing Parent   382
Homecoming   387
After a Home Birth   388
Getting Help and Advice   389
Postpartum Emotions   390
What About Your Feelings   392
Practical Matters at Home   394

11. Getting Started with Feeding Your Baby   400

Reasons for Breast-Feeding/Chest-Feeding   401
Getting Off to a Good Start   403
How to Offer Support Related to Infant Feeding
Early Concerns   405
When to Give the Baby a Bottle   414
Once Breast-Feeding/Chest-Feeding Is Established   416

PARTING WORDS   417
RECOMMENDED RESOURCES   418
INDEX   428

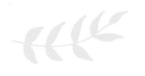

Preface

I'D LIKE TO EXPLAIN WHAT LED ME TO WRITE THIS BOOK, now in its fifth edition. The first edition was published in 1989, after I learned some truths about what it means to give birth and what it means to be a birth partner who deeply loves the person giving birth. One of these truths is this: how one gives birth matters to one's self-confidence and self-esteem, to the baby's long-term health, and to one's relationships with their partner, baby, and other loved ones.

This is as true today, with this fifth edition, as it was in 1989 and for generations (even millennia) before.

Here's another very important truth: how a person is cared for and supported during birth is a major influence, not only in how they give birth but also in how they feel about the birth for years to come. Yet, medical care before and during childbirth focuses almost exclusively on the *physical safety* of the baby and birthing person and places little emphasis on their emotional well-being, relationship with the partner, and readiness to parent. Such matters are given low priority in our very expensive health care system, which is beset by nursing shortages, pressure to increase the use of medical and surgical interventions while increasing efficiency, reduction of psychosocial support services, threats of malpractice lawsuits, and other factors that work against personalized, flexible, family-centered care.

I learned the importance of emotional care during labor when, in the late 1980s, I conducted a study of people's long-term memories of their experiences giving birth to their first child. These people had attended childbirth classes I taught between 1968 and 1974. They had sent me their birth stories shortly after giving birth. For my study, I contacted some of those people fifteen to twenty years later and asked them two things: to write their birth stories again as they remembered them and to rate their satisfaction as they looked back on their childbirth experiences.

In comparing the two stories from each person, I was astounded at how clearly they remembered their birth experiences and how consistent they were with their original stories, despite the intervening years! As we did not have copy machines in those days and they had not written their stories for themselves after the births, I possessed the only stories (which I photocopied and returned to them at the end of the study!). I then interviewed each person and discovered they had detailed memories of their doctors and nurses (there were no midwives practicing in my area at that time). Everyone vividly remembered specific things done and said to them. Many could quote the exact words! Some actually wept as they recalled some of these things—either with joy over the kindness and care they received or with sadness or anger over being treated disrespectfully or thoughtlessly.

Briefly, those who felt they had been well cared for by the professional staff reported the highest satisfaction, even if the labors had been long or complicated. Those who felt they had been treated disrespectfully or ignored reported the least satisfaction. Also, those who reported a great sense of accomplishment in giving birth were the most satisfied. They felt they had been in control and that the birth experience had been good for their self-esteem. The less satisfied women did not have these positive feelings.

The presence of husbands or other loved ones was unusual because, at the time, it was not customary for men, or even female relatives, to attend childbirth classes or the births of their babies. In fact, my classes were part of two emerging radical trends: unmedicated natural childbirth and the presence of husbands (with the marriage certificate to prove it!) to attend the births of their babies and assist their wives in giving natural births. The classes encouraged men to take the role of "coach" for the birthing person, and most played as active a role as they were allowed, although they were often required to leave the labor or delivery room for long periods.

The women's memories of their husbands were also clear and detailed. Here are quotations from some of the women:

"He was the only reason I got through it."

"It was one of the finer moments in our life and relationship."

"He was more patient and took it more seriously than I expected."

"He's a competitor. He was my coach. It was a very big deal for him."

"It hurt him to see me in pain."

"He could feel me tense immediately."

"He was there 100 percent."

"He was apprehensive, but wanted to be there."

I learned from that study that birthing persons need and appreciate loving, familiar people to stay with them, help them, and share the birth—one of life's most meaningful moments. The kind of professional care and emotional support they receive during labor largely influences how they look back on the birth experience—with satisfaction and fulfillment or with disappointment, sadness, and even anger. I realized, in this age of high-tech, high-pressure obstetrics, it is unrealistic to expect busy nurses, doctors, and even hospital-based midwives to provide continuous individualized emotional and physical comfort throughout labor and birth, along with all their other clinical responsibilities and other laboring patients.

The conclusions from my study (published in 1991 and 1992 in two parts, titled *Just Another Day in a Woman's Life?*) have been confirmed time and again by other studies of long-term memories of one's birthing experience. During the hundreds of births I have attended as a doula and with the thousands of expectant parents who have attended my childbirth classes, I have always been guided by the question, "How will they remember this?" That study prompted me to write the first edition of this book. I wanted to help partners feel more knowledgeable and confident in their support role, so their laboring loved ones would always appreciate the help.

This study helped convince me that laboring people, as well as their partners, need trained doulas to provide continuous emotional support, reassurance, and comfort throughout childbirth. I developed a training program for doulas in 1988, and with other doula advocates, founded the Seattle-based Pacific Association for Labor Support (now called PALS Doulas) and in 1992, with pediatrician/researchers, Marshall Klaus and John Kennell, psychotherapist Phyllis Klaus, and health administrator Annie Kennedy, founded the international organization Doulas of North America, now DONA International. Our goal was to ensure childbearing women get the kind of care they need and their partners the kind of practical guidance and tools they need during this challenging and unforgettable time. Extensive published research (by Klaus, Kennell, and many others) has demonstrated that the doula fills a gap in maternity care and provides benefits in medical outcomes as well as fulfillment and satisfaction as the mother or parents define it. (See Recommended Resources, page 418, for more on the benefits of doulas at birth.)

When it was time to publish the third edition of *The Birth Partner*, we realized the book had become popular with birth doulas. I decided to add extensive material for and about the doula's role during and after birth, to guide doulas and also inform parents on how doulas and partners work together with hospital staff to provide excellent support to the childbearing woman.

About the Fifth Edition

This fifth edition builds on the previous editions with updated information, added comfort measures, and new illustrations. The two major purposes in writing this book have not changed: to give readers—birth partners, doulas, pregnant people, and others—clarity, confidence, excitement, and joy about the upcoming birth of a very special child and to ensure that laboring people are not left in the care of strangers, with loved ones standing by, feeling anxious, uncomfortable, and uncertain of ways to be helpful.

Typically today, childbearing people are cared for by maternity professionals whom they hardly know or have never met. During the span of one labor, with shifts and breaks and the staff's need to look after more than one patient at a time, the laboring person will meet and adjust to numerous different professionals. This model, "care by strangers," has evolved from a need by hospitals to maintain efficiency and contain runaway costs, but sadly often results in families feeling disappointed, or even traumatized, after childbirth. While unexpected complications and extra-challenging labors cannot always be prevented, if a person is cared for with respect and kindness during such times, they are less likely to have these negative feelings and their emotional recovery is smoother and faster. Being attended by known and trusted caregivers and support people helps. Therefore, I hope to improve the chances that each laboring person will receive continuous attention, respect, and nurturing from those who accompany them in labor. I want every birthing person to be able to look back on their birth experience with the feeling of being well cared for, no matter how the labor and birth proceeded.

Introducing Katie Rohs as Coauthor for the Fifth Edition

I asked Katie Rohs to join me as coauthor in updating and adding new content for this fifth edition. As an experienced childbirth educator, a sought-after doula, an independent thinker, and an emerging leader in our field, Katie provides the fresh perspective of one who is closer to the action than I. As I age and step back from direct "in-the-trenches" involvement as a doula, I rely on Katie and other colleagues to challenge me and keep me up to date. Katie began working in my office in 2012 while parenting her busy twins and starting her career as a doula and childbirth educator. That was serendipitous. Both of us, as active childbirth educators, find our students—expectant parents—are also valuable teachers. Their needs motivate, guide, and inform us.

Katie is the person who championed the use of inclusive gender-neutral language to address the needs and interests of nontraditional families not addressed in previous editions—our nonbinary families—the lesbian, gay, bisexual, transgender, and queer (LGBTQ) communities. We hope this book ignores no one taking part in childbearing—directly or indirectly. As our society shifts toward acceptance and celebration of multiple family configurations, our language falls short of the inclusiveness needed to address everyone's needs. New words and new definitions of old words reflect the fluid nature and meaning of "gender." The language of this edition reflects where we are in 2018. A future edition may reflect more shifting as we are in the midst of rapid change.

—*Penny Simkin*

Acknowledgments

W E HAVE HAD OUR SHARE OF SUPPORT throughout the process of revising this book. We want to thank the following extraordinary people who have made it possible for us to accomplish this in the midst of our busy lives: Two people in Penny's office have been extremely helpful: Kathy Wilson has kept the office running smoothly, kept track of finances, paid the bills, handled sales and shipping, and supported Penny's birth classes, all while continuing her own career as a childbirth and parenting educator; Dolly Sundstrom, who has many talents, provided new drawings for this edition, helped with updating our Recommended Resources (page 418), and kept Penny's library up to date, all while attending university to become a clinical psychologist. Both brighten the office with their competence and good cheer!

Penny's colleagues and friends at the Simkin Center for Allied Birth Vocations at Bastyr University have challenged her to provide more culturally sensitive education. She is particularly grateful to Annie Kennedy, Carrie Kenner, Sharon Muza, Teri Shilling, Kim James, and Laurie Levy.

The Pacific Association for Labor Support, DONA International, and Great Starts Birth and Family Education, a program of Parent Trust for Washington Children, share our values and play an important role in our professional lives, as we follow our passion. Thanks especially to Linda McDaniels, associate director of Parent Trust, for her continuing support and inspiration.

We also want to acknowledge our dedicated and talented fellow board members of PATTCh (Prevention and Treatment of Traumatic Childbirth), who recognize the alarming incidence of traumatic birth and join us in seeking ways to prevent it and to treat its potential negative emotional aftermath when it occurs. Our current board, Leslie Butterfield, Annie Kennedy, Phyllis Klaus, Kathy McGrath, Suzanne Swanson, Onion Medina Carillo, Mora Oommen, Sharon Storton, and Kathleen Kendall-Tackett, have come together with us in this cause, which is also one of the causes of this book.

Lisa Hanson, Ph.D., C.N.M., F.A.C.N.M., a wonderful new friend and professor of Midwifery at Marquette University, and Ruth Ancheta, a wonderful old friend, both coauthors with Penny on *The Labor Progress Handbook*. Ruth also holds the copyright for many of the illustrations in both *The Labor Progress Handbook* and *The Birth Partner* and donated them for both books.

Phyllis Klaus, dear friend, mentor, and psychotherapist extraordinaire, and Penny's coauthor of *When Survivors Give Birth: Understanding and Healing the Effects of Early Sexual Abuse on Childbearing Women*.

Shanna Dela Cruz, the artist who drew most of the illustrations in this and previous editions, has been fastidious and reliable. We admire her simplicity, accuracy, and individuation of the people in the illustrations. Dolly Sundstrom has contributed the fine illustrations that are new to this edition.

Joy MacTavish, M.A., I.B.C.L.C., R.L.C., a lactation consultant, updated chapter 11 and assisted with appropriate gender-neutral language. We are very grateful.

Kim James, I.C.C.E., L.C.C.E., B.D.T. (DONA), birth and parenting instructor at Parent Trust for Washington Children, Swedish Doula Program, birth doula skills instructor at Simkin Center for Allied Birth Vocations Bastyr University, for allowing us to use the language about selecting a doula from her website: Doulamatch.net.

Childbirth Graphics, producers of teaching materials for expectant and new parents, has allowed me to use some of their classic drawings.

Molly Kirkpatrick for being Penny's Elder Doula and Katie's Mother Doula.

The birth partners, members of our childbirth classes, who generously shared their personal thoughts for the beginnings of each chapter, have added poignancy and realism to the text.

Bess Simkin, Eva Caldera, Eduardo Caldera, Matt Connell, and Sky Stewart, who read parts of the book and generously provided feedback on readability and appropriateness of the gender-neutral language. Their constructive feedback and encouragement of our attempts to make this book accessible and meaningful to all are very meaningful to us.

Katie thanks Todd, her partner and husband of sixteen years for holding down the fort while she attends families in labor and teaches classes in the evenings and weekends, for being the best #DoulaHusband, and for seeing Katie as an author, long before Katie believed she could do it.

Most importantly, Penny wants to thank Peter, who has been her loving, patient, and accepting partner and husband for six decades, patiently and attentively listening and giving feedback as she has struggled with phrases and concepts throughout the labor and birth of this book and others.

How to Use This Book

*T*he *Birth Partner* is intended to be both a useful guide to prepare you for your role as birth partner and a quick reference during labor. It will be most helpful if you can read the entire book before labor. Then, if there is time, you may want to review parts of it during labor.

There may be times during labor when you need immediate help and want to find something quickly in this book. Anticipating which information you may need on the spot, we have printed such topics with a dark orange background so they will stand out as you fan through the pages. Fan the pages of the book and find those with dark edges. These sections are as follows:

Chapter 1

Supplies to Take to the Hospital or Birth Center (page 33)
Supplies for a Home Birth (page 35)

Chapter 2

Signs of Labor (page 68)
If the Bag of Waters Breaks Before Labor Begins (page 71)
Timing Contractions (page 77)
Early Labor Record (page 79)

Chapter 3

When Do You Go to the Hospital or Settle in for a Home Birth? (page 95)
Normal Labor—in a Nutshell (page 138)

Chapter 4

Positions and Movements for Labor and Birth (page 169)

Checklist of Comfort Measures for Labor (page 198)

Chapter 5

The Take-Charge Routine (page 202)

On-the-Spot Coaching (page 206)

The Emergency Delivery (page 209)

Slow Progress in Active Labor and the Birthing Stage—
    with or without Back Pain (page 221)

Incompatibility with the Nurse or Caregiver (page 233)

Chapter 7

Prolapsed Cord (page 290)

Chapter 8

When Are Pain Medications Used? (page 331)

Chapter 9

Know What to Expect During Cesarean Birth (page 346)

Please also refer to Recommended Resources (see page 418) to find other recommended publications and online resources, including some videos.

A Note to Doulas

This book includes much information on the doula's role before, during, and after birth. Doulas use it as a reference and a guide regarding their role during labor and also how they interact with the birth partner, the laboring person, and the clinical care providers. Both Katie and Penny are experienced doulas (Penny now retired) and strongly believe the doula's role is uniquely different from the roles of loved ones and partners, nurses, midwives, and doctors, even though the roles overlap. Doulas' training is focused on physical comfort measures and ways to enhance labor progress. Their training also includes extensive discussion of the emotional shifts that laboring people experience throughout their labors and how to attune themselves to the changing moods and movements of the laboring person. It may be that doulas reduce stress and fear in laboring people. Those emotions increase stress hormones, which are known to impair labor progress through most of labor. Doulas help people feel safe and less afraid or anxious. They also guide and reassure partners. This nonclinical care can improve clinical outcomes (such as lower cesarean rates, shorter labors, fewer requests for pain medication, greater satisfaction with the birth, and fewer newborns who need extra nursing care).

This book explains the birth process to birth partners and pregnant people and explains the role of the doula throughout the process.

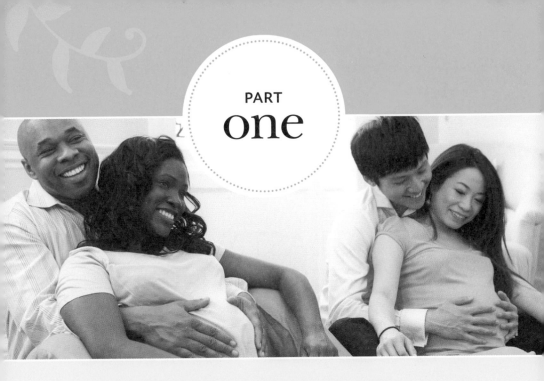

PART
one

BEFORE THE BIRTH

Your role as birth partner begins before the pregnant person is in labor. During the last weeks of pregnancy, you can learn about labor, encourage the pregnant person to continue good health habits, help with last-minute preparations for the baby and for labor itself, and figure out the role you will play as birth partner.

This is also the time for you both to make many important decisions about the birth and to discuss them with the caregiver. If you attend childbirth classes and go to prenatal checkups, you will not only become informed, but also meet the doctors or midwives and become more comfortable in your role. You can also get advice and reassurance about anything causing anxiety or uncertainty for either of you.

During these last weeks, you can prepare for your role through introspection, discussions with the pregnant person, gathering information, and practicing comfort measures.

CHAPTER 1

THE LAST WEEKS OF PREGNANCY

As the third trimester went on, I had a growing sense of wonder. The big day was coming when I would finally meet my daughter. I felt her kicks and saw Janna's belly bump around when we spoke or laughed. But, who was she? What would she be like? I couldn't wait to meet her. My spouse knew she wanted to have the baby naturally. I was worried. I thought, "Why? We have hospitals and medicines to provide comfort. Why turn it away?" She told me she just wanted the right to try. This changed my thinking forever. I would not be a roadblock because she should have the right to try to do what her body was designed to do.

—SCOTT, FIRST-TIME FATHER

Early in pregnancy, it seems that nine months are forever and there is plenty of time to do everything that has to be done. It is all too easy, especially for busy people, to postpone "getting into" the pregnancy. Now, suddenly, the baby is almost due. Time has flown by. As the pregnant person's birth partner, you realize you are being counted on you to help them through childbirth. Do you feel ready? Can you help? What do you know about labor? Do you know what to do when? What should you do now to get ready for the baby? The last months of pregnancy are a perfect time to learn these things, but you had better start right away—a month or two before the due date is truly the "last minute," especially as many babies arrive early. This first chapter is basically a checklist of things to do before labor starts, to help ensure the two of you will work well together during labor and birth.

What Kind of Birth Partner Will You Be?

Birth partners come in all shapes and sizes, and they help the laboring person in any number of ways. Most often, the birth partner is the baby's father or co-parent and/or the pregnant person's husband, wife, life partner, or lover. The birth partner may also be the pregnant person's mother, sister, or friend.

A doula is another kind of birth partner, one becoming more popular in North America. The number of doulas is increasing rapidly, especially in cities, although doulas are still in short supply in some areas. Sometimes, the doula is the pregnant person's only birth partner, but more often, the doula helps both the laboring person and birth partner. The doula is an experienced guide and support person to the pregnant person or expectant couple. (See the description of the doula's role on pages 25 through 28.) In this book, you will learn how doulas can help you and the pregnant person in the variety of labor situations you may encounter.

The role played by the birth partner varies according to many personal factors and the nature of the partner's relationship with the pregnant person. What role will *you* play? What role does the pregnant person want you to play? How much effort do the two of you want to put into learning about childbirth and practicing comfort measures? How actively does the pregnant person want to participate in decision-making, in managing labor pain, in helping the labor progress well, and in delivering the baby? Does the pregnant person prefer a more natural birth or a more medical birth?

If natural birth, both of you should acquire a basic understanding of childbirth, learn the techniques for managing pain, and plan realistically for the challenges of labor. You should expect birth to be challenging, demanding, and also fulfilling and also feel capable of meeting the challenges with help, guidance, and encouragement from the medical and support teams. The pregnant person should plan to rely more on inner strength, coping skills, and the support team and less on drugs and procedures to get through labor and give birth.

If the pregnant person prefers or needs (because of health concerns) a more medical birth, they will need to rely more on the doctor or midwife to make decisions, to use drugs and procedures to control the progress and pain of labor, and to deliver the baby.

How Will You Feel?

For a realistic idea of the situations and feelings you may encounter as a birth partner, ask yourself these questions. How will I feel if or when the pregnant person:

Asks me to take time off to go to prenatal appointments together?

Tells me we are signed up for 12 to 18 hours of childbirth classes?

Asks me to read this book or others?

Wakes up moaning every 10 to 20 minutes during the night thinking it's labor, and I am very tired?

Has a gush of water from the vagina followed immediately by long, painful contractions in the abdomen?

Does not accept my suggestions for relaxation or coping?

Needs my help with every contraction, but I am tired or hungry?

Asks me if we should go to the hospital?

Makes distressing sounds I have never heard?

Expresses discouragement ("This is so hard," "I can't keep on," "How much longer?" "Don't make me do this")?

Clings to me and says, "Help me!"?

Vomits or needs to vomit?

Is in pain and begins to cry, grimaces, and becomes very tense?

Criticizes me ("Not like that," "Don't touch me," "Don't breathe in my face," "Don't leave me")?

Needs me to press hard on their back with every contraction, until my arms ache?

Tells me, "I want an epidural."?

Has a labor that goes on for 12, 18, or 24 hours and still no baby, and I am so tired I can't keep my eyes open, but they need me?

Is told a cesarean will be necessary?

Hears the caregiver say, "Look here! The baby's head is starting to come . . . ?"

Feels and sees the baby slide out, wrinkled, soaking wet, streaked with blood, and crying lustily?

Asks if I want to cut the cord?

Hands me the little, squirming, bundled baby to hold and cuddle?

Looks at me and says, "I couldn't have done it without you."?

Although no answer is right or wrong, your role as birth partner is affected by the pregnant person's preferred approach to labor and birth and your comfort with those choices. Does the pregnant person have thoughts about what they want and need from you? Do you feel able and eager to meet those needs?

All these questions may be impossible to answer right now. But keep them in mind as you read this book and start discussing them with the pregnant person. Start imagining them in labor and the challenges you may face as the birth partner.

Use the exercise "How Will You Feel?" as a reality check. This book will help you prepare for such situations and plan good strategies to handle them. By the time labor begins, you should have a much clearer and more confident picture of yourself as birth partner.

Getting Ready for Labor

If you haven't already done the things described in the following pages, try to do so a few weeks before the due date or at least before labor starts.

Visit the Pregnant Person's Caregiver (Doctor or Midwife)

If you have not yet met the caregiver, this visit may be more important than you think—for both you and the caregiver. Even a brief meeting helps establish for the caregiver that you are an important person in the pregnant person's life. Although a substitute caregiver (another partner in the group practice) may actually attend the birth, this meeting still provides you the opportunity to ask questions, get a feel for what doctors and midwives do, and play a more active role.

Visit the Hospital or Out-of-Hospital Birth Center

Take a tour of the hospital maternity area—triage (the room where people go when they first arrive in labor) is usually where a nurse decides whether to admit patients to the hospital, birthing rooms, waiting room, nursery, kitchen, and postpartum rooms. You'll see much of the equipment used during labor. They do not usually visit operating rooms (where cesareans are done) on the tour but may show slides and describe them. You can find out when tours are available by calling the hospital. Sometimes, a tour is included in childbirth classes, or you can attend a regularly scheduled tour. Ask your caregiver how to make arrangements. This is a good time to ask questions about the hospital's usual way of doing things and any choices they offer for labor management.

Birth centers are smaller and have fewer rooms than hospitals: labor, birth, and the first hours afterward are spent in the same room. Birth centers also have fewer protocols and less equipment, but it is still important to visit and learn the usual practices in the birth center.

On the way to the tour, figure out your route to the hospital or birth center and how long it takes to get there (during both rush hour and slower traffic times). At the hospital, learn which entrances to use during the day and at night (you may have to use the main entrance during the day and the emergency entrance at night). Entrances to out-of-hospital birth centers are seldom staffed around the clock and are usually locked at night. You arrange to meet your midwife there when you call her to announce labor.

If the pregnant person is planning to give birth at home or in a birth center, be sure to tour the backup hospital so you won't be confused if a transfer becomes necessary during labor.

Preregister at the Hospital

If you're having a hospital birth, you should preregister, which involves obtaining, reading, and signing pre-admission forms and a medical consent form. By registering in advance, you save time and avoid confusion when you arrive with the pregnant person in labor.

Consider Having a Doula Help You Both During Labor

Why consider a doula? Childbirth is intense, demanding, unpredictable, and painful, and it can last for a few hours to 24, 36, or even more. Even if you are well prepared, you and the pregnant person may find it difficult to apply your classroom learning in the real situation. If you are not well prepared, all the challenges of labor are baffling and anxiety producing.

Of course, you will have a nurse and a doctor or midwife who are likely to be kind and caring, but they will probably be very busy with the clinical aspects of the birth, which are their highest priority. Hospital nurses and midwives rarely remain in the room throughout labor, as they have duties outside the room and are often taking care of more than one laboring patient at a time. They work in shifts, so over the course of labor, several different professionals are likely to be involved in each laboring person's care. Doctors rely on the nurses to manage the labor, with phone reports as necessary, and they may briefly visit from time to time and will come if problems arise during labor. And, of course, they are there for the birth.

One of the most positive developments in maternity care is the addition of the birth doula, who guides and supports women and their partners continuously through labor and birth. The doula usually meets with you in advance, is on call for you, arrives at your home or the hospital when you need her, and remains with you continuously, with few breaks, until after the baby is born. The doula is trained and experienced in providing emotional support, physical comfort, and nonclinical advice. They draw on their knowledge and experience as they reassure, encourage, comfort, and empathize with the laboring person. The doula also works with the partner, guiding and assisting you on how to help, suggesting when to use particular positions, the bath or shower, and specific comfort measures.

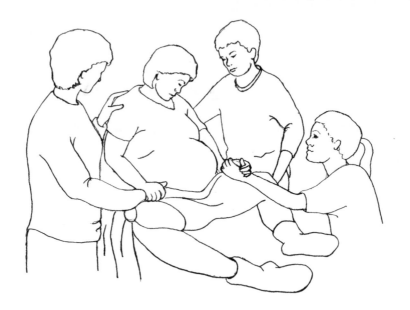

A doula cannot and does not take over your role as the birth partner because you know the birthing person better and love them and the baby as no one else does. But there are many times when the person giving birth needs more than one helper in labor, and the partner needs reassurance, advice, and help, too.

Besides helping the laboring person, a doula can help you in these ways:

- Guide you in applying the information you learned in childbirth class to the more stressful and unpredictable labor situation.

- Relieve you so you can get a meal, a nap, or just a break during a long or all-night labor.

- Bring beverages, hot packs, or ice for the laboring person so you do not have to leave to do so.

- Reassure you if you are worried about the laboring person's well-being. The doula's experience provides perspective, which can keep you from misinterpreting normal reactions to labor as signs that something is wrong or that the laboring person is not coping well.

- Help you understand what the laboring person might be feeling and interpret the signs of labor progress to you.

- Provide support and help you participate more confidently, if you do not feel comfortable as the laboring person's only constant source of support, by making sure the laboring person's needs are met.

- By getting to know the two of you before the birth, the doula can discover your priorities, fears, and concerns and help develop strategies to deal with them.

- Photograph or videotape the two of you during labor and birth or all three (or more!) of you afterward. Check hospital policies on this.

Doulas do not make decisions for you or project personal preferences on you, but rather help you get the information you need to make good decisions. A doula's goal is to help the laboring person have a satisfying birth as they define it.

One partner described the doula this way: "She was like my big sister—ready, willing, and able to help me do the best job I could. She showed me how to rub Mary's back, reminded us to try the lunge (see page 170), and got me a bagel when I was really hungry. She kept encouraging us. She seemed so confident. A lot of the time, both she and I were helping Mary. I was holding her during the contractions, and our doula was pressing on Mary's back and helping her breathe in rhythm. Our doula even gave me a shoulder rub in the middle of the night. She never left except to go to the bathroom. Without her, the birth wouldn't have been as great for both Mary and me. The doula helped me do a better job."

Numerous scientific trials have compared birth outcomes of women who had doulas and those who did not. In very "high-tech" hospitals with high cesarean and induction rates, women attended by doulas had fewer forceps and vacuum-extractor deliveries and fewer cesareans. They did not need to use as much pain medication. Also, women attended by a doula were more likely to report birth experiences that were satisfying versus those who did not have a doula. Although a doula cannot guarantee a normal or an easy labor, statistics show that having a doula results in less need for major labor interventions. Chapter 3 describes what doulas do to help during each phase of labor.

There are many organizations that train and certify birth doulas, with different methods of training and requirements for certification. When choosing your doula, it's important to consider the doula's training. DoulaMatch.net has a comprehensive guide to evaluating doula-certifying organizations, which can help guide your selection.

We agree with DoulaMatch.net's suggestions for choosing a doula trained by a high-quality training organization. They are reprinted here with permission of DoulaMatch (see Recommended Resources, page 418) for more information:

- A comprehensive doula-training program, which includes requirements for in-person classroom work, self-study, and practicum work with minimum hours for each requirement clearly stated.

- Clearly defined requirements for a doula's education.

- Demonstrated doula work experience.

- Good evaluations from clients and health care providers.

- Periodic recertification.

- Documented continuing education.

- A publicly available code of ethics outlining the doula's ethical responsibilities to clients.

- A publicly available standards of practice defining the doula's scope and limits of practice.

- A grievance procedure allowing consumers, colleagues, or care providers to lodge an objection against the organization's doula if they violate the organization's standards of practice or code of ethics. The goal of the grievance procedure is to uncover the facts of the objection and seek resolution for the injured parties or consequences for the doula, including revoking certification.

Costs of doula services vary greatly: In the United States, costs range from a few hundred dollars to as much as $2,500 or more in some large cities depending on the doula's experience. Some hospitals have volunteer or paid doulas available during labor, and some community agencies and charitable organizations employ doulas to care for clients for whom doula costs may be challenging. Some trained doulas offer low-cost services while gaining experience to apply for certification. Others offer free service to people in their own ethnic or religious communities. Some health insurers cover doula fees, and some clients can use health savings accounts to cover doula fees.

Choose and Meet with Your Doula

If you decide to have a doula, it is a good idea to start looking for one a few months before the baby is due; doulas are often fully booked for weeks or months in advance. Get referrals from your care provider, childbirth educator, or friends who have used a doula. You can also contact DONA International (DONA.org) and search their database of certified doulas or try DoulaMatch.net. Most doulas now have personal websites; take time to read their information and select three to four doulas to contact and interview. If the information isn't available on a website, ask whether the doula is available around your due date and what the fee is. If the fee is outside your budget, you can ask for a payment plan or sliding scale fee or ask for a referral to another doula. To ensure a good match, interview the doula in person.

There is usually no charge for the first get-acquainted interview with a doula, which usually lasts an hour or so. This interview is an opportunity for you to get to know the doula and for the doula to get to know you. It is important to choose a doula whose philosophy and approach are congruent with your desires for birth or who can unconditionally support your wishes for the birth. There are many lists online for questions to ask a doula, and we especially like those on the DONA.org website and on DoulaMatch.net. Some topics you might discuss:

- The doula's calendar around the pregnant person's due date (other clients due about the same time, plans to be out of town, unbreakable obligations)

- Backup arrangements (every doula should have reliable backup in case two clients are in labor at the same time, illness, or other unforeseen emergencies)

- The doula's training and certification and the reasons for choosing the training/certification organization

- The support included in the doula's package:

  – Number of prenatal visits

  – Type of postpartum support provided

  – Point at which the doula joins the client in labor

– Time limits for in-person support, including what happens in the case of a long labor

- Type of phone, email, or text support the doula provides

- Payment arrangements and possibility of health insurance or health savings account reimbursement

  Once you choose a doula, carefully read the letter of agreement or contract to make sure it reflects your understanding of the conversation from the interview. Once you've signed an agreement and paid, you will probably meet with the doula at least once more before the birth. During these prenatal visits, you may talk about the following topics:

- Any previous birth experiences the pregnant person has had and ages of older children

- How the pregnancy has progressed and any problems or concerns about it

- Childbirth preparation classes (see page 32)

- The parents' birth plan (see page 45), which the doula can help you prepare, if you wish

- Preferences regarding use of pain medication (see page 327)

- Wishes regarding photographs or video

- Concerns either of you have regarding the birth

- The kinds of things the doula can say or do to comfort and help relax the laboring person

- Things the doula should not say or do because they might bother or stress the laboring person

- How you, the partner, wish to be supported by the doula

- Postpartum plans regarding feeding, sleeping, and support

- The doula's visit to your home after the birth to see the baby, review the birth experience, and see how everyone is doing

- How to reach the doula—day and night

- Arrangements for a backup doula in case she is unavailable when needed; it is desirable, though not always possible, to meet the backup doula as well.

Some doulas offer other services, such as private childbirth preparation, massage, birth-related counseling, placental encapsulation, breast-feeding help, or postpartum doula care (see pages 57 and 389). There usually are additional charges for these services.

Consider an Alternative Support Person

Although doulas are plentiful in many areas in North America, you may not be able to find one locally. Or, you may prefer having a friend or family member play a similar role. To choose the right person, think of the birthing person's needs first. Sometimes, family members or friends assume they will attend the birth without being asked, or they will ask if they can come. It may feel awkward to say no, but if they have never given birth or have fear or a negative attitude about birth, they may be a poor choice. Here are some other things to think about when considering whom to invite to the birth:

- Does this person want to help you?

- Are they available day and night? Can they cancel all obligations on short notice, if necessary?

- Do they have reliable transportation to your home, the birth center, or the hospital?

- Are they patient, optimistic, calm, thoughtful of others, and a good listener?

- What special attributes do they bring, such as a comforting touch or tone of voice, comfort with silence, and a positive attitude toward birth?

- Do they have stamina for a long labor?

- What experience have they had with birth?

- Do they have any annoying habits or mannerisms?

- Do they recognize and accept the importance of this commitment?

In summary, think of what this person can do for the laboring person and for you. Invite this person to come, not just because they want to be there, but because the two of you want them there.

Be Reachable by Phone—Always

You can never know when labor will start and you'll be needed. Both of you should carry a cell phone, charged and turned on, whenever you are not together. If your job takes you far away or out of cell phone range, check in with the pregnant person often and have someone else available when you are not. Make sure that person can be reached at all times, too, and will come to the laborer's aid, night or day, on very short notice.

Review What You Learned in Childbirth Classes

If you have taken classes, review your handouts and notes. Rehearse comfort techniques. Gather the materials you might want to refer to during labor—this book, lists, suggestions, questionnaires, information and instructions about the hospital's services, and copies of the birth plan.

Gather Necessary Supplies

What do you pack for the hospital or birth center? What do you need for a home birth? The following lists should help.

Supplies to Take to the Hospital or Birth Center

From this list, select only those items you and the pregnant person feel will be helpful. Pack as many of these things in advance as possible. Have them on hand for a home birth as well.

For Laboring Person During Labor

☐ Oil or cornstarch for massage

☐ Lip balm

☐ Toothbrush and toothpaste

☐ Hairbrush and comb

☐ Two short gowns or long T-shirts and a robe, if preferred, rather than hospital clothes

☐ Massage device or hot or cold pack to relieve back pain

☐ Ponytail holder, clips, or bobby pins to keep long hair off the face

☐ Warm socks and slippers

☐ Warm blanket or shawl (hospital beds have only very thin cotton covers)

☐ A "labor playlist" of favorite music, including various genres such as relaxing, mellow, with and without lyrics as well as some songs that encourage movement and dance

☐ Personal comfort items (pillow, flowers, pictures)

☐ Favorite juice, frozen juice bars, or an electrolyte-balanced beverage (such as Gatorade or Recharge) in a cooler (most hospitals provide juices, but in limited varieties)

☐ Birth ball (exercise ball or yoga ball), if the facility does not have one

For Birth Partner

☐ Copy of the birth plan (see page 45)

☐ Watch with a second hand, pencil and paper to time contractions, or smartphone with a contraction timer application (see page 77)

☐ Grooming supplies (toothbrush, breath mints, deodorant, shaver)

☐ Snacks, such as sandwiches, fruit, cheese and crackers, and beverages (consider what they will do to your breath). Many hospitals have no food available at night except in vending machines.

☐ Sweater

- ☐ Change of clothes
- ☐ Slippers
- ☐ Swimsuit, so you can accompany the laboring person into the shower or bath, if desired
- ☐ Paper and pencil
- ☐ This book
- ☐ Reading materials, game apps, or handwork, for slow times when your help is not needed
- ☐ Phone numbers of people to call during or after labor
- ☐ Telephone credit card or prepaid telephone card (cell phone use might be allowed only in designated areas of the hospital; check with your hospital if this is needed)
- ☐ Camera (still or video), batteries, charger, etc.
- ☐ Smartphone and charger or computer for sending photos, texts, and messages

For Postpartum Period

- ☐ Gowns that open in front for breast-feeding, unless a hospital gown is preferred
- ☐ Robe and slippers
- ☐ Cosmetics and toilet articles
- ☐ Tasty snack foods such as fruit, nuts, cheese, and crackers
- ☐ Nursing bras
- ☐ Money for incidentals
- ☐ Going-home clothing; stretchy pants, a couple of sizes larger than pre-pregnancy size.

For Baby

- ☐ Clothing for the trip home—regular or snap-crotch undershirt ("onesie"), gown or stretch suit, receiving blanket, outer clothing (hat, warm clothing), and crib-size blanket
- ☐ Properly installed car seat (visit Seatcheck.org or call 1-866-SEAT-CHECK to locate local car seat safety check stations and learn about any car seat recalls)

**For Trip to the Hospital or Birth Center, or
in Event of Transfer During Home Birth**

☐ Full tank of gas

☐ Blanket and pillow in the car

☐ GPS to guide you on the best route to the hospital

Supplies for a Home Birth

Look over the preceding lists for ideas about what to have at home. In addition, ask the midwife for a list of special items you'll need or go over these lists together. She may recommend a source for home-birth supply kits.

Birthing Supplies

Check with your midwife before acquiring these; they may have some available or a source from which you can buy everything you need.

☐ Disposable waterproof underpads (Chux pads)

☐ Sterile 4 X 4-inch (10 X 10 cm) gauze pads

☐ K-Y jelly

☐ Bulb syringe

☐ Cord clamps

☐ Squeeze bottle to cleanse perineum

☐ Waterproof mattress cover (a shower curtain will do)

☐ Wet, folded washcloths placed in plastic bags and frozen

☐ Thermometer

☐ Basin for the placenta

☐ Washcloths, hand towels, and bath towels

☐ At least two sets of clean bed sheets

☐ Flexible straws

☐ Trash bags

☐ Birthing tub, available for rent or purchase, or a kiddie-size swimming pool at least 24 inches (61 cm) deep; ask your midwife, childbirth educator, or doula whether there is a reliable tub rental company in your area or search online for "portable birthing tubs" or "kiddie pools for birth"

Other Supplies

☐ Long, maternity-size sanitary pads

☐ Hat for the baby

☐ Food for the birthing team during labor

☐ Food and drink for a birth celebration

☐ Directions to your home for the midwife and doula
  (provide these well in advance)

For a home birth, you will want to make other preparations at the last minute:

• Turn up the water heater (to allow a long shower in labor) and make sure everyone knows by posting reminders of very hot water at every faucet.

• Clean and organize the house.

• Make the bed with fresh linens (that you don't mind getting stained) in the following way: Put a mattress pad, preferably waterproof, over the mattress. Put a cotton sheet over the mattress pad. Put a second waterproof mattress cover or plastic sheet over the cotton sheet and another cotton sheet over the waterproof cover or sheet. During labor and birth, the top sheet may become stained and wet. After the birth, the top sheet and top waterproof sheet can be quickly removed, and the other clean sheet will already be in place.

In case of transfer to a hospital, know the route, have plenty of gas in your car's tank, and include in the birth plan the pregnant person's preferences in case of transfer (see "Prepare and Review the Birth Plan," page 45).

Encourage the Pregnant Person to Drink Plenty of Fluids and Continue to Eat Well

A pregnant person should drink at least 2 quarts (1.9 L) of liquid a day—including water, fruit juices, and clear soups. This helps support the increased fluid needs during pregnancy. The pregnant person should maintain a well-balanced diet containing plenty of protein, carbohydrates, iron, calcium, vitamins, and a little fat.

Encourage Regular Exercise

Regular exercise, such as walking, prenatal yoga, water aerobics, or swimming, helps maintain or improve a pregnant person's general fitness. Prenatal yoga is especially helpful in enabling relaxation during pain and developing one's inner resources for remaining calm during labor. Encourage the pregnant person to join a class. In addition, you or a friend might take walks or swim with them.

A few special exercises can be particularly helpful during late pregnancy and labor: squatting, pelvic rock on hands and knees (called cat-cow in yoga), and the pelvic floor contraction (Kegel) exercise. These may be taught in childbirth classes. Also, see the following pages for instructions on these exercises. The information on the pelvic floor exercises includes instructions on whether and how to do this exercise.

Squatting

This may be very useful in helping the baby move down during the birthing stage. Ten squats per day, with heels on the floor and support (from you or using two doorknobs) lasting for up to 1 minute each, should increase the pregnant person's comfort and stamina with the position.

> CAUTION: If the pregnant person has joint problems in the ankles, knees, or hips or develops pain in these joints or in the pubic joint (in the middle below the abdomen), do not practice squatting.

A birth stool may give some of the same advantages as squatting, without stressing the joints in the legs. Consult the illustrations (page 174) to see how a partner supports a person while squatting.

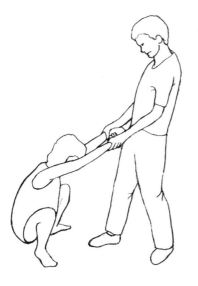 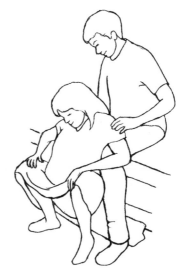

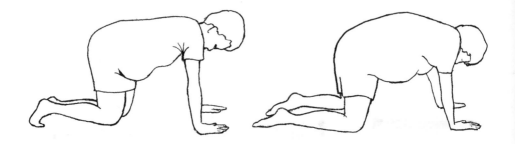

Pelvic Rock on Hands and Knees (Cat-Cow)

During pregnancy, this exercise helps strengthen abdominal muscles, relieve low back pain, and improve circulation in the lower half of the body, (see page 66). During labor, the pelvic rock also helps relieve back pain and position the baby in the favorable OA (occiput anterior) position.

On hands and knees, the pregnant person should tuck the pelvis under while arching the back, for a slow count of five, and then return to normal briefly. While arching, one should feel the abdominal muscles working very hard but should do not hold one's breath. Repeat for a total of ten times per day (see illustrations, page 176).

Pelvic Floor Contractions (Kegels)

Many people (regardless of gender) can benefit from pelvic floor contraction exercises. These strengthen the muscles that support the pelvic organs, improve urinary and bowel control, and help prevent hemorrhoids as well as increase sexual pleasure. During pregnancy, having a good resting tension in the pelvic floor muscles protects against incontinence (involuntary loss of urine or stool) and pelvic organ prolapse. In childbirth, these toned muscles help the baby rotate and descend (see page 76). The laboring person's ability to relax these muscles in childbirth, especially in the second stage as they push the baby down the birth canal, greatly assists the birth. Having established healthy function and control of the pelvic floor muscles before childbirth can help restore function more quickly postpartum.

Because pelvic floor contraction exercises are important for everyone's lifelong general health, we describe the exercise in detail here.

Everyone (regardless of gender or age) performs the exercise in the same way. Contract by squeezing and lifting the pelvic floor muscles upward. Squeeze as you would if trying to keep from urinating or passing

Should Every *Pregnant Person Do Pelvic Floor Contractions, or Kegels?*

There are some people for whom these exercises are not necessary or may even be inappropriate; these are pregnant people with very strong or overactive pelvic floor muscles. This may have been caused by long-time participation in extreme sports or exercise that places high demands on the pelvic floor and increases muscle strength (endurance exercises, dance, etc.). Excessive pelvic tension or pain might also have been caused by pelvic floor trauma (injury, surgery, sexual assault).

For those who suspect they have such a condition, there are ways to do a self-assessment. See Recommended Resources (page 418) for a link to "Pelvic Floor Self-Assessment for Women," by April Bolding, P.T., a well-known physical therapist who specializes in women's health. It explains how to evaluate one's own pelvic floor muscles and can help one figure out if one should focus on strengthening or relaxing these muscles in preparation for birth or otherwise.

gas. Do five to ten quick contractions in a row. Now, hold a contraction for up to 10 seconds. You may find it difficult, at first, to do these longer holds, but your stamina will improve with practice. If the contraction seems to fade when you have not consciously let go, reengage your muscles to tighten again. After 10 seconds, let go and rest. Try another 10-second hold, but this time try not to contract the muscles in your legs, buttocks, or abdomen. Try also to do them without holding your breath.

Do ten 10-second pelvic floor contractions a day. You and the pregnant person can remind each other to do them while riding in the car or bus, waiting in line, or talking on the telephone. Or, do one or two while washing your hands after using the toilet.

Do Some Strengthening Exercises, Too

Labor can be physically demanding for you as well as for the laboring person. A strong partner is invaluable in helping the laboring person change and maintain certain positions (see page 169), and in providing steady pressure on their low back or hips to relieve back pain (see page 194). Furthermore, you will need physical stamina to remain awake and on your feet for hours. If you are not in very good shape, you might want to begin some strength training, particularly for your core, arms, and legs. Push-ups, sit-ups ("crunches"), back and leg strengthening exercises, and weight training will all improve your strength. Search online for videos and articles on these topics.

Prenatal Perineal Massage for the Pregnant Person

Regular massage of the inside of a pregnant person's perineum (the area between the vagina and the anus) in late pregnancy helps prepare them to release tension in their perineum during birth (see illustration, page 65). While the research findings indicate perineal massage reduces the incidence of episiotomy, study results vary on whether it reduces spontaneous tearing. We feel, however, that the greatest value of prenatal perineal massage is in rehearsing the release of tension in the perineum. Prenatal perineal massage lets the expectant person experience sensations similar to those they will feel as the baby descends and emerges and to rehearse relaxing the perineum as they should during the actual birth. This massage does not permanently stretch the vagina.

Some people wish to do the massage; others do not. If the pregnant person wishes to have your help with perineal massage, we suggest you do it several times a week beginning 4 to 6 weeks before the due date. If, after several sessions, they find it quite easy to relax the perineum, even with increasing pressure, you might not need to do it more than twice a week or so; if it is more challenging to relax during the massage, the pregnant person might need to do this more often. Pushing will be less painful if they are able to relax the perineum in response to the stretching sensation.

> CAUTION: If the pregnant person has inflammation, infection, or a herpes sore in or near the vagina, perineal massage should not be done until the problem heals. If either of you has questions about the massage or find it remains painful, consult the midwife or physician or see a physical therapist who specializes in pelvic floor health.

Instructions for Perineal Massage by the Partner

While the pregnant person can do perineal massage to themselves, it might be easier if you do it together. If you decide to do this, it is important to keep clear communication with the pregnant person so they feel relaxed and comfortable with your touch (these directions are for you, the partner):

1. Make sure your fingernails are short. Wash your hands well before beginning. If you have rough skin on your fingers that might scratch sensitive tissue, wear disposable rubber gloves.

2. The pregnant person rests comfortably in a semisitting position, with legs bent and relaxed.

3. Lubricate your index finger with coconut or almond oil, any other vegetable oil you have in your kitchen, or water-soluble jelly.

    Do not use baby oil, mineral oil, or petroleum jelly, as these tend to dry the tissue; vegetable oils are better absorbed. To avoid contaminating the oil in the container, squirt a little over your finger instead of dipping your finger into the oil.

4. Start with one index finger. Place your finger well inside the vagina, beyond your second knuckle. Bend your finger slightly and pull down and out (in the same direction the baby will come out) until the pregnant person feels a slight stinging. Provide time to relax to the stinging sensation. If the pregnant person cannot relax, ease the pressure to the point that relaxation is possible.

5. While maintaining the same pressure, slowly rotate your finger in a U-shaped curve to the left, back to center, and to the right—back and forth for 3 minutes. If you think of six o'clock as straight down, you'll be moving from about four o'clock to about eight o'clock. The pregnant person should concentrate on relaxing the perineum as the pressure is felt.

6. Once they get used to the massage with one finger, use both index fingers at the same time, moving in opposite directions— from six to eight o'clock with your left finger and from six to four o'clock with your right finger.

7. As the massage becomes more comfortable for the pregnant person, increase the pressure just enough to make the perineum begin to sting from the stretching; if they tighten the perineum, reduce the pressure.

8. Ask your caregiver or your childbirth educator to answer any questions you may have after trying the massage.

Perineal massage puts a stretch on the vaginal tissue, the muscles surrounding the vagina, and the skin of the perineum. After doing the massage 3 or 4 days in a row, you will probably find the pregnant person clearly tolerates the stretching better than at first and that you have to increase the pressure to cause stinging. This is a good sign. During the birth, the birthing person will still feel the stretching as an intense stinging sensation, but by then will know how to relax despite the stinging.

Consider Tracking Fetal Movements

Although most babies have no problems during pregnancy, some do, and a major purpose of maternity care is to prevent, detect, or treat such problems. On rare occasions, there is a decline in the placental transfer of nutrients and oxygen from the pregnant person's to the baby's circulation. As a result, the baby's growth or activity may slow. Counting fetal movements sometimes detects such a problem.

An active baby is a healthy baby. If a baby is not getting enough oxygen, it slows its movements to conserve oxygen. There is usually a period of decreasing movement—enough time to act—before the situation becomes serious.

Some caregivers ask all pregnant clients, or at least those at high risk for fetal problems, to keep a daily or every-other-day record of fetal movements from about week 28 of pregnancy. If the caregiver doesn't ask the pregnant person to keep this record, you can decide together whether to count fetal movements on your own.

Many pregnant people find fetal movement counting to be fun, interesting, and reassuring. Not only do they gather helpful information, but they enjoy the time spent focusing on their babies. They learn about different types of movements, their babies' sleep and wake cycles, and other things. Others find fetal movement counting makes them worry, feeling they are just waiting for something to go wrong.

If the pregnant person decides to count fetal movements, do it together, at least some of the time. You can learn a lot about the baby, too, and offer support if it creates stress.

There are several ways to do fetal movement counting. It's easy to do using a pencil and paper or many smartphone apps include a "kick count" tool (see Recommended Resources, page 418). The "Count-to-10" method, which follows, is simple and can be started at any time in late pregnancy (after week 32).

How to Count Fetal Movements

It is most helpful if the pregnant person counts the baby's movements at roughly the same time every day. It makes sense to begin counting when the baby is awake and active. Babies tend to be most active soon after meals.

The pregnant person notes the time when the counting starts. A movement may be a short kick or wiggle or a long, continuous squirming. When there is a pause in activity, it is counted as one movement. The pause may last only a few seconds or longer. Hiccups do not count as movements. Some babies may move ten times in 10 minutes. Others may take much longer to move ten times. Once ten fetal movements are counted, the time the tenth movement occurred is noted. Now, calculate how long it took to count ten fetal movements. See the chart following.

Fetal Movement Counts

Date	Starting time	Movements	Starting time of 10th movement	Time elapsed
1/1	8:45 A.M.	//// ////	9:05 A.M.	20 min.

The important thing is not how quickly the baby makes ten movements, but whether the baby maintains the same degree of activity from day to day. The pregnant person should call the caregiver if the baby's movements suddenly slow, if over some days the baby takes longer and longer to get to ten, or if the pregnant person has not felt ten movements in 2 hours. The caregiver will evaluate the baby's well-being with a nonstress test (see page 242), ultrasound, and other tests and prepare to deliver the baby if there are problems. Most times, there are none, but once in a while, a real problem with the baby is detected, and this vigilance allows early intervention and a good outcome.

Communicate with Your Unborn Baby

Babies can hear, remember what they hear, and even have preferences in what they hear. Sing songs to your baby. One couple sang "You Are My Sunshine" to their unborn baby for weeks before he was born. The father sang it again when the baby was crying shortly after the birth, and the baby immediately calmed down. He remembered and liked the song! Many of our students now sing in this way and use it very successfully as a soothing technique (especially when the baby fusses in the car seat!). It is the baby's own song. See Recommended Resources (page 418) for the YouTube link to *Singing to Your Baby in Utero*, by Penny Simkin, to see how a baby is affected by the parent's singing.

Besides singing or playing instrumental music to your baby, you can read a simple children's book aloud to the baby during late pregnancy. It is best to read the same story over and over so the baby can become familiar with its sounds.

Some partners lie with their head in the pregnant person's lap to talk to the baby, tell stories, and make plans. One father had a lot of fun telling his unborn baby stories about his own childhood and the movies he liked.

Prepare Other Children for the Birth

Things go more smoothly if siblings are prepared in advance for the arrival of a new brother or sister. Children are reassured to know where their parent will be during the birth, where they will be, and who will be with them. Include the children, as appropriate, in preparations for the new baby. Take them on the hospital tour and to some prenatal appointments and check whether sibling preparation classes are available in your area. These classes teach about birth and prepare older siblings for life with a new baby.

Some parents consider having older children attend the birth. This can be a very good experience if the child wants to be present, is generally calm and not too needy, and has an adult support person, so the child can come and go.

See Recommended Resources (page 418) for books and videos on the subject of children and birth.

Prepare a Contact List of Key People

Make a list of the names, phone numbers, and email addresses of the people you may need to reach around the time of the birth. These may include the pregnant person's doctor or midwife, the hospital's maternity unit or the birth center, your and the pregnant person's employers, your doula, childbirth educator, family members, friends, a baby-sitter for your older children or a support person for each child who will attend the birth, dog- or cat-sitter, the baby's doctor, your postpartum doula, and a breast-feeding counselor. Enter the list into your cell phone, computer, or both and post copies in places handy for everyone. Some families like to start a group text so many people can be notified at the same time as the labor and birth progress. In this day of social media, it is important to let your family and friends know if you have preferences about who makes a social media announcement and when that should be made. This is your special day, and you might not want other family or friends to spoil the announcement before you get to share.

Prepare and Review the Birth Plan

The birth plan is a written plan that tells the caregiver and nurses which options are important to the birthing person, what their priorities are, any specific concerns, and how they want to be cared for during labor, birth, and the first few hours after the baby is born. The plan should reflect an awareness that medical needs could require a shift from the written choices, and it should include a Plan B—including preferences in case labor stalls or there are problems with the laboring person or the baby. Although most useful for birth in a hospital, where the nurses (and often the caregivers) do not know the pregnant person, a birth plan can help every couple, even those planning a home or birth-center birth, to think through their choices and priorities. And, because some planned out-of-hospital births require transfer to the hospital, a transfer plan is also a very good idea.

If you are the laboring person's life partner (spouse, husband, wife, father of the baby) as well as birth partner, the two of you should prepare the birth plan together. If you have a doula, they can help you write it to reflect your wishes clearly. If you are not intimately involved with the parents, you should become very familiar with their birth plan so you will know how best to help them.

The birth plan is most useful when short and concise—one page is best; no more than two. We suggest using bulleted sentences or brief paragraphs, with any details that seem appropriate, for each of the relevant items that follow. Find out your hospital's and caregiver's usual practices before preparing your birth plan. If you both are comfortable with those practices, you don't have to list them. Only list preferences that differ from the usual care.

Introduction to the Birth Plan

Your plan might begin with the following information:

- **Personal information (two or three sentences).** What does the pregnant person want the staff to know about them? For example, describe strongly held beliefs or preferences, relevant previous experiences with health care, trauma, fears, concerns, or other information that can help staff know them and treat them as an individual.

- **Message to staff.** Do the two of you want to express appreciation for any support, expertise, and assistance staff can provide to help you have a safe and satisfying birth experience? If you both want to be involved in decision-making regarding your care, say so here (see pages 237 and 238). Let the staff know you understand that labor sometimes requires flexibility and a change from your desired options by using phrases like, "as long as labor proceeds normally" or "unless medically indicated."

- **Making medical care decisions.** How do you like to make decisions as they relate to medical care? Do you and the laboring person need private time to discuss the situation and come to a decision? Do you prefer that the care provider offer recommendations you can accept or reject?
- **Support team.** Names of those on the support team who will attend the birth.

Labor Options

The pregnant person can consider the following options for labor. To keep the plan brief, try to condense their wishes to general statements.

- Options include a preference to rely mainly on self-help and nondrug approaches to pain (see pages 145–164) or on pain medications or epidural block (see "Pain Medications Preference Scale," pages 328–329).
- Include general preference regarding use of procedures and interventions. Is the pregnant person okay with usual routines or using them only when medically necessary (see pages 239–269)?

Birth Options

The pregnant person can consider the following options for birth:

- **Positions.** Freedom to move and use a variety of positions or to lie on their back or in one position for the duration (see pages 169–176).
- **Pushing techniques.** Spontaneous, nondirected bearing down or prolonged breath holding and straining with directed pushing (see page 164).
- **Perineal care.** Warm compresses on the perineum and other measures to help relax and push effectively; preferences regarding episiotomy or avoiding episiotomy (see page 263). If the pregnant person has been doing perineal massage to improve the chances of an intact perineum (see page 40), say so.

After-Birth Options

The birthing person can consider the following options in post-partum care:

- **Immediate care of the baby.** Contact with the baby: immediate skin-to-skin contact with the birthing parent or removed to a warmer for initial procedures and wrapping; immediate or delayed umbilical cord clamping and cutting, for a few minutes or until it stops pulsating; routine suctioning or omitting suctioning baby's nose and mouth if baby is vigorous; immediate or delayed newborn routines (eye care, vitamin K, newborn exam, weighing, and so forth) until parents have bonded with the baby (see pages 135–137).

- **Cord blood (public donation or private storage).** You may choose to have placental blood extracted immediately after birth for future use in treating a variety of serious diseases. The cord blood may be donated to a blood bank for public access. Alternatively, it may be stored privately with a for-profit company at considerable cost to the family, where it is reserved for that family's use only. If you choose private storage, say so in your birth plan. To learn more about this option, see chapter 10, pages 366–367, and Recommended Resources (page 418).

- **Your presence.** Whether you stay in the hospital with the postpartum parent and baby or return to visit each day.

- **Feeding.** Breast-feeding or formula-feeding (see pages 401 and 414).

- **Circumcision.** Yes or no if the baby is male (see page 379).

The Unexpected, or Plan B

The two of you should think through the possibility of extra challenges or complications, such as a long, exhausting labor or problems for the laboring person or baby. For safety or well-being, interventions may become necessary, and some of the preferences you list for a normal labor and birth may no longer be appropriate. Consider the following:

- **Difficult labor or complications.** Parents can leave all care decisions to the staff or they continue to participate in decision-making after receiving explanations of the situations and discussion of possible nonmedical and medical options, including waiting.

- **Transfer to the hospital during a planned out-of-hospital birth.** It is a good idea to tour the backup hospital and prepare a hospital transfer plan in the event that complications develop. Some priorities still exist, such as those mentioned in "Difficult Labor" (see previous page). Please note that a laboring person is transferred to a hospital due to a need for medications or other interventions available only in a hospital. The care necessarily changes if transfer occurs (see part 3, "The Medical Side of Childbirth," page 236). Preferences should reflect the awareness that they will have interventions not initially planned for.

- **Cesarean birth.** Options to think about if a cesarean becomes necessary: degree of information the laboring person wants before and during surgery; presence of you, the doula or both; preferences about pain medications (any sedation that causes sleepiness, along with the epidural or spinal, during the surgery); contact with the baby after birth (skin to skin as soon as possible or wrapped in a blanket in the operating room or in recovery). If the baby needs to go to the intensive care nursery, do you go with the baby or stay with the birthing person? (A doula or other loved one can stay with the birthing person while you go to the nursery.) Does the birthing parent prefer to have sleep or sedative medications afterward for trembling and/or nausea or to wait to see if it is needed in order to remain awake and hold and nurse the baby (see chapter 9)?

- **Premature or sick infant.** Possible options: Involvement by both in the baby's care and feeding versus minimal contact; involvement in decision-making and explanations of the baby's problems, the procedures to be done, and possible options versus leaving care decisions entirely up to staff. If the baby cannot breast-feed, the birthing person tube-feeds or bottle-feeds the baby with expressed colostrum or (later) milk versus giving the baby formula. Once discharged, parents to receive resources for follow-up of the baby and support for parents.

- **Stillbirth or death of the baby.** Such a tragedy, as rare as it is, leaves the parents so stunned with grief it is almost impossible to make important decisions. Discuss this possibility together and think about how you and the pregnant person want the situation handled. Weeks or months after the death of a baby, the things that were done (or not done) at the time will be very important. Consider some or all of the following:

- An opportunity to hold the baby and say goodbye in private

- A chance to dress the baby

- Mementos—photos, the baby's clothing or blanket, a lock of hair, handprints and footprints

- Help from a counselor or member of the clergy

- An opportunity to discuss the birth and the baby's problems with the doctor, midwife, nurses, and doula

- An autopsy to determine cause of death

- A memorial service or funeral—an opportunity for family and friends to acknowledge the baby's life and death and demonstrate their love, support, and sympathy for the parents

- Ongoing support from a group for grieving parents or a grief counselor (see Recommended Resources, page 418)

As difficult as it is to face the possibility the baby could die, it is wise to think through this possibility. Once you think it through, put your plan away. We hope you will never need it, but, if you do, you will be glad later that you thought about this ahead of time, when you were calm and able to think clearly. Many hospitals are very sensitive and helpful with grieving parents.

Personal Choices

Think about other choices that may make this birth experience more comfortable or memorable for the pregnant person and you. For example:

• Creating a peaceful environment with favorite music, low lighting, and minimal disturbances

• Including others—doula, relatives, friends, interpreter (if needed), or your other children

• Excluding nonessential personnel (for example, students, observers) or requesting they introduce themselves and politely ask to be present during the birth

- Determining if the caregiver is comfortable having you assist in delivering the baby or cutting the umbilical cord, as long as the birth is going smoothly

- Photographing, videotaping, or audiotaping the birth or the new family

- Welcoming the baby with private time together, by singing or playing music (see page 44), or with a religious or personal ceremony

- Incorporating traditional or culturally significant birth customs (foods, bathing, contact with baby, and so forth)

The 36-week prenatal appointment is a good time to give the birth plan to the doctor or midwife. This allows time to review it and make sure it is realistic and consistent with the options available and the pregnant person's health status. The birth plan can then be placed in the pregnant person's hospital chart, where other staff will have access to it. It is a good idea, however, to take extra copies along to the hospital to share if necessary.

Keep a copy of the birth plan with you during labor. Be ready to ask the staff to read and follow the plan and be ready to remind the birthing person of prior choices if forgotten when caught up in the intense demands of labor. Use the birth plan as a guide, but be willing to accept changes if medical circumstances require it.

Preparing for Life with the Baby

Following is a reminder list of some things to do before the baby is born. It is easier to do these things before the birth rather than afterward, when time and energy are limited.

Take a Baby Care and Safety Class

You'll want to learn about a newborn's temperament, capabilities, and needs; how they communicate needs; how to soothe newborn babies; diapering and bathing; guidelines for safe sleeping; how to tell whether a baby is sick; making your home safe for your baby; infant cardiopulmonary resuscitation (CPR); and more. Most hospitals and parent-support organizations offer such classes or can help you find them. If you can't take a class, get a good book on baby care (see Recommended Resources, page 418).

Gather Essential Supplies for the Baby

Is everything ready for the baby? Are the necessary supplies on hand? Use the following lists as a guide. The internet and other parents are great sources of advice on what to get and where. If you're on a tight budget, don't forget consignment stores and used-clothing stores for some supplies, and hand-me-downs are a real budget saver. Also, register your choices at baby stores to help friends and family members who want to give you something.

Baby Equipment

☐ Car seat (installed correctly and checked; see page 34). If you don't have a car, you should still have a car seat to use in other people's cars, taxis, or airplanes. Unfortunately, most buses do not have seat belts, which are necessary to install a car seat. Check with your baby's doctor (for information on local bus safety for infants). Also check the American Academy of Pediatrics website regarding infant car seat safety.

☐ Crib, bassinet, cradle, or baby bed that attaches to your bed (make sure it meets current safety standards)

Bedding (Minimum Requirements)

☐ Two or more snug fitted sheets for the crib, bassinet, cradle, or baby bed

☐ Two square waterproof pads to fit under the baby's diaper area

☐ Two or three lightweight swaddling blankets (about 34 to 42 inches, or 86 to 107 cm, square)

Clothing

Buy baby clothes with room for growing—nothing smaller than 10- to 12-pound (4.5 kg to 5.4 kg) or 3-month, size. Babies usually weigh close to 10 pounds (4.5 kg) by the time they are 1 to 2 months old, if not at birth. Often, babies outgrow even 6-month-size clothes by the time they are 2 or 3 months old. On the other hand, if the baby is very small at birth, you will need tiny clothes, which are widely available, Search the internet.

☐ Four onesies (pullover undershirts that snap at the crotch)

☐ Three one-piece coveralls (stretch suits, sleepers) or nightgowns

☐ Two or three one-piece footed blanket sleepers, for cold weather

- ☐ Two sweaters

- ☐ One hat for use indoors (not while sleeping alone) during the first few days

- ☐ One hat for outdoors

- ☐ One warm outfit for outdoors

- ☐ Two pairs of booties or socks

- ☐ Four Velcro-fastening diaper covers or plastic pants

- ☐ Diapers: Two to four dozen cloth diapers and a diaper pail, unless the parents plan to use a diaper service, or at least 80 newborn-size disposable diapers

- ☐ Two hooded baby bath towels

- ☐ Two baby washcloths

Health Supplies

- ☐ Blunt fingernail scissors

- ☐ Thermometer for taking baby's temperature

- ☐ Diaper-rash ointment

- ☐ Baby wipes

Breast-Feeding Supplies

- ☐ At least three well-fitting, comfortable nursing bras (the pregnant person should be fitted for these by a store clerk who knows about breast-feeding)

- ☐ Nursing pads to fit inside the bra (commercially available or homemade, from six layers of cotton flannel cut into 4- to 5-inch [10 to 13 cm] rounds and sewn together)

- ☐ Nursing cover, for nursing where modesty is preferred

- ☐ Breast pump (there are many types in a wide price range). Be sure the pregnant person needs one, such as for pumping one or more times per day (to increase a low milk supply or while working, for example); a heavy-duty fast pump is the best choice. These can be rented or purchased; check online for available sources. Contact your insurance plan about breast-feeding benefits, including coverage of breast pump costs. Your plan may require pre-authorization from the pregnant person's or baby's doctor or midwife.

Supplies for Formula-Feeding

- ☐ Formula (recommended by the baby's caregiver)
- ☐ Eight to twelve bottles with nipples and caps (or fewer, if the pregnant person plans to breast-feed mostly, with an occasional relief bottle in the middle of the night or while away from the baby)
- ☐ Nipple brush, for washing the nipples

Optional Paraphernalia

- ☐ Mobile (choose one with black and white or other high-contrast colors that attract the baby's interest)
- ☐ Infant seat (an infant car seat can double as one)
- ☐ Soft-front carrier or sling (for carrying the baby hands free)
- ☐ Stroller or carriage
- ☐ Baby swing
- ☐ Rocking chair
- ☐ Baby bathtub
- ☐ Birth ball (exercise ball or yoga ball), for sitting on and bouncing while holding the baby against your shoulder (see illustration, page 182)
- ☐ Pacifiers (in case the baby needs to suck a great deal)
- ☐ Electronic baby monitor (if the baby will sleep beyond easy hearing range)
- ☐ Recordings of soothing heartbeat sounds, nature sounds, white noise, lullabies, or other music
- ☐ Toys (the possibilities are endless)
- ☐ Books on baby feeding, baby care, and infant development (see Recommended Resources, page 418)

Choose a Caregiver or Clinic for the Baby

The baby will need a medical caregiver (pediatrician, family doctor, naturopathic doctor, nurse practitioner, or health clinic) to provide well-baby care (routine checkups, immunizations) and to treat illnesses if they occur. Check the baby's health insurance plan for a list of preferred providers and get recommendations from friends, your childbirth educator, or the pregnant person's caregiver. Many parents make the baby's first doctor's appointment based on these recommendations or from information on the doctors' websites. However, some children's doctors provide opportunities for parents to meet them before making a selection, which allows you both to discover their views on topics important to you and determine whether you feel comfortable with them. The following are important considerations when choosing a caregiver. Check the list to narrow your choices for an interview:

- **Location of the office.** How far away is it? There is a real advantage to its being close to home. Traveling a long distance with a sick child can be nerve-wracking.

- **Practical considerations.** Is the caregiver covered by your health insurance? What are the caregiver's educational and professional qualifications? What are the fees? Who covers the practice when the caregiver is not available? At which hospital(s), if any, does the caregiver have privileges?

- **Questions to ask during the get-acquainted appointment.** If you have an opportunity to meet the doctor in advance, here are some topics you might want to explore. You probably won't have time to ask about all these; select one or two topics.

  – What are the caregiver's attitudes or advice about breast-feeding?

  – Introducing solid foods?

  – Circumcision?

  – Immunizations?

  – Infant feeding and sleeping?

  – Daycare, and so on?

- **Personal attributes.** Does this caregiver seem kind, competent, and caring? Is this someone whom both of you could trust with your baby's health care? Most importantly, is the caregiver's approach consistent with your values and beliefs regarding health and medical care?

  It can be a great relief to have your child enrolled in a good caregiver's practice. Having a trusted person to consult about your child's development and health issues will bring great peace of mind. If, however, you discover you are uncomfortable with any person, you can always change to another.

Prepare a Place at Home for the Baby

Whether the baby will have a fully equipped nursery or a corner of a room, you will need to organize space for the baby—for storing clothes, diaper changing, sleeping, and for all the equipment that comes along with babies.

Investigate Parent-Infant Classes or Peer-Support Groups

Classes and drop-in or online support groups for new parents are widely available. Consult your childbirth educator, doula, or caregiver for possibilities. Also, hospitals near you may offer new-parent groups. These classes and support groups provide information about child development, emotional needs of parents and infants, and discuss common problems. Parents learn exercises, songs, massage techniques, techniques for soothing crying babies, and games to play with their newborns. If it's convenient and appealing to you, attend the classes together. You may enjoy the opportunity to form new friendships and share your questions, concerns, and triumphs.

Prepare Meals Ahead of Time

You may be surprised to find that simply going to the grocery store or even figuring out what to eat can seem almost overwhelming in the first weeks after the baby arrives. So, stock the kitchen with nutritious foods that are easy to prepare and eat. Cook and freeze food ahead for reheating later. Locate stores and delis with prepared dishes and nutritious convenience foods available (see page 398 for more suggestions about putting together quick, nutritious meals).

If family and friends want to help after the birth, you might ask them to set up a meal train—that is, to take turns bringing meals every day or two, for 2 or 3 weeks. (Most people bring enough food for more than one meal, so if you want to avoid accumulating leftovers, ask for meals every other day.) A meal train is usually a very welcome gift for new parents. Sometimes, though, a meal is delivered when the new family is sleeping or not feeling up to receiving guests. One way around this is to put a cooler on your front porch with a note thanking people for the meal, asking them to leave it in the cooler because the new family is sleeping. Do let them know you look forward to introducing them to the baby soon. Helpful people understand what it's like to have a new baby at home! Another option is a "chore sign up" to get help with grocery shopping, laundry, dog walking, light housekeeping, errands, etc. Look online for meal train or chore sign-up lists for friends and family.

If accepting gifts of help and chores makes the new parent feel uncomfortable, create a list of daily or regular chores, such as sweep the kitchen, unload the dishes, walk the dog, or take out the trash, and post it on the fridge. When a kind-hearted visitor asks what can be done to help, simply point to the list and ask them to choose whatever they feel comfortable doing.

Plan to Share Responsibilities

You will probably be astounded by the amount of work and time it takes to feed and care for a new baby—and the parents—and to keep the household running. Remember, a baby needs almost constant care for the first few weeks. If the new parent tries to do it all, they will get much less sleep than usual. Full-time newborn care is tiring enough, and as the birthing person is also recovering from the physical demands of birth, or possibly from a cesarean, it may take weeks to recover.

As the father or co-parent, plan to share the baby's care responsibilities and take over much of the housework and cooking or make arrangements for someone to help. Many partners use vacation time or family leave to stay home for the first days or weeks to share the work. The baby's grandparents or other relatives can also be a great source of help, if the birth giver's relationship with them is good. If the birth giver and parents or in-laws do not get along well, those relationships will *not* suddenly improve with the arrival of the baby. Some communities offer classes for grandparents, which may be very helpful (see Recommended Resources, page 418, for some helpful books for grandparents). Friends can be wonderful about providing meals, running errands, and doing chores. Say yes if they offer to help. See the next page for suggestions explaining what new parents may need from the baby's grandparents.

A Letter to Grandparents

Dear Grandparents (and other family members),

Congratulations on the birth of your new grandchild! This birth marks the continuation of your family into a new generation. Your support and love can ease your own child's transition into parenthood.

If your children invite you to come and help, recognize it as an honor. Ask what you may do to help: Prepare meals? Do laundry? Shop? Keep the house clean? You will work hard, sleep little, and leave tired and appreciated. But please avoid the mistakes that some new grandparents make—monopolizing the baby, criticizing the parent's decisions and actions, and giving unwanted, out-of-date, or opinionated advice. Of course, if they ask you for advice, feel free to give it or to check recent books in areas where you are uncertain.

What your grandchild needs most from you is a nurturing support of their parents. The parents need you to support and honor their thoughtful decisions about and style of parenting, even if different from yours. Discover what books they are reading on newborn care and feeding and read the same books yourself. You are needed to support them as they learn about and care for their new baby.

The new parents need to hear that you think they are wonderful parents and the very best parents your grandchild could have. They need to hear from you that parenthood is always challenging and tiring and, at the same time, one of the most important and rewarding things they will ever do. Let them know you have confidence in them.

If your relationship with the parents is strained or difficult, think of what you can and cannot do to support this new family. If being with them is too difficult for you, or for them, your presence might worsen your relationship and make this adjustment to parenthood more difficult. Instead of visiting right away, you might send help in the form of costs of a postpartum doula, diaper service, meals, or the presence of another family member. Reaching out in this way could go a long way in healing your relationship.

Be gentle with your expectations of the new family and forgiving if they forget to thank you for your presence and gifts. Memories are made in these first weeks following birth—ones never forgotten. Your children will always remember your unconditional love and acceptance.

With best wishes for joyful grandparenting,
Penny Simkin

In many communities, postpartum doulas are available to help new families for the first few weeks. These doulas come to the home, usually for a few hours each day for a few weeks, and do whatever needs to be done in the way of light housekeeping, meal preparation, errand running, and care of older children. Most importantly, they are very knowledgeable about newborn care and feeding and can teach new parents a great deal. A postpartum doula also can identify problems the new parent or baby may be experiencing and make referrals for help, if necessary. Hiring a postpartum doula can make it possible for you both to spend time enjoying the baby, to relax a bit, and even get a nap.

To help you decide whether to hire a postpartum doula, you may want to get some names, check their websites, and/or have a phone conversation to find out more. To find one, visit DONA.org, or DoulaMatch.net, or a local doula organization, if available. Search online for [your city] + doula association or ask your childbirth educator, birth doula, or caregiver for a referral. Some birth doulas are also postpartum doulas. Ideally, you should book a postpartum doula before the birth, though many are available for last-minute hires.

The services of a postpartum doula are a popular gift for distant grandparents to give their children. Many grandparents wish they could come and help, but cannot, for various reasons. If a postpartum doula is not available, a house cleaner, a baby nurse, or even a teenage helper may help ease some of the burden on new parents.

On to the Next Step . . .

Once you have prepared as much as possible, enjoy yourselves as you wait for labor to begin. Photograph the pregnant person at the end of pregnancy; share some evenings out for dinner, movies, concerts, plays, and visits with friends and family. If you have other children, plan activities with them. Make these last days relaxed before your lives change forever.

And now that you know how to really help the expectant parent *before* labor, let's go on to the next step—how you can really help *during* labor and birth.

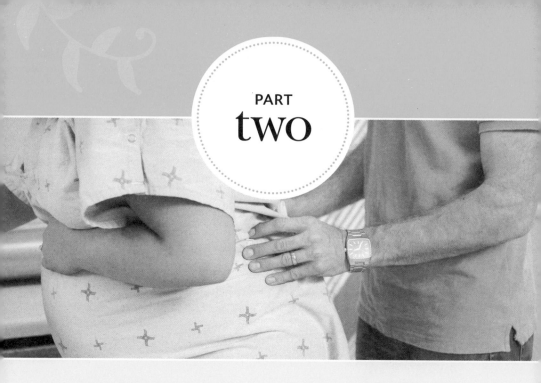

LABOR AND BIRTH

THE CLIMAX OF PREGNANCY—the birth of a baby—is an everyday miracle for the family, but just part of a day's work for the doctor, midwife, or nurse. For you, the birthing person, and those who love and support them, it is a deep and permanent memory. Your role as birth partner is to do as much as possible to *help make this birth experience a good memory for the person giving birth*. This birth is an event that will never be forgotten—including the good and the bad. The kind of care a person receives and the quality of support during labor make the difference in whether the birth experience is remembered with satisfaction and fulfillment or disappointment and sadness. This is where you come in. Being a birth partner—helping someone through labor and birth—is clearly a challenge, but it is a challenge that people like you meet all the time.

To be a good birth partner, you need:

- A bond of love or friendship with, and feelings of commitment and responsibility toward, the birthing person.

- Familiarity with the birthing person's personal preferences and quirks, the little things that are soothing and relaxing, and the things that may be irritating or worrying.

- A commitment to help continuously throughout labor, either by yourself or with the help of a doula or other supportive person.

- Knowledge of what to expect—the physical process of labor, the procedures and interventions commonly used during labor, and when these procedures and interventions are necessary and when they are optional.

- An understanding of the emotional side of labor—the emotional needs of laboring people and the changing emotions usually experienced as labor progresses.

- Practical knowledge of how to help in various specific situations— what to do when. A trained doula can help with this and the two preceding points.

- Flexibility to adapt to the laboring person's changing needs during labor—leading by following. How you help, and how much you help, are determined by the laboring person's needs and responses at the time.

If you also love the birthing person and the baby, you will care for them in the intimate and personal way only a husband, wife, or loved one can. The next few chapters cover the normal birth process and explain what happens, how the birthing person is likely to respond, what the caregiver does, how you can help, and what you can expect if you have a doula. These chapters also discuss situations that are particularly difficult for the laboring person and, therefore, particularly challenging for the birth partner, too. Read these chapters in advance and use them as an on-the-spot guide during labor.

chapter 2

GETTING INTO LABOR

I work in construction. I was at the job site early, eating breakfast with my buddy in my truck. My phone rang. I listened, said, "Hmmm, okay, okay," hung up, and went back to my breakfast. My buddy asked, "Who was that?" I said, "My wife. Her water broke . . . HER WATER BROKE! Get outta my truck, man! I gotta go!"

—CARL, FIRST-TIME FATHER

A few days past her due date, my wife started having small contractions, about three every hour. I thought this was the beginning and, anytime now, she would be in labor. Then they stopped. A few days later, the contractions became a bit more intense and very regular—one contraction every 10 minutes. I thought this was the beginning and she would be in labor anytime now. Contractions stopped. After another week passed, we went for a walk and the contractions became a bit more intense and frequent, about 4 to 6 minutes apart. At this point, you know what I thought. I asked my wife if she thought she was going into labor. She said she didn't know, but everyone says you will know when the real contractions hit. That night, at 1 a.m., she sat up in bed and said, "That was different. I'm in labor."

—SCOTT, FIRST-TIME FATHER

Everyone wonders how to tell whether a pregnant person is in labor. Even those with experience cannot usually identify exactly when labor starts. Often the labor "sneaks" up with unclear, on-again-off-again signs—like an orchestra tuning up before a performance. Over the course of many hours or days, the signs intensify, and you both come to realize that something is different—this is *it*! Step by step, the birthing person becomes mentally and physically more ready for the coordinated effort that eventually results in the birth of the baby. It is normal to experience a period of uncertainty and questioning while awaiting clear signs that labor has truly started.

The one situation in which labor is clearly starting is described in the vignette at the beginning of this chapter—the pregnant person's bag of waters breaks with a gush. Then you know. But only one or two in ten labors start this way. (**Note:** A gush of fluid is different from leaking fluid. About two in ten people have leaking of fluid before labor. In such cases, contractions may not begin for hours or days; see page 71.)

As long as the two of you eventually put the pieces together, it usually doesn't matter if the labor is vague at the beginning. There is almost always plenty of time, once labor clearly starts, to get to the hospital or birth center or settle in for a home birth. Occasionally, however, a pregnant person is caught by surprise and goes into labor earlier or more suddenly than anticipated. Because of this possibility, you will want to be able to tell the difference between the tuning up, or prelabor, and the real thing, progressing labor.

This chapter helps you recognize when labor truly starts. It explains how labor begins physically and emotionally and describes the role you should play as birth partner.

The Difference Between Prelabor and Labor

Labor is the process by which someone gives birth to a baby and a placenta. It usually follows hours or days of prelabor contractions, which are shorter, less frequent, and less intense than labor contractions. In prelabor, the cervix begins to soften and thin and is preparing to open once labor is established. The labor process involves the following:

1. Contractions of the uterus, the largest and strongest muscle in the pregnant body. These build in intensity and frequency over time.

2. Softening (ripening), thinning (effacement), and opening (dilation) of the cervix.

3. Breaking of the bag of waters (the membranes or amniotic sac) surrounding the baby and the release of water (amniotic fluid), either as a leak or a gush.

4. Rotation and molding of the baby's head and tucking of the chin, to fit into the pelvis.

5. Descent of the baby out of the uterus and through the birth canal (pelvis and vagina) to the outside.

6. Birth of the placenta.

7. The first hours when parents and baby ideally stay together with the baby, skin to skin with a parent, feeding, and getting to know each other.

Normally, labor does not begin until both the pregnant parent and baby are ready—between 37 and 42 weeks of pregnancy. The last weeks prepare the pregnant person physically and psychologically to give birth and breast-feed and nurture a baby. During this time, the baby acquires the "final touches" preparing for the stress of labor and adaptation to life outside the uterus. It is the baby who usually initiates the labor, by producing and secreting the hormones that begin the chain of events leading to the steps just listed.

In 2017, about one in ten U.S. babies was born prematurely, before being really ready. Premature birth may be due to conditions in the pregnant person—infection, high stress, poverty, heavy smoking, poor nutrition, drug use, or unknown reasons that override the mechanisms normally initiated by the baby. Multiple pregnancies (twins, triplets, and more) and some fetal abnormalities are other causes.

Sometimes, babies are born post-term, after 42 weeks. Of these, most are fine, but the chances of *postmaturity syndrome* increase with longer pregnancies. This cluster of symptoms in the newborn indicates the placenta was no longer providing adequate nourishment to the fetus. A postmature baby looks, and is, undernourished, having loose, peeling skin from having lost some fat in the uterus and long nails. The postmature baby may have yellow stains on the nails and skin, signs the baby passed meconium (fetal stool) in the uterus. Postmaturity is caused by some interference with the hormonal chain of events that normally brings on labor between 37 and 42 weeks. Because of the widespread

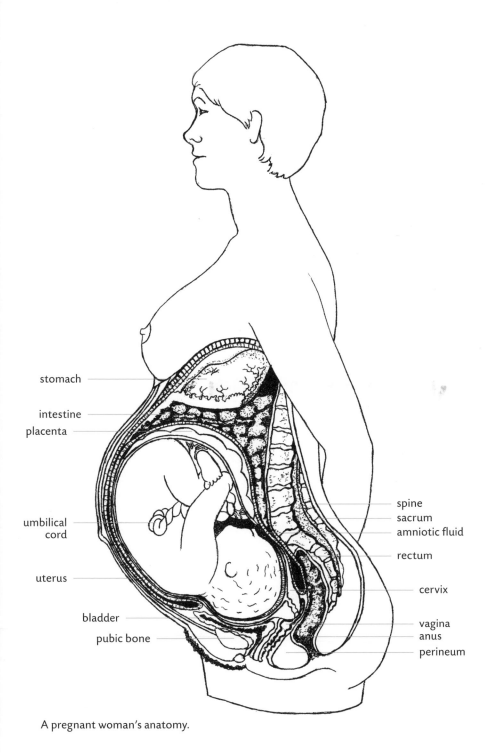

stomach

intestine

placenta

umbilical
cord

uterus

bladder

pubic bone

spine

sacrum

amniotic fluid

rectum

cervix

vagina

anus

perineum

A pregnant woman's anatomy.

policy of induction by 42 weeks, very few babies are born postmature today. When they are, they may need special care in the hospital.

How Long Will Labor Last?

It is impossible to predict how long any particular labor will last. A perfectly normal labor can take between 2 and 24 hours following hours or days of prelabor. Many factors influence the length of labor:

- Whether this is a first or later baby

- The condition of the cervix (soft and thin or firm and thick) when progressing contractions begin

- The size of the baby, particularly the head, in relation to the size of the pregnant person's pelvis

- The presentation and position of the baby's head within the pregnant person's body

- The strength and frequency of the contractions

- The pregnant person's emotional state—if lonely, frightened, or angry, labor may be slower than when the person is confident, content, and calm

Presentation refers to the part of the baby—top of the head (the vertex), brow, face, buttocks, feet, shoulders—that is lowest in the uterus. The vertex almost always *presents* first; problems may occur in delivery if any other part of the baby presents first. *Position* refers to the placement of the presenting part within the pregnant person's pelvis. The most common positions are:

- OA (occiput anterior): The back of the baby's head (the occiput) points toward the pregnant person's front (anterior).

- OT (occiput transverse): The back of the baby's head points toward the pregnant person's side (transverse).

- OP (occiput posterior): The back of the baby's head points toward the pregnant person's back (posterior).

Although babies can and usually do change position during labor and during the pushing (second) stage, at birth, the OA position is

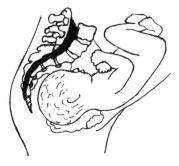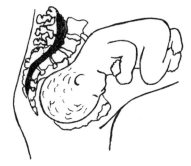

A baby in OA (occiput anterior) position (left) and OP (occiput posterior) position (right)

much more common than OT or OP. When the baby is in the OP position in labor, with the back of their head toward the pregnant person's back, labor is sometimes prolonged, and the laboring person may experience intense backache. There are many other reasons for back pain in labor, however (see page 221). Do not assume the baby is OP just because the laboring person has back pain.

Signs of Labor

How will you know labor has started? A few clues can usually help you recognize labor long before the birth is imminent. It is equally important, though, to be able to tell when the pregnant person is not in labor. There is nothing more frustrating or disappointing for someone than thinking labor has begun and discovering, after a trip to the caregiver or hospital, that the cervix is not opening (or dilating), which is the most important sign of labor (which results in going home to wait). The best way to avoid this is to know the signs of labor (see table, pages 68 and 69) and how to interpret them. Some signs are clearer than others. They are categorized as Possible Signs, Prelabor Signs, and Positive Signs.

- **Possible Signs (tuning up):** Without other signs, these signs are not clear enough to get excited about. They can fool and confuse a pregnant person because they feel different from what they were feeling earlier. However, unlike the Positive Signs, they do not indicate that the cervix is dilating and that labor has started. Rather, Possible Signs indicate the body is *getting ready* for labor. These signs may continue, on and off, for days or even weeks, before the cervix begins to dilate.

We do not recommend that you or the pregnant person go away on a trip when these signs are present because, at any time, they might turn the corner into labor. If the pregnant person has had a rapid labor with a previous birth, they should be particularly alert to the Possible Signs, as these might be all the signs that occur before suddenly going into another rapid labor.

- **Prelabor Signs:** These are more important than Possible Signs, but real labor could still be hours, or even days, away.

- **Positive Signs:** These are the most certain signs that labor has truly started—that is, the cervix is dilating.

If you know the significance of these signs, chances are very good you will correctly interpret what is happening. Sometimes, though, couples need a caregiver's help to figure out whether the pregnant person is really in labor. You should certainly call your caregiver if there are any Prelabor or Positive signs before 37 weeks, as they could indicate the onset of premature labor.

SIGNS OF LABOR

SIGNS AND SYMPTOMS	COMMENTS
Possible Signs (late pregnancy changes)	
Vague nagging backache causing restlessness—a need to keep changing positions	• Different from the fatigue-related backache common during pregnancy
Several soft bowel movements—sometimes accompanied by flu-like "sick" feelings	• When this sign accompanies others, it is probably associated with an increase in hormone-like substances in the bloodstream (prostaglandins). These substances soften and thin the cervix and stimulate bowel activity. By itself, this symptom may be due to digestive upset.

SIGNS OF LABOR *continued*

SIGNS AND SYMPTOMS	COMMENTS
Cramps, similar to menstrual cramps, that come and go; the discomfort may extend to the thighs	• May be associated with prostaglandin action and early contractions • May go away and return several times over weeks or progress steadily to Positive Signs
Unusual burst of energy resulting in great activity (cleaning, organizing)— termed the "nesting urge"	• Ensures the pregnant person will have strength and energy to handle labor (avoid exhausting activity)

Prelabor Signs

Nonprogressing contractions—that is, contractions that continue without changing; they do not become longer, stronger, and closer together over time. They sometimes last for hours and subside before restarting. These are prelabor, or Braxton Hicks, contractions (see "'False' Labor, or Prelabor," page 72, and "Timing Contractions," page 77).	• Accomplishes softening and thinning of the cervix, preparing the cervix to begin dilating • Should not be perceived as unproductive • Usually not painful, but may be tiring or discouraging if they continue for many hours
Water leaks, resulting in a trickle (not a gush) of fluid from the vagina (see "If the Bag of Waters Breaks Before Labor Begins," page 71.)	• Leaking fluid occurs before labor in about 2 of every 10 labors. • A signal: call and report to caregiver
Blood-tinged mucus discharge ("show" or mucus plug) may be released from the vagina before labor; more likely to occur once there are other Positive Signs (see following); laboring person continues passing this discharge off and on throughout labor	• Associated with thinning of the cervix • May occur days before other signs or not until after progressing contractions have begun • A discharge, often mistaken for show, may also appear within a day after a pelvic exam or sexual intercourse and is not a sign of labor. Show is pink or red; the discharge after a pelvic exam or sex tends to be brownish.

SIGNS OF LABOR *continued*

SIGNS AND SYMPTOMS	COMMENTS

Positive Signs

Progressing contractions—that is, contractions that become longer, stronger, and closer together over time. These usually continue until it is time to push. Some laboring people having second or subsequent babies, however, have periods of progressing contractions that come and go over a few days before they settle into a continuous pattern (see page 77 for instructions on timing contractions).

- The cervix is very likely to be opening if they have 12 to 15 contractions in a row that are consistently 1 minute long, occur 5 or fewer minutes apart, and feel painful or "very strong."

- It is an even clearer sign if these contractions are combined with a "show" (blood-tinged discharge).

- The laboring person cannot be distracted from these contractions.

- Contractions may be felt in the abdomen, back, or both.

Spontaneous breaking of the bag of waters (rupture of the membranes) with a pop or gush of fluid followed by progressing contractions within hours (see "If the Bag of Waters Breaks Before Labor Begins," page 71).

- Often associated with rapid labor

- The bag of waters usually breaks in late labor. Rupture of the membranes with a gush occurs before other signs of labor in only 1 or 2 out of 10 labors.

CAUTION: If the pregnant person is less than 37 weeks' pregnant and experiences four or more noticeable contractions in 1 hour for more than 2 hours, combined with any of the other Possible, Prelabor, or Positive signs of labor, they should consult their caregiver. This might be premature labor, which can sometimes be stopped if caught early. The caregiver may ask them to go in to be checked or to first drink some fluids and lie down to see if the contractions stop. If the contractions don't stop, they'll be asked to go the caregiver's office or the hospital to determine whether it is preterm labor. Catching this early often means stopping it. If the pregnant person is beyond 37 weeks and the pregnancy is normal, wait for the Positive Signs before calling the caregiver.

If the Bag of Waters Breaks Before Labor Begins

If the pregnant person's membranes rupture—if water leaks or gushes from the vagina—before labor begins, make the following observations to report to the caregiver:

1. The *amount* of fluid: Is it a trickle, a leak, or a gush? A "leak" is a squirt that occurs when a pregnant person changes position; about 2 in 10 labors begin this way. A "gush" is an uncontrollable heavy flow that may start with a popping feeling. About 1 or 2 in 10 labors begins this way.

2. The *color* of the fluid: Normally, the fluid is clear. If it is brownish or greenish, the baby may have had a bowel movement (passed meconium), which happens when a baby is stressed in the uterus. Such stress is caused by a temporary lack of oxygen. While usually not serious, the caregiver may want to check the baby's well-being.

3. The *odor* of the fluid. Normally, the fluid is practically odorless. If it has a foul smell, there may be an infection within the uterus, which could spread to the baby.

This information helps the caregiver plan what to do next—whether to stay home, with precautions, or go to the hospital or caregiver's office so some of the fluid can be collected and tested to determine whether it is amniotic fluid or something else (liquid mucus or urine). To collect fluid from the vagina, the caregiver uses a sterile speculum and a sterile swab. This test is important if the status of the membranes is not clear.

One concern with ruptured membranes is whether the pregnant person is a carrier of Group B streptococcus, a type of bacteria present in vaginal secretions of about one-third of people. If so, the caregiver may want to start treatment with antibiotics and, if labor does not begin spontaneously, induce labor in a matter of hours. For more information on Group B strep, see page 240.

Also, once the bag of waters breaks, the pregnant person should take precautions to prevent bacteria from entering the uterus, as this might increase the chance of infection. Put nothing in the vagina—no tampons; no penetrative intercourse; no checking the cervix with fingers. Taking a tub bath is okay and will not increase the chance of infection, provided the tub is clean.

Until the laboring person is clearly in active labor, the caregiver and nurses should be very cautious about doing vaginal exams to assess the cervix for dilation. Such exams tend to push bacteria through the cervix into the uterus and increase the chances of infection. Even if you're curious about dilation, do not ask for a vaginal exam. You should also question the nurse or caregiver who wants to do one. Collecting fluid for testing is an exception to this rule; because the speculum and swab do not enter the cervix, this procedure poses little risk of infection.

If precautions are followed and the pregnant person does not carry Group B streptococcus, it is probably safely to wait for labor to begin spontaneously. The caregiver probably won't think it necessary to induce labor, sometimes for a day or more. Most caregivers have a policy regarding management of ruptured membranes (broken bag of waters); some induce labor within hours after the bag breaks; others wait. It is wise to ask about this policy ahead of time. If the pregnant person is at low risk for infection (for example, having tested negative for Group B strep and has had no vaginal exams), it is reasonable to ask to delay induction for a day or more.

CAUTION: On very rare occasions, when the bag of waters breaks with a gush of fluid, the baby's umbilical cord slips below the baby or out of the uterus as the water escapes. This is called prolapsed cord and is a **true emergency** (see "Prolapsed Cord," page 290).

"False" Labor, or Prelabor

Frequently, pregnant people have contractions that are quite strong and frequent, but they are *nonprogressing*—that is, the pattern of contractions remains the same. The contractions do not become longer, stronger, or closer together over time. When examined, these people may be told they are in "false" labor, which means the cervix is not yet opening (dilating). The term *prelabor* is much more appropriate because there is nothing "false" about these contractions, and they accomplish changes that allow "true" labor (that is, dilation) to occur. Prelabor contractions are also called Braxton Hicks contractions. Many people who are examined in prelabor and told it is not labor feel discouraged and embarrassed at the error and may lose faith in their ability to recognize labor, or they may feel distressed and confused if admitted to the hospital. The support the pregnant person receives from you or a doula in these circumstances is critical to their ability to cope with "true" progressing labor later. Here is how you can help:

- Most importantly, point out that "false" labor does not mean what they are experiencing is not real. All it means is the cervix has not yet begun to open. Refer to the contractions as "prelabor" instead.

- Remind the pregnant person that opening (dilation) of the cervix beyond about 2 centimeters is one of the *last* things to happen, after the cervix has moved into position, ripened, and effaced (see page 74). The fact that the cervix is not yet opening does *not* mean there is no progress.

- If the pregnant parent becomes discouraged with a prolonged period of nonprogressing contractions, remind them of the six ways that labor progresses (see "Labor Progresses in Six Ways," page 74).

- Ask the caregiver who examines the pregnant parent whether the cervix has moved forward, softened further, or thinned more. Sometimes, the caregiver is so focused on the opening of the cervix (dilation), these other important signs of progress are not mentioned.

- If the laboring person does not want to go home, you might walk around outside the hospital or hang out in the cafeteria or lobby to see if the contractions progress further. If they don't change, you might be more comfortable at home.

See "Prelabor," page 85, and "The Slow-to-Start Labor," page 216, for strategies to help the laboring person cope with these early contractions. You can be sure that if the laboring person has either of the Positive Signs of labor listed in the table on page 68, the cervix is opening. The pregnant person cannot be in "false" labor if, over a period of time, the contractions have become longer, stronger, *and* closer together or at least two of those three things occur (see "Timing Contractions," page 77).

Labor Progresses in Six Ways

A laboring person makes progress toward birth in the following ways. Note that significant dilation does not take place until step 4. The first three steps usually occur simultaneously and gradually over the last weeks of pregnancy and into early labor.

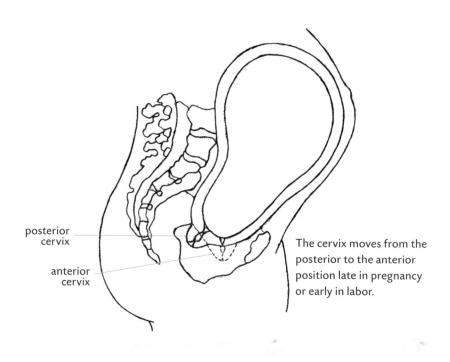

posterior cervix

anterior cervix

The cervix moves from the posterior to the anterior position late in pregnancy or early in labor.

1. **The cervix softens (ripens).** While still thick, the cervix, through the action of hormones and prostaglandins, softens and becomes more pliable.

2. **The position of the cervix changes.** The cervix points toward the pregnant parent's back during most of pregnancy and then gradually moves forward. The position of the cervix is assessed by a vaginal exam and is described as posterior (pointing toward the back), midline, or anterior (pointing toward the front).

3. **The cervix thins and shortens (effaces).** Usually about 1½ inches (3.5 cm) long, the cervix gradually shortens and becomes paper-thin. The amount of thinning (effacement) is measured in two ways:

- **Percentages:** Zero percent means no thinning or shortening has occurred; 50 percent means the cervix is about half its former thickness; 100 percent means it is paper-thin.

- **Centimeters of length:** One and one-half inches (3.5 cm) is the same as 0 percent effaced; ¾ inch (2 cm) long is the same as 50 percent effaced; and less than ½ inch (1 cm) long means 80 to 90 percent effaced. Do not confuse centimeters of cervical length with centimeters of cervical dilation!

4. **The cervix opens (dilates).** The opening (dilation) of the cervix is also measured in centimeters. The measurement is estimated by the caregiver who inserts two fingers through the cervix, spreads the fingers to the edges of the cervix, and estimates how far apart (in centimeters) the fingers are—it is not an exact science. Dilation usually occurs with progressing contractions—after the cervix has undergone the changes just described—but it is common for the cervix to dilate 1 to 3 centimeters before the pregnant person has Positive Signs of labor. The cervix must open to approximately 10 centimeters in diameter to allow the baby through.

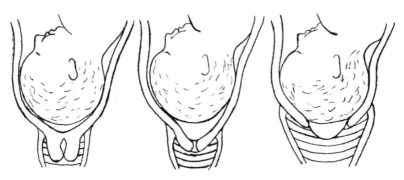

A cervix that has not effaced or dilated and is 3–4 cm (1 to 1½ inches) long

A cervix that is 75 percent effaced (about 1 cm long [½ inch] and 1 cm (½ inch) dilated

A cervix that is 100 percent effaced (or paper-thin) and 4 cm (1½ inches) dilated; the bag of waters is bulging

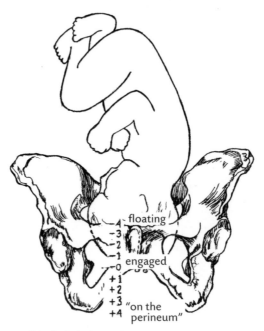

floating

-4
-3
-2
-1
-0 engaged
+1
+2
+3 "on the
+4 perineum"

Station—a measure of the baby's descent

5. **The baby's chin tucks onto the chest (called flexion) and the head rotates.** The rotation makes it easier for the baby to pass through the birth canal. (Sometimes, especially if the head is large, it must "mold" before it can rotate. This means the head changes shape, becoming longer and thinner. Molding is normal, although some babies' heads look somewhat misshapen for a day or two following birth, after which they return to a round shape.) The most favorable position for birth is usually the OA (occiput anterior) position; see page 66 for information on other positions.

6. **The baby descends.** The head continues to mold as necessary to fit and descends through the cervix, the pelvis, and the vagina to the outside. The descent is described in terms of "station," which tells how far above or below the pregnant person's midpelvis the baby's head is (or buttocks or feet, in the case of a breech presentation; see page 226); is measured in centimeters; and ranges from minus 4 to plus 4. A "zero station" means the baby's head is right at mid-pelvis. Minus 1, 2, 3, or 4 means the head is that number of centimeters above midpelvis. The greater the "plus" number, the closer the baby's head is to the outside and to being born.

Some descent usually takes place before labor begins, especially for first-time labors. When the baby "drops," it settles into the pelvis to about minus 2 or minus 1. Most of the descent occurs late in labor.

Steps 4 through 6 (dilation beyond 2 to 3 centimeters, rotation, and descent) cannot take place until the first three steps are well under way. In other words, a firm, thick, or posterior cervix won't open. It simply is not ready. And a baby won't rotate and descend significantly until the cervix is open. For many laboring people, the first three steps take place imperceptibly and gradually in late pregnancy. For others, they take place in a few days, with strong or even painful nonprogressing contractions, referred to as "prelabor" contractions (see page 72).

Timing Contractions

In early labor, one of the important jobs of the birth partner is to time contractions. Changes in the length, strength, and frequency of contractions are the all-important hallmarks of true progressing labor, so it is a good idea for you to know how to time them correctly and keep a written record. When you call the caregiver, you will have accurate and concrete information to provide.

You may use a smartphone or computer with an application for timing contractions. There are many available. Search the web or app store for "contraction timer," or something similar, or see our Recommended Resources on page 418. The laboring person indicates the beginning and end of the contractions and one of you taps the screen or presses a key. The smartphone keeps track of duration and frequency. You can enter other information such as that shown in the "Comments" column in the table on page 79. Keep track of five or six in a row to record the contraction pattern. Then, you may wait until the contraction pattern seems to have changed. Time five or six more contractions and resume timing when the contractions are clearly stronger. Continue this until it is time to call the hospital.

A note of caution: Many apps provide an "average duration" and "average frequency." Often, this can give the impression the contractions are closer together than they actually are and may cause you to leave for the hospital too soon.

portant to look for the one key rule: contractions that have ___ over time. That is, contractions have become *longer, stronger,* *r together or at least two of these criteria.* Once you meet these crite-___ the pattern reaches 4-1-1 or 5-1-1 (see page 94), it is time to go to the place of birth.

If you are not using a smartphone, use this method to track the contractions:

1. Use a watch or clock with a second hand and a written form similar to the sample "Early Labor Record," page 79.

2. You do not need to time every contraction. Instead, time and record five or six contractions in a row and then stop for a while (a few minutes to several hours depending on how quickly the contractions seem to be changing). Draw a line across the page to separate the timing periods. Later, when the pregnant person thinks the contractions have changed or is experiencing other signs of labor, time and record another five or six contractions.

3. Always note the time each contraction begins (specify when the times change from a.m. or p.m.). Record this time in the column headed "Time Contraction Starts."

4. Time the length of each contraction in seconds and record this time in the column headed "Duration." Contractions usually range from 20 to 50 seconds long in pre- or early labor and 1 to 2 minutes in late labor. Knowing when a contraction begins and ends is tricky. The best way is for the laboring person to signal that the contraction has begun or ended.

5. Determine how frequently the contractions are coming by subtracting the time at the start of one contraction from the time at the start of the next. Record the number of minutes between contractions in the "Interval" column. (For example, if one contraction begins at 7:32 and the next one begins at 7:38, they are 6 minutes apart.) Do the same for each subsequent contraction.

6. In the "Comments" column, record anything else that may be significant: how strong the contractions seem now compared with earlier, the laboring person's appetite and what they've

EARLY LABOR RECORD

DATE _____

	Time Contraction Starts	Duration (seconds)	Interval (minutes from start of one to start of next)	Comments (contraction strength, foods eaten, coping method, vaginal discharge, etc.)
sample	7:32 AM	40 sec		some bloody show
	7:38 AM	43 sec	6 minutes	ate toast
	7:45 AM	42 sec	7 minutes	

eaten, what they're doing to cope (see chapter 4), whether they have back pain or blood-tinged discharge ("show"), whether fluid is leaking, etc. Of course, if the fluid has gushed, call the caregiver or hospital as described on page 71.

When you call the caregiver or the hospital's labor floor, have the information near you and be prepared to report what you recorded. (Make sure you know whom to call. Some caregivers prefer you call them directly; others want you to call the hospital's labor-and-delivery area and talk to a nurse.)

Note: When timing contractions and considering the interval, or how far apart the contractions are, it is important to count from the *start* of one contraction to the *start* of the next. Don't fall into the trap of timing from the end of one to the start of the next, as you will go to your place of birth or call your birth team too soon!

See page 95 for the discussion "When Do You Go to the Hospital or Settle in for a Home Birth?"

Now that you know how to tell when labor is underway, you're ready to read the next chapter about what happens during labor.

CHAPTER 3

MOVING THROUGH THE STAGES OF LABOR

At home with my wife in labor, I couldn't wait to get the doula to the house. Shortly after she arrived, I wanted to get to the hospital. In the end, it was 16 hours from the first contraction that woke my wife until we went to the hospital. You may have way more time than you think.

—SCOTT, FIRST-TIME FATHER

The class described a step-by-step process and walked me through what I needed to know. Afterward, I was nervous because I did not remember the stages and how I could help. Then labor began, and it all came flooding back in one rush of a major contraction. We are told a woman has the instincts to birth and care for her child, but I think the partners during these experiences are also enabled with such gifts. We just need the knowledge and facts to go along with these instincts.

—HOWARD, FIRST-TIME FATHER

Labor and birth rate among the most intense of all normal human experiences because they are so demanding—physically, emotionally, and mentally. This is true not only for the person in labor, but also for those who love and care for that person. Labor is unpredictable, empowering, and fulfilling—and it comes with a great prize at the end!

Compare Labor to Running a Marathon

Childbirth has many similarities to a marathon or other physical endurance event. Both include pain and psychological demands for the participant. Both require stamina and patience. Both become much more manageable when the participant is well prepared and flexible and has the following in advance:

• Knowledge of what to expect

• Prior planning with a knowledgeable guide

• Good health

• Encouragement and support before and throughout the event

• Confidence that muscle pain and fatigue are normal side effects of such effort

• Fluids and adequate nourishment

• The ability to pace oneself

• The availability of expert medical assistance, in case it is needed

The meaning of the event (the race or the labor) varies among endurance athletes and childbearing people alike. For some athletes, running a marathon means not only finishing, but also trying to come in at the front of the pack. For others, finishing is the goal and the reward. For some childbearing people, labor and birth mean not only having a baby, but also doing it without medical or surgical intervention. For others, having the baby is the goal and the reward.

It is true for both athletes and birthing people that if they develop complications, or begin to worry about the tough challenges ahead, or become preoccupied with the pain, or lose confidence, or become overwhelmed, they will need to adjust. The athlete may have to slow down or drop out; the laboring person may need to change strategies and rely more on the caregiver and medical interventions to help facilitate a birth that is safe and satisfying.

The analogy between an endurance sporting event and childbirth breaks down, however, when we look further. One of the greatest differences is the matter of choice. Marathon runners do not have to run the race. They choose to do so and they can choose not to finish. Pregnant people, however, must go through labor and delivery (or another demanding and painful process—cesarean delivery) if they are to have a child. The other enormous difference between the two events is their degree of predictability. The marathon runner knows when the event will take place and how long the course is and can study the course ahead of time. The course doesn't change and is the same for all participants.

The most predictable thing about childbirth is its total unpredictability. A pregnant person does not know when labor will begin, how long it will take, or how painful it will be, or whether problems will arise that may require medical treatment. They do not know whether or how it might be similar or different from their mother's labors or the labors of other people. They cannot even be sure to get a good night's sleep beforehand! And they cannot predict what the postpartum course will be like.

This unpredictability of childbirth may be a source of frustration or anxiety for both of you as you learn what to expect and how to help. Partners in our childbirth classes often ask questions such as these:

• Once the cervix has begun to ripen, how long does it usually take before labor starts?

• After contractions begin, how many hours before we should go to the hospital?

• How long is the pushing stage?

• When should I take time off from work?

• How bad will the pain get?

• When do babies sleep through the night?

• How long do people breast-feed?

Questions like these usually receive evasive answers: "It may be hours or days. You can be sure it is a sign they are moving in the right direction." "It varies." "We can't be sure." "People experience things differently." "It's hard to say."

Birth partners want to know exactly what to prepare for, but it is simply not possible to answer these questions precisely. Variations are inherent in childbirth because each human being and each labor is unique. The key is to accept the unpredictability and pace yourselves while the labor process unfolds.

There is good news, however. Despite all the uncertainties, there are some things you can count on. This chapter gives you a broad idea of what you can expect from this mysterious process. You will learn the wide range of normal possibilities and how you can be truly helpful. The emotions experienced by laboring people constitute a large part of the discussion, along with the emotional responses you may have. Here, you'll find practical and useful suggestions to help with the challenging task of providing the laboring person emotional support as well as physical comfort. Finally, you will learn how a doula may help both of you throughout the labor for two reasons:

1. Besides being for birth partners, this book is used as a training guide for doulas.

2. Knowing the doula's role may help you decide whether to have a doula at your birth.

The following terms describe what happens during labor and how the laboring person may respond:

- *Prelabor* refers to the time before labor actually begins, when the pregnant person experiences nonprogressing contractions (see page 72) and the cervix is changing, but not yet dilating. The contractions may come and go for a period of hours to days.

- The *first stage* of labor (often simply called *labor*) is the *dilation stage*, during which the cervix dilates completely—to about 10 centimeters in diameter. The contractions progress over time, becoming longer, stronger, and/or closer together.

- The *second stage* is the *pushing and birthing stage*, during which the baby is born.

- The *third stage* is the *placental stage*, during which the placenta, or afterbirth, is born.

- The *fourth stage* is the *recovery and bonding stage* during which the birthing parent and baby get to know each other and the first feedings occur.

See the illustrations of each stage and phase of labor on page 115.

The dilation (first) and birthing (second) stages are further divided (four phases in the first stage and three in the second). With every new phase, labor changes its rhythm, and the laboring person must make an emotional adjustment. This chapter describes each stage and phase and includes suggestions for how you and a doula can help the laboring person cope. See the table "Normal Labor—in a Nutshell," pages 138–142, for a brief summary of this information you may want to keep handy during labor.

Prelabor

Prelabor is the phase that precedes actual labor. See chapter 2 for a detailed discussion of prelabor. This is the time when you and the laboring person are likely to be on your own or with an anxious relative or friend. If you understand what is happening and how to help, you have a better chance of getting to the hospital or birth center or gathering the birth team for a home birth at the appropriate time—neither too early nor too late.

Getting to the hospital too early means either that the pregnant person will be sent home or that medical interventions to start labor may be performed essentially out of impatience ("They're here; let's get labor going."). Medical interventions don't always succeed, and they tend to pile up—one intervention leading to another. If you can avoid this cascade of interventions by going to the hospital at the proper time, the pregnant person will have a better chance of a normal delivery. In fact, the American College of Obstetricians and Gynecologists, which sets guidelines for maternity care, strongly recommends NOT being admitted to the hospital too early as a way to avoid unnecessary medical treatment, including cesarean delivery. We want to help you feel confident in staying home until the right time. See page 95 for guidance on when to go and what to do until you go or your midwife joins you for a home birth.

What is Prelabor Like for the First-Time Parent?

During prelabor, the first-time pregnant parent may have very regular uterine contractions as the uterus begins "tuning up." These may continue in an unwavering pattern for many hours. Contractions may be regular and strong, and sometimes even fairly close together (every 5 to 8 minutes), for hours. However, they do not progress (by becoming longer, stronger, or closer together over a period of time), and they may even stop after a few hours. The cervix softens, moves forward, and thins, but does not dilate beyond 1 to 2 centimeters. Until the contractions are clearly progressing (which you can best discover by timing them for a while as described on page 77), the pregnant person is in prelabor, and the cervix is not ready to begin dilating significantly.

Before going on, we should mention that a small percentage of pregnant parents, first-time and not, never experience much of what we have just described. They skip the preliminaries and begin having progressing contractions as soon as they are aware they are having contractions. Sometimes, when they look back, they realize that the restless night's sleep or the crampy, soft bowel movements must have been prelabor. Others have no warm-up. They plunge immediately into labor.

What is Prelabor Like for the Pregnant Person Having a Second or Subsequent Child?

Prelabor is often different for the experienced parent. Strong contractions may continue for a while, especially at night, even progressing enough to convince them they are in labor, but then subside by morning and resume the next night. This "on-again-off-again" contraction pattern is not unusual for an experienced pregnant person. They may be 3 or 4 centimeters dilated but not yet be in labor! While such a pattern can be frustrating, think of it this way: "You're dilating, and you aren't even in labor!" Once labor actually gets going, it is usually faster than the first, though there are exceptions.

As you can see, prelabor can be a confusing time for the pregnant person, birth partner, and even the caregiver. You may find it difficult to distinguish between this tuning up and the "real thing." Then, without warning, and perhaps without either of you recognizing it, prelabor contractions become the "real thing"—getting longer, stronger, and/or closer together. The cervix begins to dilate.

How Long Does Prelabor Last?

Prelabor may last from a few hours to many hours, or it may come and go over several days.

What Will the Pregnant Person Feel?

During prelabor, the pregnant person may feel one or more of these emotions:

- Confusion about whether they are in labor or not

- Excitement and anticipation, as they realize the baby will be here soon

- Overreaction, as it's easy to assume the cervix must be dilating more than the labor signs indicate

- Fear or dread, especially if they are not mentally prepared, if labor is earlier than expected, or if the contractions are more painful than expected

    If prelabor goes on for days, the laboring person may feel one or more of these emotions:

- Frustration over not knowing what is happening and feeling tricked by the confusing signs

- Discouragement over the long wait

- Fatigue or exhaustion, if sleep has been missed

- Doubt or anxiety about their body's ability to function properly, especially if the contractions are painful but not progressing

- Worry about being too tired to handle the progressing contractions when they begin

What the Caregiver Does

Depending on your report, the caregiver may suggest that the laboring person wait at home, come into the office for a progress check, or go straight to the hospital or birth center. In addition, the caregiver may do any of the following:

- Come to your home to check the laboring person, if a home birth is planned. Depending on the midwife's findings, they may leave or stay.

- Offer advice and encouragement to help handle this frustrating phase.

- Suggest a warm bath or medication for rest or to slow contractions if prelabor has been going on for a long time; see page 311 for information about medications used for these purposes.

- Try to speed labor with medications or by breaking the bag of waters (see "Induction or Augmentation of Labor," page 256).

What Might You Feel?

As the birth partner, you may experience:

- Confusion, as you have no frame of reference against which to compare the birthing person's present behavior or verbal expression of pain ("This seems easy." or "How much harder can this get?" or "I can't believe the nurse told us not to come in yet.").

- Anxiety about packing the car and getting to the hospital or birth center in time

- Frustration that prelabor seems to be taking a long time or that the signs of labor are not clearer

- Concern over whether you are helping the laboring person enough or that they are not handling it very well

- Excitement that the big day is here (or near)!

- Eagerness to help the laboring person and see the baby

- Worry, if the laboring person is tired and discouraged

- Exhausted, if you have missed a lot of sleep

- Guilty, if you slept and the laboring person didn't

How You Can Help

Assist the laboring person with prelabor in these ways:

- Realize that a long prelabor, though challenging, is not a medical problem in itself. Therefore, it is mostly up to the two of you to handle it, perhaps with the help of a doula, friends, or family members.

- Recognize prelabor for what it is. Help the laboring person determine whether the contractions are progressing by timing them occasionally. If they are not progressing, point out that labor will feel clearly different from what is currently happening (see "Timing Contractions," page 77; "Signs of Labor," page 67; and "'False' Labor, or Prelabor," page 72).

- Check with the caregiver for advice and reassurance and possibly to arrange an examination.

- Encourage the laboring person to eat when hungry and drink when thirsty.

- Do projects or activities together to help get your minds off the contractions. You might give a massage, or the two of you might prepare food, play games, go for a walk, visit with friends, or read a book aloud to each other. If the laboring person likes to color or do crafts, have the necessary materials on hand.

- Consult "The Slow-to-Start Labor," page 216, for specific coping techniques if prelabor continues for a long time.

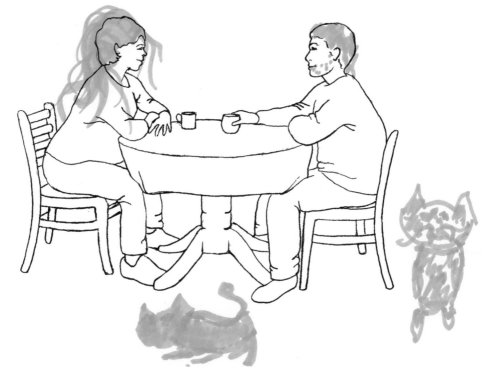

How Does a Doula Help?

If you have a doula, give them a heads-up call during prelabor even if you do not need extra support yet—especially if prelabor goes on for a long time. Depending on the situation and the pregnant person's needs, the doula may simply talk with you by phone or may join you at this time. The doula will listen to both of you describe what is going on and give concrete suggestions for raising your spirits if you are discouraged, pacing yourselves if progress is slow, and getting some rest, even if neither of you can sleep.

The doula may review how you will know when labor is progressing and remind you of comfort measures that help during prelabor. If they live close enough to come to your house, the doula can go for a walk with the laboring person, suggest and help with activities such as packing the car and baking cookies or bread, or just stay a while so you can run errands, take a nap, or shower. The doula may go home if contractions slow and you no longer feel the need for their company. If the doula leaves, they will make sure you know how to reach them immediately when you are ready for more support. The doula can also help you decide when to call the caregiver or go to the hospital.

The Dilation, First, Stage

Dilation, or the opening of the cervix, occurs in the first stage of labor. Dilation begins about when the prelabor contractions change from their nonprogressing pattern to becoming longer, stronger, and closer together (or at least two of those three). The first stage ends when the cervix has dilated completely (to approximately 10 centimeters). The dilation stage can proceed very quickly, unevenly, or slowly. It has distinct phases: the latent phase (also called early labor), the active phase (or active labor), and the transition phase (or just transition; see illustrations, page 115).

The change from prelabor to the dilation stage may be gradual, so don't expect that either of you will know the moment the cervix begins to open.

In a "textbook" labor, the contractions gradually and steadily increase in intensity and duration and come closer together. Early contractions may last from 30 to 40 seconds and come anywhere from 5 to 20 minutes apart. Although there are exceptions, these early contractions are usually painless. As they progress in length, frequency, and duration, they become more intense and painful. By the time the cervix opens to 8 or 9 centimeters, the contractions may last 90 seconds or more, feel very intense (almost surely very painful), and come every 2 to 4 minutes. The pain of labor usually reaches its maximum by 7 or 8 centimeters. Second-stage contractions are different and may not be painful or may be painful in a different way (see pages 121–123).

How Long Does the Dilation Stage Last?

The dilation stage lasts from 2 to 24 hours, although for first-time labors, it rarely lasts fewer than 4 hours.

You cannot know in advance how long dilation will take, but the way labor starts may give you some clues. If the labor starts right off with contractions that seem very long or very painful and close together, you may wonder whether these are the relatively easy ones you've been expecting. You must trust the laboring person's perceptions and yours. Their labor might be one of those uncommon, very fast ones. Call the caregiver or the hospital, give an accurate idea of what is happening, and get the caregiver's or nurse's advice. Try not to worry; a very fast labor usually means everything is normal (almost too normal!). Turn immediately to chapter 5, page 207, for a discussion of the very rapid labor.

In a slow labor, contractions continue as quite manageable and progress very gradually over a long period of time. This can lead to discouragement, fatigue, and worry. You'll both need to pace yourselves through an extra-long labor (see "Arrest of Active Labor [Dystocia]," page 286).

When to Call the Caregiver or Hospital?

Make sure you have the correct numbers to call (see chapter 1, page 45) and call under any of the following circumstances:

• Signs of labor before 37 weeks—a premature labor (see "Signs of Labor," page 67)

- Leaking or a gush of fluid from the vagina (see "If the Bag of Waters Breaks Before Labor Begins," page 71)

- Contractions clearly becoming longer, stronger, and closer together (see "Signs of Labor," page 67; "The 4-1-1 or 5-1-1 Rule," page 94; and "Timing Contractions," page 77)

- You or the laboring person has questions or concerns

- If the pregnant parent has given birth before, call the caregiver or hospital when the contractions are progressing and the pregnant person thinks or knows labor has started. A second (or later) labor is usually faster than a first one.

Early Labor

This first phase of the dilation stage lasts until the cervix is dilated to 5 or 6 centimeters. Medical professionals call this the *latent phase* of the first stage.

The big difference between prelabor and early labor is that during early labor, the cervix begins to open gradually. For the laboring person, birth partner, and doula, this shift to early labor is signaled by clearly progressing contractions. The caregiver uses vaginal exams as necessary to determine changes in the cervix during this phase.

How Long Does Early Labor Last?

Typically, early labor takes from two-thirds to three-quarters of the total time of the dilation stage. In other words, it could take from a few hours to 20 hours or so for a person in labor to reach 5 or 6 centimeters of dilation. The length of early labor depends largely on the state of the cervix, the position and station of the baby within the pelvis at the time labor begins, and the strength of the contractions. Chances for more rapid progress are increased if the following conditions exist:

- The cervix has moved forward and is very soft and thin (see page 74).

- The contractions are intense and close together.

- The baby is in the occiput anterior (OA) position, with head down, chin on chest, and the back of the head toward the pregnant person's front (see page 66). You and the pregnant person really can't tell the position of the baby; it is also difficult for the caregiver to tell.

• The baby's head has begun to move down into the pelvis (see page 76).

These favorable conditions increase the likelihood of an average or shorter-than-average early labor. Under any other conditions, early labor is likely to take longer than the rest of labor. Labor is not a race against time, however. A normal early labor can last from a few hours to many hours.

How Will the Laboring Person Feel?

The laboring person's response to early labor will probably not be that different from the response to prelabor. They are still likely to feel somewhat uncertain as the Positive Signs of labor become clear.

How the laboring person adjusts emotionally to being in labor depends on the circumstances—whether labor is early, on time, or late and whether early contractions are hard and fast or vague and slow. It also depends on their self-confidence, understanding of what is happening, knowledge of self-help comfort measures to manage the pain, and the support from you, the staff, and a doula.

Reactions to labor range from relief, elation, or excitement to denial, disbelief, worry, fear, or panic. As labor settles into a rhythmic pattern, the laboring person usually settles down emotionally, pacing themselves and finding routines for handling each contraction.

Sometimes, in the excitement of early labor, the laboring person rushes the labor along in their mind. You may do the same thing. You both may overreact to these relatively mild contractions. If they concentrate hard on each one, they can feel it for a longer time, and so it seems longer and more intense than if they are distracted by some other activity. This results partly from the desire for labor to go quickly and partly from not knowing what level of intensity to expect. Without this frame of reference, it is easy to become convinced that labor is progressing more rapidly than it really is.

When the laboring person rushes labor mentally, they may want to go to the hospital too early, start using rhythmic breathing and other labor-coping measures before they are really needed, and speculate that the cervix is dilated much more than it really is. Then, after a vaginal exam reveals that labor is not as advanced as thought, the laboring person becomes discouraged and may lose confidence in their ability to cope.

How can you tell whether the laboring person is overreacting to early labor, reacting appropriately, or having a particularly difficult or rapid labor? Without vaginal exams, you cannot really know whether labor is progressing quickly or not. The best you can do is make an educated guess. Refer to "Signs of Labor" (see page 67), time the contractions, and see whether the laboring person can be distracted. Try a walk outside or phone or visit with friends or relatives. If labor seems to "slow down" or become easier when distracted, they may have overreacted. Keep up the distractions (see "How You Can Help" page 88, for other ideas for handling overreaction to early labor). Above all, try not to overreact yourself. It is just as easy for you to make this mistake as it is for the laboring person.

If distraction doesn't help or if labor does not slow down when the laboring person is distracted, then they are not overreacting. Stop the distractions and help them cope instead. Encourage them to focus on the contractions and begin using their prescribed (or planned) ritual—slow breaths combined with relaxation and positive mental focus (see page 158). If strong contractions are coming one on top of another and nothing helps them cope, they are likely having a fast, intense labor (see page 207).

What the Caregiver or Labor-and-Delivery Staff Do

During early labor, the caregiver or hospital staff can help in the following ways:

• Giving advice over the telephone; when you call, be prepared to provide the information recorded on the Early Labor Record (see page 79).

The 4-1-1 or 5-1-1 Rule

Before going to the hospital or birth center, wait until the contractions have been 4 to 5 minutes apart and 1 minute long for at least 1 hour. Whether you use 4-1-1 or 5-1-1 depends on the caregiver's preferences, the laboring person's preference, whether this is a first or subsequent labor, how far you are from the hospital or birth center, and whether there is considered high risk of complications.

- Helping the laboring person decide when to go to the hospital or having a home birth, when to settle in at home for the labor. If it is not yet time to go, they may advise some things to do until it is time.

- Advising when to go to the caregiver's office or hospital for assessment of the contractions and, perhaps, a vaginal exam for an idea of how dilation is progressing.

When Do You Go to the Hospital or Settle in for a Home Birth?

Under most circumstances, the first-time laboring parent should go to the hospital or birth center or settle in for a home birth when they have had 12 to 15 consecutive contractions that:

- Last at least 1 minute

- Are 4 to 5 minutes apart (or closer)

- Are strong enough they cannot be distracted from them

- Are strong enough they *must* use a breathing, relaxation, or attention-focusing ritual (see page 147) to get through them

Usually, it takes about an hour to time the contractions and determine whether they fit this pattern. If they are less than 4 minutes apart and advancing quickly, however, do not wait an hour before going to the hospital or birth center.

Sometimes, there are reasons for going to the hospital earlier than described here. For example:

- The pregnant person lives a long distance from the hospital.

- There are medical problems that require early admission. The caregiver will advise whether these problems exist.

- The pregnant person has given birth before (especially if the first labor was very rapid) and recognizes that labor has started. A second (or later) labor usually goes faster than the first one.

- They are anxious and really want to be at the hospital or birth center.

Note: If the plan is to give birth in an out-of-hospital birth center, do not go there without calling the midwife to set a time to meet at the birth center. The facility may be locked and unstaffed, especially at night.

Because early labor can take a long time, it is often a good idea to spend the time relaxing together or with friends until the contractions fit the pattern described here. It is usually best not to arrive at the hospital (or call the caregiver to the home) too early because:

- The laboring person may feel "performance anxiety"—pressure to start producing some good contractions. They may feel watched by the caregiver or nurse, who seems to be waiting for something to happen, and may feel something is wrong because labor is so slow.

- The laboring person may become unnecessarily preoccupied with the contractions and the apparent lack of progress, and this may make labor seem longer or more difficult than it is.

- The laboring person may become bored, anxious, or discouraged.

- The staff may offer or suggest medical interventions to speed up this normally slow part of labor. You and the laboring person should ask the key questions (see page 237) before considering these interventions. They all carry some risks, including the possibility they will not succeed and then other interventions may be required. Without a medical need, these interventions may carry more risk than benefit.

Sometimes, the caregiver will recommend that you and the laboring person leave the hospital or birth center and come back later. For a home birth, everyone except you may have to leave for a while. Although discouraging, this measure allows the labor to settle into its own pattern and takes pressure off the laboring person.

How Might You Feel?

You may have many of the feelings described for prelabor, plus:

- Hope and elation, now that the contractions progressing

- Concern, especially if the laboring person is tired, discouraged, or having trouble dealing with the pain

PART TWO: LABOR AND BIRTH

- Eager to get word from "the experts" that this is labor, that it is time to go to the hospital or birth center, or for the midwife and others to arrive for a home birth

- Tired, if you have missed sleep

How You Can Help

Your role now is very similar to the role you played during prelabor. Remain close by; supply the laboring person with food and drink; time five or six contractions, as described on page 94, when the pattern seems to change; and help the laboring person pass the time with pleasant and distracting activities (see "The Slow-to-Start Labor," page 216).

Talk with the laboring person if you feel you must leave for work, errands, or other activities. Whether you go depends on their feelings and the following considerations:

- Can you be reached by phone at all times?

- How far will you have to travel to reach the laboring person? How long will it take?

- Is there someone else available (friend, relative, doula, neighbor) to help if the laboring person needs someone right away?

- What are the pressures on you—from work, school, or other responsibilities?

- Will a few more hours really let you clear up pressing obligations?

If you still feel you should leave and the laboring person agrees, make sure someone else stays there until you can return. Consider this a last resort, as labor can change suddenly.

At some point, the labor pattern will intensify and the laboring person will become preoccupied with the contractions, no longer able to walk or talk through them without pausing; the contractions "stop them in their tracks." From this point on, it is not appropriate to leave or to distract them. Instead, do the following:

- Give the laboring person your undivided attention throughout every contraction. Stop what you are doing and stop talking so you can focus. Do not ask questions during contractions.

during the contractions and, if you notice tension, help the
~ng person relax their entire body during each one (see "Relax-
~," page 147).

- ~~ggest using the planned ritual ("relax, breathe, and focus")—slow, rhythmic breathing while focusing on something pleasant or positive, such as letting go of tension with each exhale (see page 161).

- Encourage slow, rhythmic breathing through comforting touch and verbal encouragement during each contraction ("That's good. . . . Just like that.") and helpful comments when the contraction is over ("You relaxed very well that time," or "I noticed you tensed your shoulders with that contraction; with the next one, focus on keeping your shoulders relaxed.").

- Help decide when to call the caregiver.

- If you have hired one, but not yet called your doula, call now, either to alert them that you expect to need them soon or to ask them to join you.

What does a doula do? Beginning with your phone call, the doula will probably:

- Ask what's happening. Tell the doula about the signs of labor, the contraction pattern, and how you both feel and are coping.

- Ask to speak to the laboring person and assess their distractibility.

- Listen to the laboring person through a contraction to get an idea of how they are coping (does the breathing or moaning sound relaxed or tense?) and to encourage them in their planned ritual, perhaps by breathing audibly with them through the contraction. This will help the laboring person relax and breathe rhythmically.

- Ask the laboring person the all-important question: "What was going through your mind during that contraction?" As the doula listens to the laboring person's response, they assess whether the laboring person is positive and coping well or feeling distressed.

- Be sure you and the laboring person know if the doula can or will come to your home in early labor. Sometimes, it is not realistic due to distance; some doulas have a policy of joining you at the hospital or birth center. Be sure you know in advance.

If the laboring person is coping well and you do not indicate otherwise, the doula will probably decide not to come yet, but will remind you of things to do and make a plan for staying in touch.

If the laboring person is distressed or asks the doula to come, the doula may suggest some coping strategies to try until they arrive and will hurry to join you. The doula should tell you when and where they'll arrive—at your home, the hospital, or the birth center.

When the doula joins you, they will:

- Wash their hands, and, if you are at the hospital or birth center, meet the staff

- Assess the laboring person's needs and your feelings

- Assist as appropriate, keeping in mind your planned support role, which you, the laboring person, and the doula discussed in a previous meeting

- Sit quietly through a contraction or two to observe the two of you working together so their role will fit with what you are doing

- Help you determine when to go to the hospital or birth center, if you are still at home

Early labor eventually evolves into a more intense pattern of progressing contractions.

Getting into Active Labor (3 to 5 Centimeters Dilation)

For years, based on studies from the 1950s, normal labor progress was said to speed up at 3 or 4 centimeters of dilation, to a rate of 1 centimeter per hour. This was identified as the onset of "active labor." If progress fell behind that rate, it was said to be "prolonged" and interventions were started to increase the contractions, for example, breaking the bag of waters or giving intravenous Pitocin (see chapter 6). Older childbirth books still contain that information. However, recent research on dilation patterns in labors with normal outcomes has found that dilation may begin to speed up as late as 6 centimeters; this means interventions to speed labor may not be needed. The normal active phase of labor can start as late as 6 centimeters.

This may feel like a mixed blessing to the laboring person, who may be glad to know nothing is wrong if dilation is slow after 3 centimeters (1 inch), but is tired and worried about having to manage longer and more intense contractions without apparent progress in dilation.

You need to know that during the time from 3 to 6 centimeters an emotional shift takes place in many laboring people, and the support they need from their partner and doula changes. We call this period the "3 to 6 phase," or "getting into active labor." This is also likely to be when contractions reach the point when you should go to the hospital or birth center or that your home birth midwife should be called (see 4-1-1 or 5-1-1, pages 94).

It is not unusual for the laboring person to have a cervical exam and be told the cervix has not dilated much. This is discouraging. The explanation is that even though the contractions have increased in intensity and duration, the cervix may not yet be ready to dilate. It may require time to ripen, thin, or move forward enough to begin dilating (see pages 74–77). We sometimes say "3 to 6" is the time when the laboring person turns the corner into active labor. Your help with comfort measures (see chapter 4), along with guidance and reassurance from a doula or other knowledgeable person, help the laboring person understand what is happening and manage the more intense contractions. And, if necessary, pain medications are available in the hospital (see chapter 8). Note that "3 to 6" may take 2 to 4 hours or possibly more.

How Will the Laboring Person Feel?

We sometimes refer to this phase as the "moment of truth," when the laboring person realizes, in a new and powerful way, they cannot control this labor. Earlier optimism may give way to a temporary loss of confidence or a struggle to remain "in control." They may worry that labor is too difficult or weep from discouragement and a sense of a long way to go. They may want pain medications, even if that wasn't the original plan. As they struggle with the lack of control, the laboring person comes to realize they can't do it with will or determination alone and may give up trying to control it. One woman said, "I can't do this; I'm done." As she stopped "thinking her way through the contractions," things changed for the better. This time is often a turning point. If the laboring person doesn't feel judged and feels emotionally "safe," they are likely to become more instinctual and find their "spontaneous ritual"—their own way to cope during the contractions (see pages 151–153).

What the Caregiver or Labor-and-Delivery Staff Do

If the laboring person has not already been admitted to the hospital or birth center, they will be now. If a home birth is planned, the midwife will try to get there at this time.

How Might You Feel?

You may feel worried or helpless that you can't make it better, especially if the laboring person finds this harder than expected. You may think the laboring person should have pain medications, even if the plan was to postpone or avoid them.

How You Can Help

Recognize the change in mood; don't try to distract the laboring person—no jokes or games any more. Don't minimize their worries. Stay calm, use a soothing "labor voice," and murmur soothing, encouraging words. Help them maintain a rhythm (see pages 147–164). Use comfort measures (slow dancing, massage, visualizations, rhythmic breathing, and moaning). Acknowledge that this is difficult, but don't give up. Offer support using the 3 Rs (relaxation, rhythm, and ritual) through the contractions (page 147). Support their original preferences regarding the use of pain medications (see pages 327–329). If the original plan was to use pain medications, this might be a good time to get them. If the plan was to minimize or postpone medications, encourage the laboring person to continue. Try a change in ritual for a few contractions: Walk, use light breathing (see pages 163–164), try a massage (see pages 187–196), or the Take-Charge routine (see pages 202–207). The good news is that once the laboring person gets through this phase, they will have found a way to cope, and the contractions will likely be more manageable.

3Rs

How a Doula Helps

A doula reassures you both that these are normal challenges and feelings during this phase and encourages the laboring person that this can be done. The doula's calmness can transfer to and help both of you. Doulas know this is the way labor unfolds and remain patient and upbeat. Their quiet confidence, based on training and experience, along with specific suggestions and help with comfort measures, can make you more effective at this challenging time. If you feel unsure, the doula can step in and demonstrate a technique or help with such measures as massage or the Take-Charge routine. Or, if needed, the doula can give you a break.

Active Labor

The active phase of labor begins when the cervix is thin and soft and contractions are closer and stronger. At this point, the cervix has dilated to about 6 centimeters and now begins to dilate faster (although in some labors the cervix is ready to dilate quickly before 6 centimeters). Active labor lasts until cervical dilation reaches about 8 centimeters.

During active labor, contractions intensify, still lasting more than 1 minute and coming every 3 to 4 minutes. The contractions are usually very intense, and most laboring people describe them as very painful, but manageable.

It is important to recognize the positive meanings of active labor. As demanding as the contractions are, they mean labor is progressing well and the laboring body is doing exactly what it needs to do. The pain is not a danger sign; rather, it is a side effect of the strong contractions, the pressure in the uterus, and the stretching of the cervix that will bring the baby into the world. It is possible for many laboring people to cope with these intense contractions when they have had good support through the "3 to 6" phase; that is, they know ways to reduce the pain and stay relaxed; have continuous feedback from positive partners; and experience a reasonably normal labor pattern.

How Long Does Active Labor Last?

Normally, active labor is much shorter than early labor and the "3 to 6" phase. For first-time laboring people, active labor usually ranges from 3 to 7 hours. It is usually much faster for those who have had babies before—from 20 minutes to 3 hours.

What the Laboring Person Feels

The person in labor must make an emotional adjustment to the changing rhythm and sensations of labor, becoming focused on coping with the more frequent and intense contractions, and may not even realize the pace of dilation is picking up or will soon. Response to the changing rhythm of labor may include:

- Feeling tired and discouraged as they realize the tough part is just beginning, or they may have found a ritual and be very focused during each contraction. With support and encouragement, their mood will likely turn to acceptance, and they will discover their own way to handle the contractions.

- Extraneous conversation becomes annoying. The laboring person may feel very alone if you and others do not recognize this change and continue trying to distract or, worse, ignore them and talk to one another.

- When the laboring person lets their body take over, they become serious and focused on the contractions. They devote all attention to maintaining a rhythmic ritual—releasing tension, breathing, moving, or moaning during contractions. When a contraction ends, conversation, if any, is likely to consist of reviewing it with you and talking about what to do for the next one.

- With your understanding and good support, the laboring person will be able to get past this crisis, let go of the need to be in control, and work with, not against, the contractions, by letting the body take over. We call these unplanned coping techniques *spontaneous rituals*.

At this time, the laboring person benefits from a quiet room, freedom to move around in and out of bed, and as little disturbance or interruption as possible. They may want to be held or stroked or, conversely, not touched at all. This is when laboring people become more instinctual, more focused, and less verbal. You might think when labor is steadily advancing, people would find it more and more difficult to cope. But this is not the case when laboring people feel well supported. They actually find it easier to cope once they release the need to be in control because they let their bodies take over, become more instinctual in their behavior, and discover what works for them.

What the Caregiver Does

In a hospital birth, generally, the doctor isn't in the birth room very much during active labor but is available nearby or by telephone. A nurse provides most of the direct clinical care, following the doctor's orders. If the caregiver is a midwife, they are likely to provide more care than a doctor, but the nurse is a major figure in carrying out the midwife's orders.

As labor advances, the midwife or nurse becomes more actively involved. Now that progress is faster and the contractions are more intense, closer surveillance is needed. The nurse or midwife checks the laboring person's:

• Blood pressure, pulse, and temperature

• Fluid intake and urine output

• Length, intensity, and frequency of contractions

• Dilation of the cervix

In addition, the nurse or midwife also checks the baby's heart rate and position and station (see page 76).

Routines vary, depending on the management style of the caregiver. Some obstetricians rely heavily on routine interventions and medical technology. For example, breaking the bag of waters, restricting the laboring person to bed, giving intravenous (IV) fluids, using electronic fetal monitors to continuously check the fetus and the contractions, giving the laboring person medications to speed the labor and relieve pain, performing an episiotomy (a surgical incision to enlarge the vaginal opening just before birth), and, if the birth is taking too long and progressing too slowly, use forceps, a vacuum extractor, or cesarean surgery to deliver the baby.

Other obstetricians and most midwives and family doctors rely on simpler methods. They might encourage a healthy person at low risk for complications to drink liquids and move around. They might listen to

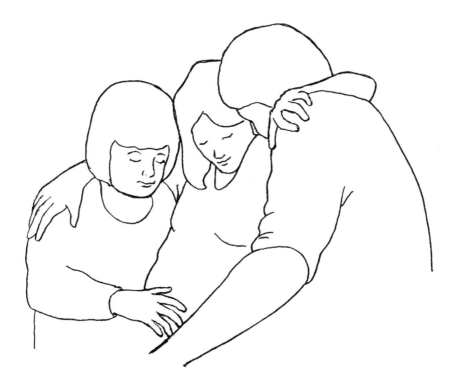

the fetal heartbeat with a handheld Doppler ultrasound device or use the electronic fetal monitor off and on through the labor rather than continuously. They might suggest comfort measures (see chapter 4, page 143) to relieve pain before offering an epidural or other drugs.

Midwives and family doctors tend to intervene less than most obstetricians, partly because of training, but also because midwives and family doctors are more likely to care for people with healthy pregnancies and few risks of medical problems in labor. Obstetricians care for people at both low and high risk for problems, and many tend to use procedures for all patients that are really only needed for high-risk pregnancies. See both the introduction to part 3, page 236, and chapter 6 for information about commonly used tests and procedures and also for key questions to ask and alternatives to consider.

The nurse or caregiver may offer helpful advice and reassurance. Having someone there with expertise and experience—someone you both trust—can be immensely reassuring. Don't hesitate to ask for help or advice if you feel uncertain about the labor or about how you can help the person in labor.

How Might You Feel?

Although you may be excited to recognize that labor is progressing faster, active labor may be hard for you in several ways:

• Seeing the laboring person in pain, weeping, or asking you for more help may make you feel ineffective, helpless, worried, or even a little guilty they have to go through so much.

• If you do not recognize that labor progress is speeding up, you may worry about how long the labor is taking, especially because it is so intense.

• You may feel cruel if you encourage the laboring person to endure the pain, even if that is what they want to do. You may feel anxious to relieve their pain and be tempted to request that an anesthesiologist administer an epidural, even if they are not asking for it.

• If you recognize the laboring person is making good progress, you may feel encouraged and confident they can get through labor as they prefer and that you are being helpful.

How You Can Help

Your role during active labor is very important. How you respond to the laboring person's needs determines, to a large extent, how well they cope and will feel later about the birth experience. Here are some guidelines for helping during this phase:

• **Take care of yourself.** How long has it been since you ate? If labor has gone on for a long time, do you need to freshen up with a shower, brush your teeth, or change your clothes? Do you need a rest? If you're exhausted, hungry, or feeling grungy, you may need a break. Do not to be gone for long and make sure the laboring person is not left alone. A doula or loved one can stand in while you are gone.

• **Make sure staff are aware of the birth plan**, especially with regard to preferences for pain medications and other interventions. See chapter 1, page 45 and chapter 8, page 304.

• **Follow the laboring person's lead.** Take your cues from them; match their mood. If serious or quiet, you be serious or quiet. Don't try to jolly them out of this mood or distract them at this time. Labor takes almost all their attention, and they need you physically and emotionally.

- **Acknowledge feelings.** If the laboring person says, "I can't do this," you might reply, "This is rough. Let me help you more. Keep your rhythm."

- **Offer liquid to drink after each contraction or two.** Don't disturb the laboring person by asking what they would like to drink; just hold the beverage where it can be seen. It will be taken if wanted, ignored if not, or a different beverage may be requested. Don't pressure them to drink more, unless the caregiver is concerned about fluid intake. Otherwise, they should drink when thirsty.

- **Give the laboring person your undivided attention** throughout every contraction, even when their eyes are closed and you think it's not needed. Do not ask questions during contractions as they may interrupt or disturb the coping ritual. Do not chat with others in the room and discourage others from engaging in nonessential or loud conversation. Such talk could make the laboring person feel very alone and ignored, even when coping well.

- **Help with comfort measures.** Hold the laboring person and slow dance; rub their shoulders or press on their back; walk with them; stay beside the shower or bathtub or get in, too, (bring a swimsuit for this purpose). For more suggestions, see chapter 4.

- **Support their "ritual."** Help maintain a rhythm through each contraction; see "Relaxation," page 153, and "Rhythmic Breathing and Moaning," page 161.

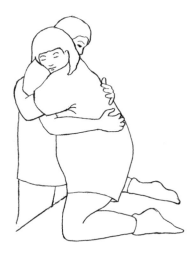

- **Remember, rhythm is everything.** Rhythm is key to coping in the dilation stage. If there is rhythm in whatever the laboring person does during contractions (moaning, swaying, tapping, rocking, chanting, even silent self-talk) or whatever they want you to do (holding them, stroking them, swaying together, talking, nodding your head, moaning together), they are coping. Being "in their rhythm" means matching or mirroring their rhythm with your words, movements, or touch. It is a way to share the experience closely and provide strong appropriate guidance.

If the laboring person loses rhythm and tenses, grimaces, writhes, clutches, or cries out, they need your help (or the doula's or nurse's) to regain the rhythm they had or to find a new one. If you have been in their rhythm, it's much easier to help them get it back. At times, you might help by making eye contact or by rhythmically talking, stroking, or swaying along with laboring person (see "The Take-Charge Routine," page 202).

Do give rhythm top priority to keep the laboring person from feeling overwhelmed and to help maintain a sense of mastery during this challenging part of labor. Let them stick with the same rhythmic ritual as long as it helps. Don't be afraid to suggest something new, though, if the laboring person loses the rhythm and has real trouble getting back to it. Labor sometimes becomes so stressful that they will need to follow someone else's lead. They will let you know when it's time to return to the previous ritual.

How a Doula Helps

It is a good idea for the doula to join you before the laboring person rounds the corner into the active phase. Once they are in active labor, the doula does the following:

- Recalls the laboring person's preferences, the birth plan, and pain medication preferences and use these to guide their actions and suggestions accordingly (see "Pain Medications Preference Scale," page 328)

- Remains calm and model patience and confidence

- Reminds the laboring person that labor is progressing and make other positive comments and suggestions

- If the laboring person wants to use little or no pain medication but is worried they cannot continue to cope, the doula offers more assistance in avoiding the pain medication. The doula will remind them to stay in the present and not look hours into the future. ("Let's take the contractions one at a time. Your job is to keep a rhythm during the contractions, and you're doing it. We'll help you.") Also see the discussion of a code word (page 330)—a way to prevent suffering.

• If the laboring person has planned to use pain medications and now acts distressed or frightened, the doula encourages them to request the medication.

• Guides you to become a part of the laboring person's ritual by using appropriate comfort measures (see chapter 4); holding or stroking them or moaning, walking, or swaying with them.

• If the doctor, midwife, or nurse suggests an intervention, the doula assists you both in asking the right questions (see page 237) so you can make informed decisions. *The doula does not make decisions for you.*

• Knowing the birthing person will always remember this birth experience, doulas ask themselves frequently, "How will they remember this?" Doulas use this thought to guide what they say and do.

• Photograph some tender moments in labor, if you have requested this beforehand

With your love and understanding of the laboring person, the knowledge you've gained from childbirth classes and this book, your dedication to the baby, combined with the doula's guidance, reassurance, experience, knowledge, and commitment to a satisfying birth as the birthing person defines it, the birthing person will have a terrific support team.

Transition

The transition phase is another turning point in labor—from the dilation to the birthing stage. In this phase, the laboring person's body seems to be partly in the dilation (first) stage and partly in the birthing (second) stage.

During transition, the cervix dilates the last 1 to 2 centimeters; (from about 8 or 9 centimeters to about 10) and the baby begins to descend. The head moves from within the uterus through the cervix and down into the vagina (see illustrations, page 115). Contractions have reached maximum intensity, each lasting 1 to 2 minutes and occurring very close together.

Sometimes, a "lip" of cervix delays the last bit of dilation. A "lip" occurs when a part of the cervix remains thick after most of the cervix has completely dilated. This may be caused by the position of the baby's head, which may press unevenly against the cervix. Several contractions or more may be needed to draw the cervix out of the way so the baby's head can come through. Changing the laboring person's position, using hands and knees, open knee–chest, or lunging may help reduce the lip. (See also chapter 4.)

The uterus may begin its expulsive action even before the cervix is completely dilated. We call this the "urge to push." It causes the laboring person to catch their breath, grunt, or hold their breath and strain; this is what is meant by the terms *pushing* and *bearing down.*

The urge to push is an involuntary reflex; the laboring person does not make it happen and cannot prevent it from happening. Yet, if the cervix is not completely dilated, they may begin bearing down very slightly. We call this "grunt-pushing." This may happen instinctively or the nurse or caregiver may instruct the laboring person to strain just enough to satisfy the urge. Pushing very hard before the cervix is dilated could cause the cervix to swell and the labor to slow (see "Avoiding Forceful Pushing," page 164).

How Long Does Transition Last?

The transition usually takes between 5 to 30 contractions or from 15 minutes to a couple hours. If the cervix has a lip or the baby's head is not well positioned (or both), the transition phase will likely take longer.

What the Laboring Person Feels

For many people, the peak intensity of contractions in the dilation stage seems to occur at 8 centimeters or so. This informal observation is based on recordings of contraction intensity by intrauterine pressure catheters (see page 249) that one of us (PS) would follow while attending numerous labors as a doula. After 8 centimeters, contractions do not seem to increase in intensity, though they sometimes come closer together. In other words, the contractions do *not* continue to become more painful until dilation is complete or the baby is born. It might reassure the laboring person to know that the contractions are unlikely to get much worse, especially if they are managing them well.

Transition poses new challenges and sensations, however. The frequency of contractions, combined with the sensations of the baby's head moving down, may cause the laboring person's legs, or even whole body, to tremble. They may feel nauseated and vomit; vomiting usually brings relief from the nausea. They may feel pressure in the thighs or pelvis. Their skin may be sensitive. They may feel the need to have a bowel movement. They may have hot flashes, then bouts of cold. They may weep or cry out, feeling they cannot handle any more—that labor will never end. They may feel overwhelmed and frustrated and react by saying, "Don't touch me! My skin hurts!" or "I can't go on!" or "Stop doing that!" or "I want an epidural right now!" Or, they may withdraw and turn inward, dozing between contractions and moaning, groaning, or whimpering during them, all the while relaxing their body quite well. Transition affects laboring people differently, but all are relieved when this phase is over.

Many of these symptoms are caused by a normal outpouring of adrenaline (also called epinephrine) and other stress hormones that occurs late in labor. Stress hormones cause the "fight or flight" response, which gives people great strength and stamina when they must exert themselves—for example, when afraid, in danger, or about to take part in competition or a demanding feat—such as pushing a baby out. Thus, the unpleasant symptoms of transition are followed by a second wind, brighter spirits, and the strength needed for the hard work of pushing a baby into the world. It helps to know that the transition symptoms mean the laboring person is getting close to the birthing stage.

Even though stress hormones help the birthing person in late labor, if they are produced as a result of great fear, anxiety, or unmanageable pain in early or active labor, they can slow progress and put stress on the baby. This is why calmness and relaxation, rhythm, and ritual are so important in early and active labor—not only to give the laboring person a sense of mastery during contractions but also to help prevent excessive production of stress hormones.

What the Caregiver Does

During the transition phase, a nurse or a midwife is in almost constant attendance. The doctor is not necessarily with the laboring person, although when informed that delivery is very close, the doctor soon comes.

The nurse or the midwife may do any or all of the following:

- Check the cervix to confirm the progress of labor

- Ask the laboring person not to push or to push only gently, with little grunts, if the cervix is not fully opened

- Reassure the laboring person that all is right and labor is moving rapidly

- Help you in your birth partner role and reassure you that the laboring person is all right and behaving normally

- Begin arranging the room, bringing in equipment for the birth, setting up the warmer for the baby (see page 374)

This is an exciting moment, when everyone begins preparing for the infant. At last, even the staff act as if a baby is really coming!

How Might You Feel?

You may feel as if you are caught up in a flurry of activity and intense feelings. You may:

- Feel surprised and excited that the laboring person is finally reaching complete dilation

- Be tired, especially if the labor has gone through the night

- Feel helpless in the face of the laboring person's pain and wish you could do something to ease it

- Feel frustrated or hurt, if the laboring person seems to find fault with everything you do to help

- Want a break (but be told, "Don't leave! I need you!")

- Worry whether such a demanding labor is normal

How You Can Help

Your role during transition is all-important. You can truly relieve some of the laboring person's burden if you know what to do:

- Help the laboring person maintain or resume the rhythmic ritual (see page 151). With all these challenges, it helps to know that transition is much more manageable if the laboring person has developed a spontaneous rhythmic ritual earlier in the labor (see page 103) because you can help the laboring person resume the ritual.

- Stop worrying about relaxation during contractions. It is unrealistic to expect the laboring person to relax when labor is this intense.

- Stay calm. Keep your touch firm and confident and your voice calm and encouraging. Maintain a confident expression on your face (not worried or pitying).

- Stay close to the laboring person, with your face near theirs.

- If the laboring person is panicky and afraid, use the Take-Charge routine (see page 202). This may be the most important way you can help.

- Remind them that this difficult phase is short and that the birthing stage is imminent. Help them through one contraction at a time.

- Remind yourself it is normal for the transition phase to be difficult, that the laboring person's mood will improve when the cervix is fully dilated, and that you must not worry. Their behavior is not abnormal and the pain is not more than one should expect at this time.

- If the laboring person wants to avoid pain medications (see "Pain Medications Preference Scale," pages 328–329), do not mention them. Instead, help the laboring person get through this phase without them, as tough as it may be. If, however, they cannot maintain any rhythm and seem panicky, even though you and others are helping all you can, and the nurse or midwife says it will be some time before the baby arrives, this might be a good time to consider pain medication or for you to give a reminder the about the code word (see page 330). If they do not use the code word, continue to help them cope without pain medications.

- If the nurse or caregiver isn't in the room when the laboring person has an urge to push, summon help immediately (see page 109). The caregiver will observe the laboring person's behavior or check the cervix to determine whether pushing is appropriate.

- If the caregiver says it isn't time to push yet (because the cervix isn't fully dilated), help the laboring person avoid pushing or push with little grunts (see page 110).

- Try not to take it personally if the laboring person criticizes you or tells you to stop doing something you expected to be helpful. Just say, "Sorry," and stop doing it. Don't try to explain why you did it or express frustration. You are just being told that labor is so difficult right now that nothing helps. You are the safest person to lash out at. Later, they will likely apologize.

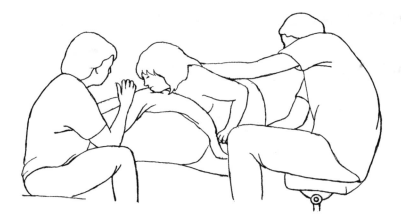

How a Doula Helps

Transition is a time when doulas are particularly helpful to both of you. With their training and experience, doulas understand the normal distress that often comes with transition. They are there to reassure and coach the birthing person through it and can be very helpful to both of you by explaining what is happening and suggesting what to do to manage it.

- If you are tired or anxious or if you lack confidence in calming the laboring person, the doula can step into your role or show you what to do.

- The doula can reassure you and the laboring person that the intense reactions are not signs of danger but of good progress and that this phase will not go on forever.

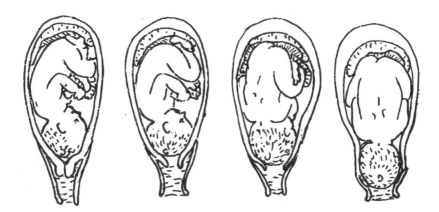

Prelabor and dilation (first) stage
The cervix effaces (thins) and dilates; the baby rotates.

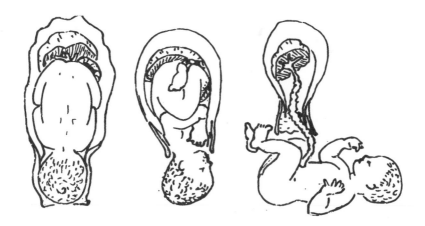

Birthing (second) stage
The baby's head enters the vaginal canal; there may be a "rest" while the uterus tightens around the baby's body; the baby descends and rotates and then is born.

- The doula can also assist if the laboring person needs two people to help through the contractions—one person holding or pressing on their sore back while the other is in front, making eye contact and helping maintain a rhythm.

- The doula models calmness and confidence during the Take-Charge routine (see page 202) and between contractions.

The laboring person may at times respond better to the experienced doula than to you, especially when you feel tired, uncertain, anxious, or frustrated and need a break.

The Birthing, Second, Stage

This stage begins when the cervix is fully dilated and ends with the birth of the baby. During this stage, the baby rotates, descends through the vagina (birth canal), and is born. Medical professionals call this the *second stage.*

During the birthing stage, the birthing person works very hard, bearing down—actively pushing—by holding their breath and straining or breathing out forcefully and vocally with the urge to push that comes several times in every contraction. In this way, they work *together* with the uterus to press the baby down and out.

The birthing stage has three distinct phases: resting, descent, and crowning and birth phases. Each phase is characterized by different physical developments and each requires the laboring person to make an emotional adjustment.

Care of the birthing person and baby during the birthing (second) stage varies among caregivers. Some are guided by patience and assessment of the birthing person's and baby's well-being. These caregivers feel it is best to let the birth unfold spontaneously, without interference, if the birthing person and baby are doing well. Instead of rushing the birthing person to push, these caregivers await the birthing person's spontaneous urge. The caregiver may encourage breathing through the contractions and bearing down when the urge to push compels them to do so (see page 110). If the resting phase lasts a long time, the caregiver may encourage the birthing person to change positions.

Other caregivers are not as patient. They want to speed the baby's descent as much as possible and so coach the birthing person to push (holding their breath and straining) during contractions while they count to 10. Then, they instruct to quickly take another breath and push for 10 more counts and to repeat this pattern until the contraction ends. These caregivers tend to place a time limit on the second stage (usually 2 hours or fewer for a first-time labor and 1 hour for the second or later births) and use drugs, instruments, and episiotomy to meet this limit.

How Long Does the Birthing Stage Last?

A normal birthing stage may last from 15 minutes (three to five contractions) to 3 hours or more. For most first-time birth-givers, the birthing stage is completed in up to 3 hours; for most people who have given birth before, in less than 1 hour. A longer birthing stage may be due to the position of the baby's head in the pelvis. One possible side effect of an epidural is a greater chance of a malpositioned baby at this time (see page 319). Also, some babies need time for the gradual molding of their head or for tucking the chin and wiggling or rotating into the best-fitting position. Other reasons for a prolonged birthing stage are described on page 287.

The Resting Phase

The resting phase is an apparent pause in the labor. Although not all laboring people experience this phase, you and the person in labor should be ready for it.

The resting phase is a "catch-up break" for the uterus; it comes after the cervix is completely dilated and the baby's head has passed through the cervix into the birth canal. The uterus had been tightly stretched around the baby before the head slipped out. Now, suddenly, only the baby's body remains inside the uterus, and the uterus fits more loosely around the baby. The uterus needs time to tighten around the rest of the baby (see illustration, page 115).

During this phase, the muscle fibers in the uterus shorten, making the uterus smaller, without noticeable contractions and without having an urge to push. After the tumult of transition, the resting phase provides a welcome break. The late Sheila Kitzinger, a famous childbirth educator and prolific author, termed this the "rest-and-be-thankful phase." Birthing persons become alert and clear thinking after the tumult of transition. One woman Penny worked with looked up at her husband during this phase and asked, "Did you feed the cats?" Only 10 minutes before she had been moaning and tensing during contractions. (Incidentally, he had fed the cats.)

How Long Does the Resting Phase Last?

The resting phase usually lasts from 10 to 30 minutes. If it lasts longer than that, the caregiver may ask the person in labor to change position or to try pushing (bearing down), in the hope this will bring on stronger contractions or an urge to push and so speed the labor along. Some caregivers are more patient than others at this time if the baby is doing well, as indicated by the baby's heart rate. Others don't want labor to slow down at this point.

What the Laboring Person Feels

The start of the birthing stage is always a milestone. The laboring person will probably welcome this rest, especially after the tumult of transition. They get a second wind. If they were confused, their head is now clear. If discouraged, they are now optimistic. If withdrawn, they are now outgoing and aware of the surroundings. Sometimes, the laboring person feels anxious if the resting phase seems to go on for too long or if staff implore them to push before feeling an urge to do so. The birthing person may also feel inadequate or apologetic if everyone is commanding them to push—making them feel as if they're not pushing correctly or well enough. In fact, no one should expect them to push if there is no urge. They should rest.

Even people who do not experience a pause in contractions feel an improved mood and greater alertness at the beginning of the birthing stage.

What the Caregiver Does

During the resting phase:

- The midwife or nurse remains close by, offering encouragement, praise, and positive suggestions.

- The nurse will probably call the doctor to come soon. If the birthing person has had a child before, the doctor will try to arrive soon after pushing begins. If this is a first child, the doctor will probably not rush.

- The midwife or nurse may become more directive at this time, telling the birthing person what positions to try or coaching how or when to push.

- The midwife or nurse listens frequently to the baby's heartbeat and continues assessing the birthing person's welfare.

- The midwife or nurse may do a vaginal exam to assess the progress of the baby's descent.

- The midwife or nurse may apply warm compresses on the perineum to help relax the pelvic floor muscles and improve their sense of how and where to push. The midwife may also pour some oil over the perineum to lubricate the vaginal outlet.

How Might You Feel?

- You may be excited by the birthing person's lifting mood as they enter the birthing stage, and you will probably be relieved that they seem more like their usual self.

- You may be baffled that the labor has apparently stopped. Do not worry. The pause is temporary and gives the birthing person renewed energy.

- You may feel overwhelmed at the realization you are about to witness a miracle, the birth of this beloved baby, and become a parent!

How You Can Help

The birthing stage is an exciting time. Even though you have your own powerful emotional reaction to the birth, if you are the birthing person's major source of support, you must remain calm and continue to encourage and assist. Here are some guidelines:

- Be patient during the resting phase. Don't rush the birthing person through it or make them push too soon.

- If the nurse or caregiver wants the birthing person to push without a contraction or an urge to push, ask whether it can wait until they feel the urge.

- Match the birthing person's mood. As they leave the emotions of transition behind, you do the same.

- If you are confused, ask the midwife, nurse, or doula what is happening.

How a Doula Helps

During this resting phase, the doula encourages the birthing person to take advantage of the break. Doulas can help in these ways:

- Remind you both about the resting phase if you are puzzled over this pause

- Point out that this break will be short and prepare both of you for the next step—pushing the baby down and out

- While patiently awaiting the next step, the doula may suggest you remind your nurse of items in the birth plan that pertain to the birthing stage, such as the kind of bearing-down efforts and positions the birthing person wants to use and their feelings about episiotomy.

- If the resting phase goes on for a long time, the doula may suggest that the birthing person change position to see whether this helps bring on an urge to push.

The Descent Phase

This phase is the longest of the three phases of the birthing stage. During the descent phase, the uterus resumes contracting strongly, and the birthing person usually feels an increasingly strong urge to push. The baby descends through the birth canal to the point where the top of the head is clearly visible at the vaginal outlet. The birthing person alternately pushes and breathes lightly during contractions and rests between contractions.

By *pushing*, we mean that the birthing person takes in a breath and strains (bears down) for 5 to 6 seconds at a time. While bearing down, they either hold their breath or let air out with a moan or bellow. The pushing may be directed, which means they push when told, regardless of whether there is an urge; this technique is used for people who have had epidurals, as they usually feel no urge to push. Or, the pushing can be spontaneous, which means the birthing person bears down with the reflexive urge to push. By this time, a rhythmic ritual is no longer possible or desirable, as the birthing person's behavior is being guided by their reflexive pushing urges, which come three or four times over the peak of each contraction. The urges last about 5 or 6 seconds, with 3 to 5 seconds in between.

Many birthing people tell us that the term *urge to push* does not come close to describing the feeling. One woman cried out during this stage, "It's like a vomit in reverse!" That, crude as it is, is a much better description. The urge to push can be as involuntary and as uncontrollable as vomiting, except that all the force moves downward instead of upward (and the result is a lot more rewarding!).

Sometimes, especially early in the descent phase, the urge to push is a much milder sensation, like a catch in the breath and a grunting sensation. Occasionally, a person who hasn't had an epidural lacks the urge to push. They may simply be having a long resting phase; a change of position and some patience usually result in an urge to push. Or perhaps, the uterus is not contracting with enough intensity to bring on an urge to push; synthetic oxytocin might be used in such a case. If the birthing person is having good contractions and no urge to push, the caregiver instructs when to push.

It can take a few minutes to an hour or two of pushing before the baby's head is visible at the vaginal opening. Before it becomes visible, there is progress in rotation and molding of the baby's head and some descent, but these changes are undetectable from the outside. It can seem as if nothing is happening, but your job is to remain optimistic and supportive, knowing that changes are happening on the inside.

Then, the birthing person's perineum bulges with bearing down. Soon thereafter, the labia part and the tiny vaginal outlet gradually enlarges as the baby moves down. Next, the head becomes visible, though at first it looks more like a wrinkled walnut. The walnut seems to grow bigger with the bearing-down efforts. But rather than moving steadily downward the baby moves down when the birthing person bears down and slips back during the pauses between the bearing-down efforts. If you watch this incredible process, you will likely find yourself totally engrossed. You almost hate to see the baby slip back each time because you're so eager to see them born. You must remember that progress is being made, and this gradual stretching is easier on both baby and birthing person than constant pressure on the baby's head and continuous stretching of the vagina.

The birthing person may change positions during the descent phase. The most common positions are semi-reclining, lying flat on one's back, side lying, on hands and knees, and squatting. Supported squatting, lap squatting, "the dangle," and sitting on the toilet are also useful at times. See "Positions and Movements for Labor and Birth," pages 169–176, for illustrations of each of these positions and descriptions of their benefits.

How Long Does the Descent Phase Last?

The descent phase usually takes up most of the total time of the birthing stage—from a few minutes to as long as 4 hours. The average is about 1½ hours.

What the Birthing Person Feels

The birthing person, especially without an epidural, has an adrenaline rush at this time, which gives a renewed strength and determination during the descent phase, even after a long labor. The imminence of the birth heartens them, and they will be receptive to suggestions and praise. Birthing persons often say they feel better during this phase because they are doing something active—working hard—to help their baby be born.

The birthing person may have other feelings as well:

- Early in the descent phase, especially, the birthing person may feel uncertain about what to do and how to do it. They may ask how to push and may need reassurance that the sensations are normal and that everyone is doing fine. They will feel better after a few contractions, as they get the hang of how to push with the guidance of a doula or caregiver.

- Many people tighten the pelvic floor, feeling afraid to let go. For some, the sensations of descent and of the large head stretching the birth canal may be gratifying but also alarming and painful. It is scary to let the baby come *because it hurts*. Alarmed by the pressure in the vagina, they may instinctively "hold back," that is, tense the pelvic floor against the baby's downward movement. It may take several contractions before they let go of the tension in the vagina. The good news is, when they do let go, it feels much better to push. If they have done perineal massage (see page 40) during pregnancy, it is often easier to relax to the stretching sensation of birth.

- If the baby's descent is extremely rapid, the birthing person may feel shocked and frightened by the intensity of the pain, the total lack of control over their body, and the suddenness with which it is all over and the baby is born.

- If the baby's descent is very slow, the birthing person may become discouraged. It may be that the baby's head is molding gradually or rotating to fit through the pelvis. This may be the most demanding work of one's entire life, and the birthing person needs much encouragement and reassurance to feel as though progress is being made.

What the Caregiver Does

During the descent phase:

- The midwife or nurse continues as before, encouraging the birthing person's efforts and offering reassurance. This may include coaching the birthing person to breathe lightly during the contraction until the urge to push is stronger and then coaching them to hold their breath and strain.

- The doctor usually arrives during this phase, sometimes to everyone's great relief.

- The doctor, midwife, or nurse performs occasional vaginal exams to confirm the baby's progress through the birth canal. They check the baby's heart rate and the birthing person's vital signs periodically.

- When birth is imminent, they scrub their hands and don surgical gloves, special hospital clothing, and a mask.

- They may place drapes beneath the laboring person, cleanse the vaginal area, and massage the perineum or place warm compresses on it.

- Many caregivers, including most midwives, are in favor of the birthing person using many positions— side lying, hands and knees, semi-reclining, or others (see illustrations of positions for labor and birth, pages 169–176). However, some caregivers prefer that the birthing person be on their back with their legs in stirrups for pushing and/or the birth. If so, the nurse, doctor, or midwife prepares the bed for delivery by removing the foot section and placing the birthing person's legs in supports attached to each side of the bed. They then sit close to the birthing person's perineum. This setup is helpful if medical assistance is needed for the birth (with forceps, a vacuum extractor, and/or an episiotomy), but many doctors prefer it for all births. It is uncomfortable and restrictive for most birthing people. If the birthing person prefers not to be in this position unless necessary, say so in the birth plan.

- The doctor or midwife uses their hands to control the emergence of the baby's head.

How Might You Feel?

You may react in various ways:

- Your fatigue may disappear and you may feel excited and ready to do whatever you are asked to do.

- You may feel divided between wanting to remain at the birthing person's head to offer support and wanting to watch the birth (or even catch the baby, with the help of the midwife or doctor).

- You may find yourself holding your breath right along with the birthing person!

- You may find yourself in an awkward position as you support their upper body or leg. Your arms or back may tire. (This is one reason to improve your fitness before the birth; see page 39.)

- Your initial excitement may fade to discouragement if progress seems slow.

How You Can Help

If there are more people around during the descent phase, you may feel less vital to the birthing person than you felt earlier. It is true that they now receive much of the direction and praise from the professionals. This may be a relief as it allows you to become absorbed in your own experience of the birth. You are, however, still the birth partner—the one who has seen the birthing person through this—and they still may rely on you despite all the attention from others.

Suggestions to consider:

- Don't leave at this time if you want to see the baby's birth. Things can change quickly.

- Stay close to the birthing person, where they can see, feel, and hear you. You may support from behind or by their side.

- Don't try to keep a rhythm now because the urge to push takes over and they must respond to that.

- Praise them on how well they are doing—after every contraction.

- Mop their brow and neck with a cold washcloth. Pushing is hard, sweaty work!

- Stay calm. Maintain a steady, reassuring tone of voice and a confident, firm touch. (Don't rub or squeeze too hard in your excitement.)

- Do not tell the birthing person to push harder; you only make them feel inadequate. Instead, offer encouragement like, "That's the way! Come on, Baby."

- Help the birthing person get in and out of positions for pushing, such as squatting or hands and knees, or the less common dangle or lap squatting (see pages 175 and 174). If they're on their side or semisitting, hold a leg up (someone else will need to hold the other leg; see page 173).

- If progress is slow, be patient; suggest a different position and help the birthing person change positions every 30 minutes, or more often, if needed. Be ready to support them in these positions.

- Using whatever suggestions work, remind them to relax the perineum: "Let go," "Relax your bottom," "Let the baby out." You might remind them to relax the same way as during perineal massage (see page 40).

- Request warm compresses to be placed on the perineum.

- Remind the birthing person that the baby is almost here! Sometimes, believe it or not, they almost forget this is all for the baby.

- Remember that during the first few contractions after the baby's head becomes visible at the vaginal opening, the head may appear wrinkled and spongy. One birth partner thought he was seeing a brain without a skull or scalp! Pressure on the head by the vaginal wall squeezes the skin of the scalp toward the top of the head until the head moves down more. Then, it looks more as you expect—hard and smooth, bluish gray, and bald or hairy.

- If the descent phase seems slow, remember that sometimes more time is needed for the baby's head to mold or to get into the best position in the birthing person's pelvis. If you are discouraged, don't let the birthing person know.

How a Doula Helps

If you and the birthing person wish, the doula can stay at the birthing person's head to offer encouragement while you watch or even help with the birth, take photos, or take a break if you are tired or feel squeamish.

Sometimes, partners worry about feeling faint or sick with the intense emotion, sights, sounds, and smells of birth. Couples want to be sure the birthing person's needs for support are met while the partner participates as is comfortable. Most of the time, partners feel swept up in the excitement of the moment and feel fine, but some have had to sit down and put their heads between their knees or take a break now and then. Attending a birth can be demanding and stressful. If you have any of these concerns, consider having a doula, so you can take care of yourself. Here are ways that doulas help:

- They encourage the birthing person through every contraction and help them feel more comfortable between contractions

- Doulas assist you in your role as needed—for example, by guiding you on positions, getting cold cloths, and taking photos of the two of you

- They help the nurse or midwife by getting blankets for the birthing person, fetching hot water and cloths for compresses to apply to the perineum, and doing whatever else needs to be done to get ready for delivery

Few people are prepared for the power of the moment: the birthing person's superhuman effort, the sounds they make, the bulging of the vagina and the sight of a wet and wrinkled scalp as the baby moves down with the pushing efforts of the birthing person, and the charged atmosphere of the room as everyone anticipates the birth. It is impossible to describe the awe, excitement, and tension you will feel as you await the moment of birth.

The Crowning and Birth Phase

The crowning and birth phase is when the baby is actually born. This phase begins when the baby's head crowns—that is, when it remains visible at the vaginal opening even between contractions, no longer sneaking back between the bearing-down efforts—and ends when the baby is born.

During the crowning and birth phase, the baby's head stretches the vagina and perineum, which may cause feelings of burning and stinging. Because the vaginal and perineal tissues might tear at this time, protecting the perineum now becomes a major focus of the caregiver's role.

Until now, the baby's head has appeared wrinkled and spongy. Once the head crowns, the skin evens out over the scalp. The head seems to lurch forward a few times, and then it emerges—first the top of the head, then the brow and ears, and then the face. The head rotates to one side; one shoulder appears; and the rest of the baby slides out with a gush of water.

The baby may immediately cry and appear vigorous or may appear bluish and lifeless at first. Under normal circumstances, babies begin breathing within seconds usually with a gurgle and then a lusty cry. Immediately, their color begins to turn, and very soon their skin becomes its normal color.

How Long Does the Crowning and Birth Phase Last?

The crowning and birth phase takes only a few contractions.

What the Birthing Person Feels

The birthing person's body gives mixed messages during the crowning and birth phase: On one hand, they know the baby is almost here and are eager to push hard to finish the birth quickly. On the other, they feel the stretching and burning (the "rim of fire") that are signals to stop pushing. To prevent the vagina or perineum from tearing, the birthing person should pay attention to this feeling and listen to the caregiver, who will tell them to stop pushing in order to ease the baby out. They should *not* push hard.

Although the crowning and birth are quick and exciting for everyone else, this phase is painful and requires that the birthing person devote all attention to getting the baby out. By the time the head is about to slip out, the pain may have disappeared because gradual stretching of the vagina sometimes causes numbing. If this happens, the birthing person may become alert, calm, and totally engrossed in greeting the baby. If not, they'll will be relieved and surprised to have the pain go away the moment the baby is born.

Some birthing people watch the birth in a mirror or touch the baby's head or body as it emerges. They may glow with joy or withdraw their hand in surprise if the warm, wet, and slippery baby doesn't feel like what was expected.

After the birth, it may take a few moments for the birthing person to realize labor is over (or nearly so) and shift attention to the baby. This may take longer for some than others. One woman yelled, as soon as the baby was out, "Yay! It's over! I did it!" Then, "Hi, little baby! Oh baby, oh baby!" and then kissed the baby and her partner. Others may need time (hours or even days) to let it sink in that they're not in labor any more, before they become engrossed in the baby.

What the Caregiver Does

During the crowning and birth phase, the caregiver:

- Supports the perineum and controls the passage of the baby's head as it crowns

- Tells the birthing person to stop pushing as the head emerges, or earlier, when they begin to feel the burning and stretching. The uterus will still contract and there will still be an urge to push. To help avoid a tear, the birthing person should keep from holding their breath and straining as much as possible. To do this, they raise their chin and blow lightly throughout the contraction (see "Avoiding Forceful Pushing," page 164).

- May consider doing an episiotomy (see page 263 for a discussion of this uncommon procedure)

- Holds the baby's head as it emerges; the caregiver may encourage both of you to touch or even hold the baby during the actual birth.

- Dries and places the baby skin to skin on the birthing person's abdomen or in a heated crib nearby, depending on the caregiver's routine, the baby's condition, and your preference

A nurse or doctor checks the baby quickly and gives an Apgar score (see page 244) at 1 minute of age and again at 5 minutes. Five signs are evaluated in order to decide whether the baby needs extra immediate care, close observation, or no extra attention at all. A total score of 7 points or above is very good. If the score is below 7 at 1 minute, the baby may need extra observation and care. By 5 minutes, problems such as sluggish movement, slow pulse, or uneven breathing are usually corrected with stimulation or an oxygen mask.

How Might You Feel?

The suspense mounts as the baby's head becomes more and more visible:

• You may be barely able to contain your excitement.

• You may feel more love and awe for the birthing person than you ever thought possible.

• You may feel stunned, overwhelmed with emotion, or even queasy—with so much going on at once.

How You Can Help

During the crowning and birth phase, you can help the birthing person in the following ways:

• Stay close by.

• Help with their position by holding a leg, lifting their shoulders for pushing, or letting them lean on you in a squatting position; see pages 171–176 for illustrations of positions for pushing and ways to support a person while pushing.

• If the midwife or doctor tells the birthing person to stop pushing so as not to injure their body or the baby with too rapid a delivery, the birthing person may find it difficult to comply. Help them avoid pushing by getting them to follow your directions: "Lift your chin, look at me, blow . . . blow . . . that's the way . . . blow . . . " and so forth.

• Participate in this miracle in the way that is most comfortable for the two of you. Stay at the head of the bed and focus on the birthing person's face if that's where you're needed or if you feel squeamish about watching the baby come out. Or, take it all in by watching in the mirror or by moving so you can watch closely. Please don't get so caught up in the birth that you ignore the birthing person!

• Remember, although the baby's initial appearance may be dusky (bluish) and almost lifeless, it will begin to change within seconds as the baby breathes and cries.

How a Doula Helps

The doula is right there, assisting and supplementing your efforts to help you and the birthing person physically and emotionally as needed.

- If there is a crowd around the birthing person at this time, the doula steps aside, knowing it is important that you be where you want to be and that the nurse and doctor or midwife have room to do their jobs.

- If the birthing person is tired and ready to give up, the doula may step in and give a pep talk to get them back on course.

- They may take photos or a video, if you have asked them to do this and the staff allows.

- If the birthing person has planned to have particular music playing as the baby is born, the doula starts the music.

- They will share in your excitement when the baby is born!

The Placental, Third, Stage

The placental stage begins when the baby is born and ends after the placenta, or *afterbirth*, is born.

This stage is usually anticlimactic when compared to the baby's birth, and many people barely notice the few contractions and the emergence of the placenta. Others feel sharp cramps. The two phases of the placental stage, the separation of the placenta and the expulsion of the placenta, are usually indistinguishable to the birthing person. Medical professionals call this the *third* stage of labor.

How Long Does the Placental Stage Last?

The placental stage is the shortest stage of labor. It usually lasts 15 to 30 minutes.

What the Birthing Person Feels

A flood of deep emotions sweeps over the birthing person during the placental stage. The apparent end of labor, the new baby, the rest of the job to be done—all vie for attention.

- The birthing person may be caught off guard when the caregiver says, "Now, push for the placenta," having thought the birth was over. Pushing out the placenta, however, is nothing compared to pushing out a baby—there are no bones in the placenta!

- They may be so caught up in the baby and you that they hardly notice when the placenta comes out.

- Some people are unable to pay much attention to the baby for a few minutes immediately following the birth because all they can feel is relief that the ordeal is over: The pushing, the pain, and the contractions have stopped. Once this sinks in, they can focus on the baby.

- They may marvel at their new shape and now very soft abdomen.

- They may become preoccupied with the baby or establishing suckling at the breast.

- They may begin to tremble all over and feel weak.

What the Caregiver Does

During the placental stage, the caregiver:

- Attends to the umbilical cord, clamping it and either cutting it or inviting the partner to cut it. It is usually best for the baby to wait a few minutes before clamping and cutting the cord (see page 369). The caregiver withdraws some blood from the cord, to analyze for the baby's blood type or, if the parents wish, to donate it or to store it privately in a blood bank. (Umbilical cord blood is a rich source of stem cells that can be used for children or adults with certain cancers or blood disorders, as an alternative to a bone marrow transplant. Consult your caregiver to learn more about this procedure and the options in your area. Also check page 418, Recommended Resources.)

- Dries and checks the baby

- Checks the birthing parent's birth canal to see whether stitches are needed

- Attends to the placenta. When the placenta has separated from the uterine wall (the caregiver can tell by feeling the uterus and putting gentle traction on the cord), they may ask the birthing person to gently push to deliver the placenta.

- Carefully inspects the placenta to make sure all of it has been delivered. If fragments remain in the uterus, the caregiver must remove them by hand (see page 296).

- Palpates the abdomen to feel whether the uterus is firm. If it is "boggy," the nurse or midwife vigorously massages the uterus through the abdominal wall. This is uncomfortable for the birthing person, but is very effective in contracting the uterus and protecting against excessive blood loss. The nurse can teach the birthing person to do this on their own abdomen (see page 366).

How Might You Feel?

At this time, you will probably be engrossed with the baby and birthing person and letting out your emotions—pride, joy, relief and love. You may find yourself weeping with joy and relief and showering kisses on your co-parent and baby.

How You Can Help

During the placental stage, you can do the following:

- Cut the cord, if you want to; the caregiver will likely invite you to do this. The symbolism of separating the pregnant person and the baby appeals to many new parents and their partners. You may be surprised at how firm and slippery the cord is. When you cut it, don't snip gently; make a decisive effort.

- Enjoy the baby and help the new parent do the same—this is your main role now. Make sure your partner is comfortable, can see the baby, and is warm enough.

- Make sure the baby stays warm. The warmest—and happiest—place for the baby is skin to skin against the birthing parent, with the two of them covered by a warm blanket. Unfortunately, many hospitals customarily keep a baby in a warming unit while the nurse does all the newborn procedures (see page 368). Then, the baby is wrapped and given a hat. If the baby is presented to the new parent all wrapped up, ask whether the baby can be placed naked against their skin with a warm blanket over both. Babies stay perfectly warm when held and covered in this way. Do not leave the baby uncovered or remove the hat unless the room is very warm. If a newborn becomes chilled, it may take a long time (often in the nursery, away from the parents) to return to normal temperature.

- Go along if the baby has to go to the nursery (either because of a health problem or because it is hospital policy), unless the birthing parent needs you to stay behind. Soothe the baby by talking and singing their song (see page 44).

- Jump at the chance, when it's your turn, to hold the baby close. If your partner and baby are both healthy, it's a good idea for them to be together, skin to skin at first, and for you and the baby to get together later in the fourth stage (see following). Talk or sing to the baby and begin getting acquainted. The baby already knows and loves your voice (see pages 44, 354, and 363).

- Congratulate yourselves on a job well done and start making those phone calls, as the after-birth care (see page 363) of your partner and baby begins.

How a Doula Helps

Once the baby is born, the doula may:

- Support the birthing parent during the birth of the placenta and the caregiver's massage of the uterus and inspection of the vaginal canal, as these can be painful. The doula's help allows you to focus on the baby.

- Remind you to ask the nurse to bring your baby to your partner, if the nurse is keeping the baby in the warmer

- Remind you both to talk or sing to the baby, keep the baby warm against your partner's (or your) skin, and keep the baby's hat on and a blanket over both of them

- Stay with your partner to hold the baby if your partner can't. If the baby must go to the nursery, you can go along, knowing the doula will remain with your partner.

- Assist your partner with initial breast-feeding, especially if the nurse or midwife is too busy with other tasks to help (see chapter 11)

- Photograph the first precious moments of the baby's life and the new family

- Point out some of the baby's capabilities—feeding cues, attention to parents' familiar voices, alert state, and more

The Recovery and Bonding, Fourth, Stage

For the birthing person, the fourth stage refers to the first few hours after birth, when the birthing person's condition stabilizes.

If the birth has been without medications or interventions, the birthing person's own oxytocin, which began to surge during the baby's journey down the birth canal, is now at high levels; endorphins are also flowing, and these combine to give the birthing person high spirits and feelings of love and gratefulness. These hormones also help override the fatigue, pain, and discouragement that may have been felt earlier. Epidural analgesia reduces oxytocin and endorphin production, which may moderate the positive feelings.

The baby, during these first hours of life, undergoes an enormous physiological shift from dependency on the pregnant person and placenta for survival and growth to dependence on themselves for such basic survival functions as breathing, taking in food, regulating body temperature, and adapting to the new surroundings. Before birth, the lungs were not important to the baby, so most of the baby's blood bypassed the lungs. Immediately after birth, however, the structure of the baby's heart changes so all the baby's blood is rerouted through the lungs to pick up oxygen and carry it wherever needed. Within minutes, the birthing parent no longer provides oxygen to the baby, who is now breathing and can get their own oxygen. You will witness these profound changes in the baby if you are present at the birth!

How Long Does the Recovery and Bonding Stage Last?

This stage usually lasts 2 to 4 hours.

What the Birthing Parent Feels

They will probably cycle through a variety of feelings, depending on the birth experience itself, the care received, and the health and well-being of birth parent and baby. It is common to feel exhausted, euphoric, loving, talkative, excited, worried, curious—anything really. It's one of life's most intense and meaningful moments. It is important to honor this time with respect and kindness.

What the Caregiver Does

The caregiver checks the birthing parent's vital signs (pulse, blood pressure, temperature, respiration rate) and the firmness of the uterus to be sure it remains contracted (which minimizes blood loss). If the uterus is "boggy" or soft, the caregiver massages it to make it contract. This can be quite uncomfortable but is very important to prevent excessive blood loss. Ask the caregiver to show the birthing parent how to do it. They may be able to get a good result without massaging as hard.

The caregiver also checks the perineum to see if the stretching during birth caused damage that requires stitches. If yes, they go ahead with the repair (using local anesthesia, if your partner did not get an epidural or other anesthetic earlier in labor). The caregiver also helps get feeding established, placing the baby skin to skin on the birthing parent's chest. The caregiver also checks the baby's Apgar score, which assesses five vital indicators of the baby's condition to determine whether the baby needs extra medical attention (see page 244 for details on the Apgar score).

How Might You Feel?

You have had your own unique experience—very different from your partner's. Anything is possible—pride, excitement, indescribable joy, love for your partner and baby, relief, gratefulness, exhaustion, shock, insignificance, loneliness, fear, trauma. Any or all these feelings may be felt, but partners often say little about them; you may feel this is not about you, but about the birthing person and baby. If you do wish to talk about your experience during the birth, you might find it very helpful. Sharing your feelings with a trusted friend, family member, doula, counselor, or midwife lets you share your joy, but also helps relieve worries or troubling feelings.

How You Can Help

Keeping birthing parent and baby together skin to skin in the first hours after birth, as long as both are healthy, helps get the family off to a good start. Not only is your partner providing everything the baby needs—warmth, colostrum, familiar heartbeat and voice, touch stimulation, smell, and more—but the baby reciprocates by giving your partner some stimulation to promote shrinking of the uterus, successful breast-feeding, and bonding.

The baby's squirming on your partner's abdomen and nuzzling and suckling at the breast releases oxytocin that stimulates the uterus to contract. The baby's actions also stimulate the birthing parent's pituitary gland to secrete prolactin, the key to both the production of breast milk and to altruistic behavior (i.e., putting the baby's needs ahead of their own), which is essential for the baby's survival. When unrushed and undisturbed, both of you can become acquainted with your child and discover all your baby's little mannerisms and sounds at your own pace.

How a Doula Helps

The doula can answer some of your questions, give tips on feeding, and help you recognize some of your baby's cues. When it is time for the three of you to have privacy, the doula will step out. Doulas usually plan to get together with the family to review the birth, admire the baby, and make referrals, if necessary. You can give feedback, ask questions, and finalize your relationship. The postpartum appointment is a special time for you both and the doula; you've shared one of life's most demanding—and meaningful—experiences.

NORMAL LABOR—IN A NUTSHELL

The following table summarizes the events in a normal labor and the ways you can help. You may find this table useful as a quick reference during labor.

WHAT HAPPENS	HOW YOU AND A DOULA CAN HELP
Prelabor	
Off-and-on or constant nonprogressing contractions for hours or days	
• The cervix softens, thins, and moves forward.	• Encourage normal, but not strenuous, activities during daytime; rest, if possible, at night.
• The pregnant person has some possible or preliminary signs of labor (see page 68), or both.	• Distracting activities are appropriate.
• The pregnant person may become anxious, discouraged, or tired if it lasts a long time.	• The pregnant person eats and drinks as needed.
• You both may overreact and be preoccupied with every contraction.	• Time the contractions off and on. Use the "Early Labor Record" (see page 79) or your smartphone app.
	• Be patient; do not get overexcited or preoccupied with the contractions.
	• The pregnant person can use music, massage, or a shower to relax.
	• Check chapters 4 and 5 or call the doula if you need coping suggestions.
Dilation (First) Stage (2 to 24 hours)	
Early labor (a few hours to 20 hours, to about 3 centimeters dilation)	
• The cervix continues ripening, thinning, and opens to about 3 cm (1 in).	• Use distraction if it works.
• Contractions increase in frequency, intensity, and/or duration.	• Start a planned ritual if the pregnant person can't walk or talk through the contractions without pausing: slow breathing, relaxation, focusing on a visualization, counting breaths, etc., releasing tension through the body on exhales.
• The pregnant person has one or both positive signs of labor (see page 68).	• The doula should join you.
• Dilation is usually quite slow at first.	• If the bag of waters breaks, take precautions (see page 71); call the caregiver.
• The pregnant person is clear-headed, may be excited and confident or anxious and distressed.	• Help calm the laboring person; offer coping technique reminders.
	• Explain that this part is often slow; model patience and optimism.
	• Give helpful feedback and relaxing reminders (see page 97).

Getting into Active Labor (3 to 6 centimeters)

The birthing person's "moment of truth," as they realize they cannot control the labor (see page 100).

- Contractions are close and intense by the end of this phase. There's often a temporary lag between contraction intensity and progress in dilation.

- The laboring person becomes more instinctual, less communicative.

- They may seem discouraged, weep, or feel labor will never end.

- They may struggle to remain "in control."

- They may want pain medication

- They may "give up" ("I can't do this; my body will have to")— a good sign that control is being released.

- Use a soothing, calming tone of voice.

- Remain with the laboring person and stay encouraging.

- Match their mood. If serious and quiet, be calm and quiet yourself.

- Give feedback, help establish a rhythmic ritual with the 3 Rs (see page147).

- The doula can reassure the laboring person about the potential length of the first stage and help the two of you focus on the present rather than hours from now.

- Do not ask questions during contractions.

- Using the 4-1-1 or 5-1-1 rule (see page 94), call or go to the hospital or the midwife and report symptoms and contraction pattern.

- Encourage movement to find comfort.

- Do not criticize; use positive language.

- Remind yourself of the pain medication preferences (see pages 328–329) and act in accordance with those preferences.

Active Labor (30 minutes to 6 hours)

- The cervix dilates from about 5 to 8 cm (2 to 3 inches).

- Contractions become intense or painful, last 60 seconds or more, and come closer—every 4 minutes or fewer.

- Progress speeds up.

- The laboring person becomes quiet, serious, and focused on labor.

- They may find a spontaneous ritual involving the 3 Rs (see page 147).

- The pain of contractions peaks by about 8 cm (3 inches) of dilation.

- Present the birth plan to the nurse or midwife on arrival in the labor ward (see page 45).

- Give the laboring person your total, undivided attention for every contraction.

- Match their quiet, serious, focused mood.

- Encourage the ritual. Point out the more rapid progress.

- Use comfort measures (see page 143). For backache, use cold or heat, counterpressure, and positions (see page 198). Use the Take-Charge routine (see page 202), if necessary, to help maintain the rhythm. Suggest a long bath in warm water.

- If worried or uncertain, ask the doula, staff, or caregiver for help, explanations, or reassurance.

- If you're exhausted or hungry, let the doula give you a break for a nap or meal.

- Remind the laboring person to urinate every 1 to 2 hours.

- Offer a beverage after each contraction, but do not insist they drink if not interested.

WHAT HAPPENS	HOW YOU AND A DOULA CAN HELP

Transition phase (10 to 60 minutes)

- The cervix dilates from about 8 cm (3 inches) to complete (10 cm, or 4 inches). This usually takes 5 to 20 contractions, but the presence of a cervical lip (see page 109) may prolong this phase.
- The laboring person has long, painful contractions, with short breaks.
- The baby may begin descending, causing pressure in the laboring person's rectum and, possibly, the urge to push.
- They may feel glad about the progress, but also restless, tense, overwhelmed, irritable, and in despair. They may weep, cry out, want to give up, or fight contractions. They may doze during the few seconds between contractions.
- The laboring person may tremble and vomit; their skin may hurt when rubbed; they may feel hot, then cold.
- The good news: They are close to the pushing and birth stage!

- Continue the same rituals as in the active phase.
- Stay very close.
- Focus on one contraction at a time.
- Let them doze or relax between contractions. It is okay if they do not relax during these contractions.
- Remind them the transition is short, they're almost ready to begin pushing the baby out.
- They need help. Use the Take-Charge routine (see page 202), if necessary; talk through contractions. Remember: Rhythm is everything.
- A firm touch usually helps; rubbing or touching may be annoying.
- Call the nurse or caregiver if they begin pushing.
- Help them push or keep from pushing (see page 130) according to the advice of the caregiver or nurse.

Birthing (Second) Stage (15 minutes to more than 3 hours)

Resting phase (10 to 30 minutes)

- The baby's head may be in the birth canal.
- The cervix is fully dilated. The birthing person becomes clearheaded, optimistic, and determined.
- Contractions may subside or seem to stop for up to 30 minutes.
- The uterus is "catching up" with the baby.
- The resting phase may not occur if the baby is very low.
- The birthing person gets a second wind and may ask questions and be more their "usual self."
- The staff may want the laboring person to begin pushing even without contractions.

- Be patient; remind them of the lull of the resting phase.
- If a staff member says to push without the urge, ask whether they can wait for the urge to push.
- Encourage the birthing person to relax and take advantage of the rest.
- If 20 minutes pass without pushing contractions, suggest a change of position.
- Try hands and knees, squatting, a supported squat, or standing (see pages 171–176).
- Join in the excitement. Review what happens, after the rest.
- Ask the staff if the birthing person can rest until they begin grunting or holding their breath reflexively (pushing).

Descent phase (30 minutes to 3 hours)

- The strong contractions resume.
- The baby moves down the birth canal.
- The urge to push becomes stronger and more frequent with each contraction.
- The birthing person cannot avoid pushing because the urge is strong and involuntary; it comes from inside. They cannot make the reflexive urge happen, although they can push without the urge.
- The birthing person may be alarmed at feeling the baby's head in the vagina. They may "hold back" by tensing the pelvic floor.
- The baby moves down during each pushing effort and slips back between pushes.

- Remind the birthing person to relax the pelvic floor. Say, for example, "Open up," or "Let the baby come."
- Encourage them to bear down and push when they feel the urge.
- Suggest they sit on the toilet for a few contractions if they seem to be holding back.
- Many find it feels good to push when they feel the urge and to breathe between the urges.
- Reinforce their efforts. Tell them how well they're doing.
- Warm compresses may help relax the perineum.
- Suggest they touch the baby's head (they may or may not want to do so).
- The baby's head appears wrinkled; do not be alarmed.
- Help with position changes (see page 168) when needed.

Crowning and birth phase (2 to 20 minutes)

- The baby's head no longer slips back between pushes.
- The birth of the head is imminent (it will emerge within a few contractions).
- The birthing person feels intense burning or stinging in the vagina ("rim of fire"). They may be confused, wanting to push very hard to get the baby out right away but feeling they may split if they push.
- The baby's head emerges and rotates; then, the shoulders and the rest of the body are born.

- Don't rush the birthing person; remind them to stop pushing and "breathe the baby out," or pant (chin up) to keep from pushing (see page 165).
- Help them tune in to the caregiver's instructions.
- Apply warm compresses.
- Help your partner hold the baby, preferably skin to skin.
- Keep the baby warm, covering both the birthing person and the baby with blankets.

Placental (Third) Stage (5 to 30 minutes)

- The birthing person may be very shaky, tired, curious, and in wonder of the baby.
- The birthing person may feel mild cramps with expulsion of the placenta.
- The caregiver massages the birthing parent's abdomen, which causes the uterus to contract and protects from excessive bleeding. It may be quite uncomfortable. Luckily, the massage does not take long.
- The placenta separates from uterus wall.
- The cord is clamped and cut.

- Sing or talk to the baby—a song sung often during pregnancy. Watch your baby's response!
- Use the Take-Charge routine (see page 202) to help them tolerate the pain.
- Ask the nurse to show the laboring person how to massage their own abdomen, which should be done frequently during the first days.
- Make sure both the birthing person and baby are warm and comfortable.
- Cut the cord, if you wish, after a few minutes to allow blood in the placenta to transfer through the cord to the baby.
- Hold the baby if your partner is not ready or having pain during stitching.

Recovery and Integration Phase (2 to 4 hours)

- The uterus starts to shrink in size.
- The nurse or midwife checks your partner's and baby's vital signs.
- Breast-feeding/chest-feeding begins—preferably unrushed, allowing baby to set the pace.
- Skin-to-skin contact facilitates hormones that promote bonding and milk production.

- Stay close by and appreciate these uniquely special moments.
- Greet visitors but be mindful of your partner's physical and emotional state and fatigue.
- Make calls to family and friends.
- Take photos or video as desired.
- Arrange for a delicious meal for both of you.

CHAPTER 4

COMFORT MEASURES FOR LABOR

I'll tell you, while practicing that Take-Charge routine in class I thought, "Is Penny trying to make us look stupid?" It seemed so phony—"conducting" Lynn's breathing. . . . Well, in labor, I used it a lot. It helped Lynn stay on track with her rhythm.

—JEFF, FIRST-TIME FATHER

That rhythm rocks!

—GREG, FIRST-TIME FATHER

The pain of labor has many physical causes. In the first stage, pain is caused by:

- Contractions of the uterus—the strongest muscle in the human body—which reach maximum intensity during this stage. (Try doing several chin-ups for 1 minute at a time. The muscle pain in your arms is similar to the kind of pain caused by uterine contractions, but less intense.)

- Stretching of the cervix as it opens. (Try sitting on the floor with your legs out straight and bending forward as far as possible with your hands grasping your lower legs. This will give you a sense of the nature of the pain caused by the cervix stretching.)

- Stretching of pelvic ligaments from the pressure of the baby's head within the pelvis. This causes mild to severe back pain. One-fourth to one-third of laboring women have back pain during labor.

In the birthing stage, pain is caused by uterine contractions, pressure in the pelvis, and also by stretching of the pelvic floor muscles, the vaginal canal, and the skin of the vaginal outlet.

Labor pain also can be increased by fear, worry, shame, or exhaustion. These can affect the laboring person as much as physical causes and can turn pain into suffering.

Pain versus Suffering

Although the terms *pain* and *suffering* are often used interchangeably, there is a big difference between the two. Labor, even when long and painful, does not inevitably cause suffering. Pain is an unpleasant physical sensation that may or may not be associated with suffering. For example, the pain people feel when working out at the gym or jogging uphill is not suffering. Consider the motto, "No pain, no gain." Suffering is a distressing psychological state that may include feelings of helplessness, anguish, remorse, fear, panic, or loss of control and may or may not be associated with pain. For example, being jilted by a lover or emotionally abused (ignored, insulted, or humiliated) or witnessing another person being hurt or injured may cause one to suffer, even though one may feel no physical sensation of pain.

Many people tell us that what worries them most about labor pain is they will be overwhelmed, helpless, and out of control. They worry the pain will take them beyond their limits and make them behave in a shameful way. This is a fear of suffering. If they carry this fear into labor, the fear will augment the pain, and they will likely suffer in the ways they fear. These pregnant people do not have confidence that labor pain can be manageable and that it does not inevitably lead to suffering.

When pregnant people recognize that labor pain is really a side effect of a normal process, not a sign of damage or injury, fear cannot increase the pain. Most of us have had pain that we did not understand, and it frightened us. For example, when I (Penny) turned my ankle with an awful crunching sound, I was terrified I had broken it. In great pain, I was rushed to the emergency room where I was told there was no break, only a bad strain that should clear up if I wore a stabilizing boot for a couple of weeks. I immediately felt better and was able to walk (or limp) out of the hospital I had entered in a wheelchair. Once knowledge replaced fear, my pain diminished.

Some laboring people will cross from pain to suffering if they become exhausted or if something interferes with their confidence or way of coping, such as frequent disturbances, rigid hospital routines, thoughtless or demoralizing remarks, lack of emotional support, or clinical complications. If a laboring person understands why contractions hurt and are continuously nurtured and encouraged by humane, caring, confident people in a peaceful and safe environment; if they are free to move about to find greater comfort; and if they know effective ways to respond to contractions, fear gives way to mastery, confidence, and a sense of well-being. Even though the contractions become very intense, the pregnant person does not suffer—they cope.

We discuss the difference between pain and suffering in our childbirth classes. After giving birth, one of our students said when she was considering an epidural she asked herself, "Am I suffering?" and answered herself, "I'm in a lot of pain, but I am not suffering." She decided she could manage without the epidural, and she did so without suffering.

How to Decrease Pain and Prevent Suffering in Labor

There are many ways you and the laboring person can reduce labor pain. Through childbirth education (classes, this book, video, media, and internet resources), you can learn about the birth process, self-help comfort measures, the wide range of other measures to relieve labor pain, and other options regarding the laboring person's care in labor. Laboring persons can use relaxation techniques, rhythmic breathing or moaning, attention focusing, movements, and positions. You can help by never leaving them alone in labor, attending to their emotional needs, comforting with massage, hand holding, and hot or cold packs, by suggesting a shower or bath, and by assisting them in the use of other self-help comfort measures, which we discuss here.

This chapter tells you more specifically what you can do to ease the laboring person's pain. These numerous techniques do not take away all pain, but, when combined with caring and skilled labor support, they enable many people in labor to cope successfully with the pain. Some people in labor use these techniques in combination with pain-relieving medications; others rely on the techniques alone.

Make sure, before labor begins, that you know and respect the pregnant person's preferences regarding the use of pain medications. Use the "Pain Medications Preference Scale," pages 328–329, to help describe their feelings and whether your feelings are different. Then, you will know how to react if and when they approach their pain tolerance limits. You will either ask for pain medication (see chapter 8) or redouble your efforts in encouraging, guiding, and helping the laboring person continue to handle the pain. For the latter, many of the comfort measures described here are highly effective.

The techniques described in this chapter work in different ways, by:

• Eliminating or reducing factors causing the pain

• Increasing other pleasant or neutral sensations to dampen the awareness of pain

• Involving the laboring person in activities that focus attention on something other than the pain

• Showing the laboring person they are cared for, respected, and heard

Using a variety of techniques seems more helpful than doing the same thing for the entire labor.

Learn the following techniques before labor so you can suggest them when appropriate and help the laboring person use them. Along with the lists in chapter 1, the information in this chapter will also help you choose comfort items to take to the hospital (or have ready in your home) to use during labor.

As you learn these techniques and positions, keep in mind there are other ways to help a person through labor. Sometimes, the best thing to do is simply to be there, quietly standing by, while labor unfolds and the laboring person searches within for the best way to respond. If they seem withdrawn and incommunicative, do not be concerned. You don't need to engage them in discussion. Let them discover what they need from you. Take your lead from them in the moment rather than trying to plan it all in advance.

The Three Rs:
Relaxation, Rhythm, and Ritual

Coping well with the pain and indeterminate length of labor involves the use of the Three Rs: relaxation, rhythm, and ritual. The concept of the Three Rs arose from my (Penny's) observations as a doula for hundreds of laboring women. I learned some people cope well with pain and stress in labor; others are overwhelmed. I noticed these three responses to contractions are shared by most people who cope well:

- The person can *relax* during or between contractions or both. Relaxation often involves remaining still, with limp limbs (passive relaxation) while breathing slowly and fully. It really helps reduce discomfort if the laboring person releases tension, remains still, and goes limp throughout the body. Alternatively, it is also soothing and relaxing to sway, rock, moan, chant, or sing rhythmically. This is called "active relaxation" and can be very helpful, especially with the intense contractions of later labor or if passive relaxation is no longer doable. Between contractions, the laboring person rests or resumes normal activity until the next contraction.

- The use of *rhythm* to cope

- The discovery and use of *rituals*—personally meaningful rhythmic activities repeated with every contraction

Using Rituals During Labor

In prelabor and very early labor, a laboring person coping well uses distracting activities until the contractions become intense enough they can no longer continue walking or talking through them. When they must stop everything for 30 seconds or so at each contraction's peak, the laboring person stops trying to use distraction and begins using a ritual.

During early labor, the ritual is usually one rehearsed in advance, perhaps in childbirth class. If they haven't learned a ritual in advance, the nurse or doula may teach one in the moment. This "planned" ritual usually involves sighing (breathing slowly, audibly, and rhythmically), releasing muscle tension with each exhale, and focusing attention in some positive way (for example, letting go of tension in one muscle group at a time: brow, shoulders, arms, buttocks, legs or counting breaths through the contractions).

As labor intensifies, the laboring person may adopt another planned ritual. They may change to a lighter, quicker, rhythm of breathing (4 to 6 shallow breaths every 10 seconds), move rhythmically (sway, rock, slow dance with you, their partner, [see page 170], or tap or stroke themselves, you, a pillow, or other object), and focus their attention by staring into your face, counting their breaths, using imagery, or chanting, singing, moaning, or self-talking, audibly or not.

By this time in labor (around 5 centimeters in dilation), however, many laboring people stop thinking and behave more instinctually as they give up trying to control the labor. Their planned ritual gives way as they discover their own spontaneous rituals. These become very powerful aids in getting through each contraction. Once laboring people discover these rituals, they repeat them for many contractions. Then, as labor changes, they may change rituals spontaneously once again.

It is a good sign when a laboring person goes into a more instinctual state, almost a reverie. It means the thinking part of their brain, the neocortex, is calm; this allows the more primitive parts of the brain—the midbrain and brain stem, which guide all basic bodily functions—to prevail. Michel Odent, a French obstetrician, has explained the need to avoid stimulating the neocortex in laboring people. When in a state of reverie, being asked questions or touched unexpectedly, having bright lights come on, or having people coming and going is a disturbance that tends to activate the neocortex and inhibit the primitive brain. When a person in labor finds their own spontaneous ritual, they have found a way to deal with the pain of contractions. If anyone disturbs the ritual, they become more aware of the pain, and it might take a while to reestablish the ritual.

Of course, disturbances are common in modern hospitals. We often marvel at how well some laboring people block out interruptions and disturbances for long stretches without appearing to notice the busyness around them.

What do labor rituals have in common? As already described, they always seem to involve rhythm in some way. In fact, rhythm is the most essential element in the Three Rs. Sometimes, the rhythm is supplied by someone or something else, in the form of murmuring, rhythmic stroking or pressure, pouring water over the contracting belly, or moaning or swaying together.

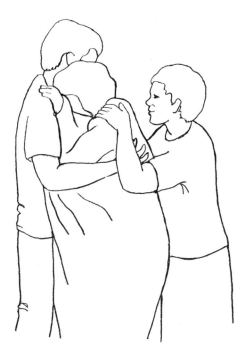

This person's ritual: burying their face in their partner's chest with the doula rubbing their shoulders and all three swaying together

Internal and External Rituals

Some people in labor close their eyes and either become very still or rock, tap, or sway and moan during contractions. Their rituals are *internal*; they involve relaxation, rhythmic breathing or moaning, and some kind of mental activity. These people seem hardly aware of those around them.

Other laboring people keep their eyes open and focused, move their bodies, vocalize rhythmically, and depend on someone else to be a part of the ritual. These are *external* rituals, in which the laboring person receives help from outside.

It is quite common for a laboring person to use an internal ritual early in labor and shift to an external one later or vice versa.

How to Help with Labor Rituals

As birth partner, you can help a laboring person develop or continue their ritual. First, observe their behavior during contractions. Are they still, with relaxed muscles? Or, are they moving or vocalizing in a rhythm? If doing any of these, they are coping well, even if the ritual involves moaning loudly or swaying vigorously. If they have lost the rhythm, your job (or the doula's) is to help them find or regain a rhythm (see "The Take-Charge Routine," page 262, and "How You Can Help," page 106). Do not interrupt the ritual during a contraction by asking a question or suggesting something other approach.

Your assistance will probably be more active with the use of an external ritual than an internal ritual. For example, with an external ritual you might:

• Maintain eye contact

• Help keep a rhythm by moving your head or hands, stroking, or murmuring soothing words in the rhythm of their breathing or moaning

• Press firmly on their upper arms, hands, thighs, or feet to anchor them

• Press on their hips or low back (see "Counterpressure for Back Pain," page 194)

• Hold them close, walk, sway, or slow dance together

If they use an internal ritual, you might:

• Remain close by, holding their hand quietly and calmly

• Refrain from, and ask others to refrain from, disturbing them during contractions

If you have prepared for a very active support role, you may feel useless if the laboring person uses an internal ritual. You may want to do more, to have them look at you or allow you to stroke or talk to them. You must realize, however, they need you, but more as a calm, caring presence than an active helper. If they are coping (relaxing during contractions and remaining still, with eyes closed), engaging with eye contact or following your rhythm will be disruptive.

Even if the laboring person does not seem to need much help from you at the moment, continue to observe and be in their rhythm during contractions. If they begin to wince or tense or vocalize or lose rhythm, get their attention and help them regain the rhythm.

If there are continual interruptions—examinations by a nurse or caregiver, checking their pulse, taking their temperature or blood pressure, drawing blood, general monitoring—the laboring person may become too unsettled to be able to keep a rhythm or regain their ritual. In this case, you might tell the nurse, "If they could get through a few contractions without interruption, I think they could feel more in control. Is this possible?" If the procedures cannot be postponed, you may need to play a more active "coaching" role. Use the Take-Charge routine (see page 202) and tell the laboring person, "All that matters during this contraction is that you keep your rhythm. Let me help you through this." Help them with their rhythm until they have some quiet, undisturbed time to resume or develop another ritual.

Once the cervix dilates completely and the laboring person is in the birthing stage, they will become more alert and focused. They are less likely to use the same ritual now, and their rhythm will give way to the powerful urge to push. The contractions will now dictate whether, when, and how they push, and they will approach birth in a crescendo of emotion, excitement, and sensation. Instead of helping maintain a ritual during the birthing stage, help them maintain a good position for birth and encourage them to relax the perineum during pushes (see "The Birthing Stage," page 116).

Examples of Spontaneous Rituals

The following examples illustrate some spontaneous rituals developed by people in labor and their birth partners. You can see how people add their personal touches to get the most out of the comfort measures.

One couple found themselves handling the contractions with the birth partner scratching the laboring person's back during each contraction while she knelt on the floor and leaned forward onto his lap. She had always loved having her back scratched, and she found that, during contractions, it really helped for him to scratch lightly, moving gradually upward from the left buttock to the left shoulder, over to the right shoulder, and down to the right buttock. Following the changes in her breathing, he timed his scratching so when he reached her right shoulder, the contraction had peaked, and when he reached her right buttock, it had ended. This back scratching was a helpful focus for the laboring person; she could tell where she was in the contraction by where her birth partner was scratching! Later she said, "He cut my contractions in half! I knew I just had to cope until he got to my right shoulder. Then, I knew I was on my way out of the contraction."

Other birth partners have helped birthing persons know when a contraction has passed the halfway point by counting breaths. Once you know about how many breaths it takes the birthing person to get through a contraction, you can tell when it is more than halfway through—"on the downside." In active labor, if you listen carefully to the rhythmic breathing or moaning, you'll notice it sounds more strained at the peak and seems to relax and sound easier once they are over the peak. You can then say, "It's peaking now," and, when you are sure the contraction is well past the peak, "You're on the downside," or "You're on the way out. Good job."

In another case, the ritual involved hair brushing. The woman had long, straight, silky hair, and she found she could cope well as long as her mother brushed it rhythmically during the contractions. If her mother stopped, the woman felt more pain. It happened that her mother had often brushed the woman's hair when she was a child and teenager, and during those times, they had felt very close to each other. The daughter had felt safe and content, and these same feelings surfaced during her labor.

An example of the importance of detail is the laboring person who found herself staring at a hole in her partner's T-shirt during every contraction and repeating to herself, "Blow out the hole and you're in control. Blow out the hole and you're in control." When her partner turned away to get a drink of water during a contraction, she fell apart. She said, "You can't do that!" He thought she meant he couldn't drink water: "I'm thirsty! I need something to drink!" Her reply, "I need your hole!" He had no idea how important the hole in his T-shirt was in keeping her focused.

Here is a heartwarming ritual. A laboring person and her partner pace slowly between contractions. When a contraction begins, they face each other and slow dance (see page 170), swaying together silently. When the contraction ends, they resume the pacing. Later, at the childbirth class reunion, he described this ritual with tears in his eyes: "I've never felt so manly in all my life. Holding her close, I could feel every contraction while she pressed against me."

One last ritual shows how relaxation can give way to rhythm: The woman was having a very rapid, painful labor. While reclining in the tub, she discovered it really helped to slam her open hand against the wall in the rhythm of her moaning. Slam! Slam! Slam! Her doula worried she would injure her hand, but knew it was best not to stop her. Soon the slams began to turn the bathroom light off, then on. This went on for an hour. Apparently, there was a faulty connection in the electrical system. Later, the nurse told the doula, "I thought you were doing that—some fancy new ritual!" (Incidentally, the woman did not injure her hand. We assume the hospital fixed the light.)

The development of rhythmic rituals is a truly creative aspect of labor, although it is largely unrecognized by caregivers and by childbirth educators and authors. It is not the comfort measures by themselves that reduce pain; rather, it is the laboring person's unique adaptation of these measures to suit their personality and needs at the time.

Self-Help Comfort Measures

Self-help comfort measures are skills the pregnant person masters before labor to help manage pain and enhance labor progress. Many are taught in childbirth classes, on audio or video media, online streaming sites such as YouTube, or in books. Plan to learn and use these. They can make the difference between feeling overwhelmed by the pain and coping in a positive way. This section covers many self-help comfort measures. Practice them together and adapt them to work best for the pregnant person.

Relaxation

Relaxation, rhythmic breathing, and attention focusing have long been the cornerstones of childbirth preparation. Relaxation is the goal of most comfort measures. If a laboring person lets their body go limp during contractions (passive relaxation) or if they sway, rock, moan, or murmur rhythmically (active relaxation), they will feel less pain or be less overwhelmed. The laboring person's attempt to relax, even if not completely successful, is helpful in itself because it serves as a positive focus away from the pain.

In active labor, passive relaxation during contractions may be more difficult than in early labor; the laboring person may need to keep moving in rhythm. At this phase, the goal is to relax passively between contractions and carry on an active ritual (see page 149) during them.

During the last weeks of pregnancy, help the pregnant person learn to recognize and release tension in all parts of their body. By practicing with them, you learn what tone of voice, which words, and what sort of touch helps them relax. Try the following:

- While the pregnant person lies still, as they breathe slowly and deeply, state which body parts to focus on and relax. Start at the toes and gradually go through the parts of the body up to the head.

- Help the pregnant person identify any "tension spots" and release the tension at will. A tension spot is a part of the body where tension seems to settle when they are stressed. This same spot (or spots) is likely to be the seat of tension during labor. Tension spots might be the shoulders, neck, brow, jaw, low back, or buttocks. Help them let go of tension when you touch the spot with your whole hand or when you say, for example, "Relax your right shoulder," or "Let go right here." If the pregnant person has difficulty relaxing, they can learn to let a particular part of their body go limp by first tensing it (for example, tightening the arm or leg as much as possible) and then relaxing it. Repeating this exercise trains both of you to recognize when their body is tense and trains the pregnant person to relax.

- Try "floating" an arm or a leg. While the pregnant person sits or lies comfortably, gently lift their arm with one of your hands just above the wrist joint and the other just above the elbow. Gently move the arm up and down and around in circles. Encourage them to "let go," to avoid helping or resisting your movements. They can try to imagine being a rag doll, loose and floppy. This exercise teaches trust as well as the difference between tension and relaxation.

Good childbirth preparation classes emphasize passive and active relaxation techniques. DVDs and YouTube videos are also available to help people master the skill of relaxation for childbirth. See Recommended Resources (page 418) for a description of some helpful aids for relaxation.

During labor, you can help the laboring person relax in the following ways:

- When they feel a contraction start, remind them to begin their ritual immediately (if it doesn't begin spontaneously), using rhythmic exhales to release tension. Remind them that each exhale is a relaxing breath.

- If you notice tension in any part of their body as the contraction intensifies, use soothing words or touch (or both) to help them let go of tension in those places. Don't just say, "Relax." Be more specific. Instead say, "Let go right here," as you touch a hands, brow, shoulder, and so forth. Your touch should be comforting, not tense or tentative. When they releasing tension, say, "Good," or "Just like that."

- Try "floating" a limb between contractions, if this was helpful during your relaxation practice.

- Use the comfort measures in this chapter and verbal reminders to help the laboring person relax during and between contractions. Trial and error will tell you what works best. Once you find something that works, stick with it.

- If labor becomes so intense that the laboring person is unable to relax *during* contractions despite your efforts, help them relax and rest *between* contractions while keeping a rhythm during them. Use soothing words, touch, and other comfort measures.

Hypnosis

Many laboring people can achieve a trance state during which they are able to remain deeply relaxed, with a reduced awareness of pain. The use of self-hypnosis during labor requires proper training and practice in advance. The hypnotic trance can be induced during labor by the laboring person or by a trained birth partner or doula. (Hypnotherapists do not accompany clients during labor, though there are some "hypno-doulas" trained to assist with hypnosis.)

Hypnosis classes and DVDs are popular adjuncts to conventional childbirth education. Certified hypnotherapists or childbirth educators with additional training work intensively with pregnant people and their partners, using hypnosis to reduce fear and anxiety, build confidence, and foster mastery of pain-relief techniques (see Recommended Resources, page 418). Recent research studies that compared self-hypnosis with more conventional comfort techniques in labor found less need for

The Perfect Parent—Relaxation Exercise
Script for Passive Relaxation

Read this script to the pregnant parent calmly and slowly, letting them spend two or three breaths releasing tension in each area of focus, offering time to allow the tension to slip away.

1. Yawn or exhale completely.

2. Focus on your toes and feet. Imagine you are breathing away any tension there. Feel how warm and relaxed they are.

3. Now, focus on your ankles. Think about how floppy and loose your ankles are. They're relaxed and comfortable.

4. Now, focus on your lower legs. Let those muscles become loose and soft. Good.

5. And now, focus on your knees. They're supported and relaxed—you're not holding your legs in any position. Wiggle them to see how relaxed they are.

6. Think about your thighs. Those strong muscles are soft and relaxed because they have no work to do right now, and they're fully supported. Good.

7. And now, think about your buttocks and perineum. This area needs to be especially relaxed during labor and birth, so just let it become soft and yielding. When the time is right, your baby will travel down the birth canal, and the tissues of your perineum will spread to let your baby out. You'll release, letting your perineum relax and open for your baby.

8. Focus on your lower back. Imagine someone with strong, warm hands giving you a lovely back rub. It feels so good. Your muscles are relaxing, and your lower back is comfortable. Notice the tension leaving your back.

9. Let your thoughts turn to your belly. Let those muscles relax. Let your belly rise and fall as you breathe in and out. Good. Now, let's move your focus deeper, to your baby within your uterus, floating or wiggling and squirming in the warm water of your womb—a safe place meeting all your baby's needs for nourishment, oxygen, warmth, movement, and stimulation. Your baby hears your heartbeat, your voice, my voice, music, and other interesting sounds. What excellent care you're giving your baby. You're the perfect parent—meeting all the baby's needs!

10. Now, focus on your chest. As you inhale, your chest swells easily, making room for the air. As you exhale, your chest relaxes to help the air flow out. Breathe easily and slowly, letting the air flow in and out, almost as though you're asleep. Good.

11. Take a moment to focus on your breathing again—inhaling through your nose and exhaling through your mouth—slowly and easily, letting the air flow in and out. At the top of an inhalation, notice that little tension in your chest, which you can release with an exhalation. Listen as you exhale. Your breath sounds relaxed and calm, almost as if you were asleep. Every exhalation is relaxing. Use your exhalations to breathe away any tension. Good.

12. And now, focus on your shoulders and upper back. Imagine you've just had them massaged. Breathe any tension away and feel the warmth and softness as the tension slips away.

13. Focus on your arms. Exhale and let your arms go limp—from your shoulders all the way down your arms to your wrists, hands, and fingers. Let them become heavy, loose, and relaxed.

14. And now, focus on your neck. All the muscles in your neck are soft because they don't have to hold your head in any position. Your head is either comfortably balanced or completely supported, so just let your neck relax. Good.

15. Focus on your lips and jaw. They're slack and relaxed. You're not holding your mouth closed or open. It's comfortable—no tension there.

16. And now, focus on your eyes and eyelids. You're not keeping your eyes open or closed. They're the way they want to be. Your eyes are unfocused and still. Your eyelids are relaxed and heavy.

17. Focus on your brow and scalp. No worries there! Think about how warm and relaxed they are. You have a calm, peaceful expression on your face, reflecting a calm, peaceful feeling inside.

18. We've gone all the way from your toes to the top of your head. Take a few moments to enjoy these feelings of calmness and well-being.

    You can relax this way anytime—before bedtime, during an afternoon rest, or during a quiet break. This is how you'll want to feel in labor.

    Of course, during labor, you won't lie down all the time. You'll walk, sit up, shower, and change positions. But whenever a contraction comes, you'll let yourself relax all the muscles you don't need to hold yourself in a particular position, and you can let your mind relax, giving you a confident, peaceful feeling. This feeling will help you yield to contractions, letting you focus on breathing and finding comfort through each one.

19. And now, it's time to end the exercise. Gradually open your eyes, stretch, and tune in to your surroundings. Take your time. There's no need to rush.

pain medications among women who used self-hypnosis. The drawback for some is the intensive practice time required to master the technique and use it successfully in labor.

Attention Focusing

This technique diverts the laboring person's mind from the pain by having them concentrate on something else. During contractions, attention can be refocused in several ways:

- The laboring person can *look* at you or a meaningful picture, figurine, flowers, or another object. One woman hung a baby's outfit on the wall and focused on it and the fact that she soon would fill the suit with a baby. Another person made an inspiring collage to hang on the birthing room wall; it included beautiful scenery and images of powerful people doing impressive physical and artistic feats. Another posted pictures of her older child's artwork. Still another hung pictures of her many pets—her horse, three dogs, and a cat. Like the person who focused on a hole in her partner's T-shirt (page 152), all these laboring women used objects to ground or inspire them. Focusing on an object can become an all-important part of a laboring person's ritual.

- The laboring person can *listen* to your voice, to music, or another soothing sound (see page 196). Many people like to hear rhythmic murmuring with each contraction.

- They can focus on *feeling* your touch, your massage, or your caress. Match their rhythm with your stroking.

- They can *concentrate* on a mantra or mental ritual such as counting breaths or repeating words throughout each contraction. For example, they might chant, "Ooopen . . . , ooopen . . . , ooopen . . ." or say, "I think I can . . . , I think I can . . . , I thought I could . . . , I thought I could. . . ." (from *The Little Engine That Could*); or repeat, "Be still like the mountain and flow like the river." One laboring person even loudly repeated the word *epidural* over and over while swaying through the contractions. The doula asked whether an epidural was needed. The person replied, "No, if I can say it, I don't need it!" Usually, these rituals are unplanned and emerge spontaneously. You might join them if they are counting, chanting, or moaning aloud. Certainly, whatever you do, do not interrupt their rhythm. Help them maintain it.

Visualization

The laboring person can visualize something positive, pleasant, or relaxing, using the contractions, focus, or breathing as a cue. For example, they might visualize their exhalations or your soothing touch or massage as drawing the tension and pain away. They might imagine being in a special, safe, comfortable place, where the contractions are cues to relax more deeply into the comfort of the place. They might visualize each contraction in various ways: as a wave and floating over the crest or as a mountain, climbing up and down as the contractions come and go. They might use the onset of the contraction as a cue to imagine soaring like a seagull above the waves of contractions below. Several people from our childbirth classes have told us that during labor they visualized the opening of the cervix of the knitted argyle uterus that we use during classes to demonstrate contractions and dilation.

Some visualizations are planned; others emerge spontaneously in labor. Spontaneous visualizations are usually very creative and personally helpful.

Sometimes, couples plan visualizations together during pregnancy, so the partner can guide the laboring person through them during labor. We recommend recalling some positive or empowering experiences you have shared or that they have gone through. Following are guidelines for two personal visualizations: one for early labor and one for active labor.

To plan a visualization for **early labor**:

1. Think of an event in which the two of you were relaxed and content (for example, a trip you took, a beautiful afternoon, a warm conversation).

2. Take a walk together or have a delicious meal together and recall as many details of that experience as you can.

3. Weave the details into a brief description with a beginning, a middle, and an end. During contractions, you will narrate the visualization, varying the details with each contraction.

For example, one couple had taken a canoe trip early on a cold misty morning. The river was still; the mist was rising; birds were soaring overhead; a ramshackle barn was visible in the distance; a fallen tree partly blocked the river; and so on. In labor, the woman was in a large tub and a friend was pouring water over her back in rhythm with her breathing. With each contraction, her partner told, "Now, let's get in the canoe and glide over the contraction. Birds fly overhead. See the barn with the caved-in roof. There is no one else in sight. It's all so still and beautiful. Now, take your rest." The partner varied the details but repeated them often. Later the woman said, "He took me back there. My breathing became the strokes of my paddle. The sound of the water being poured over my back became the drips off the paddle when I took it out of the water."

For **active labor**:

1. Ask the pregnant person to describe a time they were challenged—physically, mentally, or artistically—and met that challenge.

2. Weave the event into a brief description that can be narrated during contractions as a reminder of their ability to meet challenges.

3. Plan to vary or intensify the description as labor becomes more intense.

For example, one person recalled regularly riding a bicycle on a trail that had one very steep, long uphill stretch. For a long time, they were unable to make it to the top without walking the bike partway. With persistence, though, they could eventually pedal to the top before coasting down the other side. In active labor, they pictured each contraction as that hill and recalled the persistence it took, with shortness of breath and aching muscles, to get to the top. Their mantra became, "Keep it up. Keep it up." The partner encouraged the laboring person by repeating the mantra and then, "Almost there—a little more—that's right. Now you're over the top. Coast your way down." The laboring person said later that each hill became higher and tougher to climb as the contractions intensified, but the memory of successfully pedaling up the hill helped with every contraction.

Rhythmic Breathing and Moaning

Every method of childbirth preparation has used rhythmic breathing as its mainstay. It is the most widely used comfort technique for childbirth. In a large U.S. survey, 49 percent of laboring people who responded used breathing techniques. A large Canadian survey found that 74 percent used breathing. In fact, success in every demanding physical activity, or sport, as well as meditation and stress-reduction techniques, requires breath awareness and rhythm. Rhythmic breathing or moaning (which is actually vocal breathing), along with relaxation, have tremendous value and offer unique pain-relieving capabilities:

- Breathing or moaning in steady rhythm helps one relax, especially when having learned to release tension with each exhalation.

- Rhythmic breathing or moaning is calming, especially when a person feels anxious or overwhelmed.

- Rhythmic breathing or moaning gives the person some measure of control over their responses to the contractions, even though the uterus, with its involuntary and all-encompassing contractions, is completely outside one's conscious control.

- When institutional policy or the laboring person's own condition does not permit comfort measures such as a bath or shower, massage or movement, rhythmic breathing or moaning is always available. (Many comfort measures are impossible, for example, when the person cannot get out of bed, if electronic fetal monitor belts or an intravenous line are in the way, or they have received pain medications; see "When the Birthing Person Must Labor in Bed," page 224, for specific suggestions for such circumstances.)

The laboring person will be able to use breathing rhythms most effectively and with the least effort during labor if the techniques are mastered beforehand.

There are two basic breathing rhythms to use during the dilation (first) stage: *slow breathing and light breathing.* We suggest that you and the pregnant person learn each, adapt their speed and rhythm so you feel comfortable with them, and use them during labor. The laboring person's preferences and the nature of the contractions should guide the two of you in deciding how and when to use these rhythms.

Slow Breathing or Moaning

We suggest beginning with slow rather than light quick breaths because this is the easier of the two rhythms. Start this when distracting activities no longer keep the laboring person comfortable; that is, when contractions become so intense that the laboring person stops in their tracks and is unable to continue walking, talking, or whatever they are doing, through each contraction. From this point, they should use slow breathing for as long as they can relax well with it, perhaps moaning or sighing audibly with each exhale.

For slow breathing to be most relaxing and calming, the key is for the laboring person to breathe easily and fully and not work to keep it slow: "Easy in, easy out." If they are working too hard, their breathing will sound tense and strained and their bodies will show tension.

This is how to use slow breathing during labor:

1. When the contraction begins, the laboring person focuses their attention as described on page 158.

2. They take a big, relaxing sigh, releasing tension throughout the body and, if desired, make a low moaning sound as they breathe out.

3. They breathe in slowly—preferably (though not necessarily) breathing in through the nose and breathing out through the mouth—with each exhale a long sigh or moan. At the end of each exhale, they pause and wait a moment, rather than rushing to inhale. The rate should be somewhere between 5 and 12 breaths per minute. With each exhale, they relax, releasing tension all over or from a different part of the body (such as the brow, jaw, shoulders, or right or left arm). Some people find it relaxing on each exhale to make "horse lips" sounds, which horses sometimes make by letting their loose lips vibrate as they breathe out through their mouths, also called a "nicker."

4. When the contraction ends, normal activity resumes and you do not think about the breathing.

The laboring person should use slow breathing for as long as it helps. Some people use only slow breathing throughout the entire labor. For most, however, the contractions become too intense and close together to maintain the slow breathing. In that case, switch to light breathing. If the laboring person switches to light breathing early in labor, they might be able to return to slow breathing later.

Light Breathing

Mastering the light breathing rhythm takes some practice, just as it takes time to learn to breathe rhythmically while swimming the crawl stroke. And, just as rhythmic breathing when swimming enables one to swim better, the light breathing rhythm enables the laboring person to manage pain better. (Light breathing is much easier to master than breathing while swimming.) Once mastered, light breathing is as easy to do as slow breathing. This is how to use light breathing during labor:

1. When the contraction begins, the laboring person focuses their attention.

2. They begin breathing in short, light breaths through their mouth, with a silent inhale, an audible exhale, and a brief pause after each exhale. The rate is about 1 breath every 1 or 2 seconds or 30 to 60 breaths per minute. With each exhale, they breathe out tension.

3. The breathing continues at this rate until the contraction begins to subside. Then, they either slow their breathing rate, if desired, or continue at the same light breathing rate until the contraction is over.

4. When the contraction ends, they can rest or resume whatever they were doing before it started. With the next contraction, they repeat the light breathing.

Encourage the pregnant person to practice this rhythm enough to master it before labor starts. It requires only a few practice sessions. At first, light breathing may be uncomfortable (it may cause dry mouth, lightheadedness, or a feeling of not being able to get enough air). By adapting it and working with it, however, the person can become relaxed and comfortable doing it. Light breathing may become their best friend in labor (besides you).

Practice light breathing until the pregnant person is able to breathe at the rate of 30 to 60 breaths per minute for a full 1 to 2 minutes without stopping or feeling lightheaded (from hyperventilating). If they feel lightheaded, slow the pace slightly, pause a bit longer at the end of each breath, or breathe more shallowly (so as not to move as much air in and out). The lightheadedness is annoying and uncomfortable, and it will not occur once the technique is mastered. If the pregnant person masters light breathing before labor begins, it is very unlikely they will hyperventilate during labor.

As the pregnant person practices rhythmic breathing, see that they relax all over, especially in the shoulders and trunk. If tense, it is more likely they'll hyperventilate. Remind them to relax. It is helpful if you "entrain" yourself to them by being "in their rhythm." If you sway, bob your head, count their breaths, or move your hand up and down in the rhythm of their breathing, it seems to help them continue in that steady rhythm. Keep your hand and wrist relaxed and floppy while conducting, remembering to stop briefly at the end of each exhale. Your own relaxation is contagious and will help them relax.

Once light breathing without hyperventilating is mastered, the laboring person will be able to adapt these breathing rhythms during labor in whatever way is most comfortable. They may want to combine slow and light breathing; for example, they might begin and end the contraction with slow breathing and use light breathing over the peak.

Do remember, however, that rhythmic breathing is most beneficial if the laboring person can use it easily—without thinking much about it and without tensing. Rhythmic breathing should be relaxing; it becomes an attention-focusing aid in itself once the pregnant person has mastered it.

Pushing (Bearing-Down) Techniques

There are four techniques for handling the urge to push:

- One is used to help the laboring person *avoid forceful pushing* (or bearing down) when this would be nonproductive or harmful.

- The others are used during the birthing stage, when the birthing person *should* be pushing; they are *spontaneous bearing down, self-directed pushing*, and *directed pushing*.

Avoiding Forceful Pushing

There are three occasions during labor when the birthing person should *not* push (holding their breath and straining) even though they feel like doing so. These are:

1. Before the cervix has completely dilated, as determined by a vaginal exam. A premature urge to push sometimes happens as early as 6 centimeters, if the baby's head is positioned so that it puts abnormal pressure on the vaginal wall.

2. During transition (between 8 and 10 centimeters dilation), if there is still a firm lip, or rim, of cervix remaining (see page 109). The caregiver detects this with a vaginal exam.

3. During the birthing stage, as the baby's head crowns and emerges.

Forceful pushing during dilation or transition might increase the pressure of the baby against the cervix, cause the cervix to swell, and, thus, slow the progress of labor. With a strong urge to push long before the cervix dilates, changing to the open knee–chest position or side-lying position may help (see page 173). During transition, until the lip disappears, the laboring person should push only enough to satisfy the urge (see "Transition," page 109).

If the laboring person is told not to push because of a lip, "grunt pushing" can help keep them from straining too hard. Grunt pushes are quick but gentle breath holds followed by forceful releases of air, which make a grunting sound. You might talk them through each contraction, helping them breathe or do grunt pushes.

During the crowning and birth stage, pushing hard might cause stretching that is too rapid and injures the vagina or a delivery that is too rapid. The laboring person can avoid holding their breath at this time by raising their chin and blowing or panting lightly whenever they feel the urge to push. This is sometimes easier said than done because the urge can be very strong. You can help by keeping eye contact and breathing with them, talking them through it, or nodding your head in the rhythm of their panting.

Don't expect too much from these techniques; they do not take away or diminish the birthing person's urge to push. All they do is minimize additional pushing in excess of what their body is already doing.

Spontaneous Bearing Down

Once the birthing person feels like pushing and the cervix is fully dilated, the caregiver will give the go-ahead. Usually, the birthing person should push spontaneously. Spontaneous bearing down works like this:

1. The contraction begins. The birthing person focuses their attention as described on page 158.

2. They use whichever breathing rhythm—slow or light—seems best, until the urge to push is so strong they cannot resist bearing down.

3. The urge to push comes in waves or surges—three to six in each contraction. These surges of the uterus sweep the birthing person along into an involuntary bearing-down effort (holding the breath or grunting, moaning, or straining) that lasts 5 to 7 seconds. Do not worry that they lose rhythm while pushing. In the birthing stage, the urge to push is the guide, not the rhythm.

4. Once each surge subsides, they breathe lightly again until the next surge. This pattern continues until the contraction is over.

5. When the contraction ends, they rest until the next one.

Self-Directed Pushing

This is reserved for times when the birthing person's spontaneous bearing down is ineffective. Their eyes may be clenched shut and they may be wincing, arching their back, tipping their chin up, as if fighting against the contraction. (We sometimes call this diffuse pushing, as the pushing efforts are not directed to move the baby down the birth canal.)

If progress is being made while pushing this way, do not worry. If the baby is not coming down, however, consult the caregiver and try this:

1. Between contractions, tell the laboring person to keep their eyes open and look toward where the baby will come out during the next contraction. This helps focus the pushing efforts downward.

2. You may need to remind them to open their eyes if this seems to improve progress.

3. If there are visible signs of progress, you might hold a mirror so the birthing person can see the baby coming. (Do not be surprised if they do not want to look. This should be their choice.)

4. The laboring person should bear down spontaneously, while looking toward where the baby will emerge.

5. If still bearing down ineffectively, suggest a change of position. Any change of position may help focus and push more effectively.

6. If these measures do not succeed, try directed pushing.

Directed Pushing

Until the late 1980s, directed pushing was the only bearing-down technique used in virtually every hospital. With this technique, the birthing person would be coached to hold their breath and strain as hard as they could for a count of 10 and then grab a breath and repeat this throughout every contraction. Research has shown that using forceful prolonged breath holding and straining may exhaust the birthing person, cause distress in the baby (because the breath holding decreases oxygen for the baby), and cause extreme stretching of the pelvic floor muscles and ligaments supporting the bladder and uterus, which can lead to later bladder and bowel problems.

Today, directed pushing is used under the following circumstances:

• When the baby's descent is too slow with spontaneous bearing down and the caregiver is considering assisting the delivery with instruments—forceps or a vacuum extractor (see pages 266–267)—or episiotomy (see page 263). The birthing person should try directed pushing before the instruments are used.

• When the birthing person has been given an epidural and cannot fully feel the urge to push and so cannot use the spontaneous bearing-down pattern. In this case, however, some side effects may be eliminated if they can use the modified form of directed pushing described following.

• When directed pushing remains the routine in the institution. Ask the birthing person's caregiver in advance whether the staff advocate spontaneous bearing down or directed pushing.

Modified Directed Pushing

Except when needed to avoid the use of instruments, the directed-pushing technique can be modified to resemble spontaneous bearing down to reduce undesirable effects:

1. The contraction begins. The birthing person focuses. You, the nurse, or doula says what to do: "Breathe in and out, two to four

times, letting the contraction build. Now, hold your next breath and strain—1, 2, 3, 4, 5, 6. Now, breathe for the baby. Take several quick breaths in and out and repeat the breath holding and straining."

2. The birthing person continues in this way until the contraction subsides.

3. The contraction ends. They rest until the next one.

Movement and Position Changes

When free to move and change positions, the birthing person:

• Is more comfortable and labor may even speed up

• Can find positions or movements that feel right

• May stand, walk, sit, recline, squat, kneel, lie on one side, get on hands and knees, or lean on you, the wall, a birth ball, the bed, or the nightstand (see illustrations, page 169)

• May walk, rock, or sway rhythmically

Encourage the birthing person to try a change in position or movement if they are restless, discouraged, or in a lot of pain, or if labor has slowed. A change every 30 minutes or so may make a positive difference. During the birthing stage, too, the birthing person may use several different positions, especially if this stage takes more than an hour.

Just before the actual birth of the baby, the caregiver may ask the birthing person to assume a position where the caregiver feels more confident "catching the baby," such as semisitting or lying flat on their back with legs drawn up to the chest. Some caregivers, however, are comfortable with the birthing person in a variety of positions; see pages 171–176 for a list of useful positions and the possible benefits of each.

Most hospitals have birthing beds that can be raised or lowered and that have moving sections and add-ons that can be configured to support a birthing person in a variety of positions, such as semisitting, sitting upright, kneeling and leaning forward, and squatting with a bar for support. Most of these beds have electronic controls. When you first arrive at the hospital, push all the buttons to see how the bed works and try the many possible positions.

POSITIONS AND MOVEMENTS FOR LABOR AND BIRTH

POSITION/MOVEMENT	UNIQUE BENEFITS

Standing

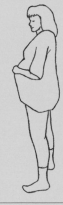

- Takes advantage of gravity during and between contractions
- For some people in labor, it's more comfortable than sitting or lying down.
- Shortens contractions and helps them be more productive
- Helps position the fetus to enter the pelvis
- May speed labor if the laboring person has been lying down
- May increase the urge to push in the second stage

Walking

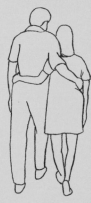

Same as standing, plus:

- Causes slight changes in the pelvic joints that encourage rotation and descent

Standing and leaning forward on the partner, the bed, or a birth ball*

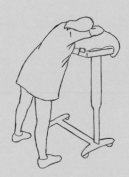

Same as standing, plus:
- Relieves backache
- Makes it easy for the partner or doula to give a back rub
- May be more restful than standing upright
- Can be used with an electronic fetal monitor (the laboring person must stand by the bed unless wireless monitors are used)

* These positions are particularly helpful for slow labor or back labor.

POSITION/MOVEMENT	UNIQUE BENEFITS

Slow dancing: The laboring person leans against the partner, resting their head on the partner's chest or shoulder. The partner's arms are around the laboring person, with fingers interlocked at their low back. The laboring person can tuck their thumbs into the partner's waistband or belt loops for comfort. They sway, perhaps to music, and breathe in rhythm.*

Same as standing, plus:

• Causes changes in the pelvic joints that encourage rotation and descent

• Being embraced by a loved one increases the laboring person's sense of well-being.

• Rhythm and music add comfort.

• Pressure from the partner's hands relieves back pain.

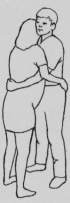

Standing lunge: Standing beside a chair and facing forward, the laboring person places one foot on the chair seat, with the raised knee and foot turned out. Bending the raised knee and hip, they "lunge" sideways repeatedly, slowly, and rhythmically during a contraction (either in the direction that is more comfortable, or to the right for two or three contractions and then to the left). They should feel the stretch in the inner thighs. Secure the chair and help keep them balanced.*

• Widens the side of the pelvis toward which they lunge

• Gives room for the baby to change position, if necessary

• May ease backache for a few contractions

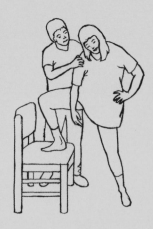

POSITION/MOVEMENT	UNIQUE BENEFITS

Kneeling lunge: From starting position: (a) slowly raise their knee and hip and "lunge" sideways, as in (b), and return to position (a) repeatedly during a contraction in the direction that is more comfortable, or if they feel the same, lunge to the right for 2 or 3 contractions and then to the left for 2 or 3. They should feel the stretch in the inner thighs.*

Same as standing lunge

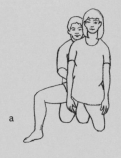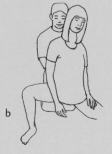

a   b

Sitting upright

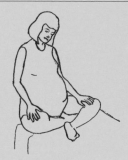

- Gives the laboring person a rest between contractions
- Uses gravity to help the baby descend
- Can be used with an electronic fetal monitor

Sitting on a toilet or commode**

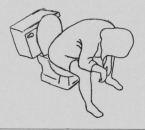

Same as sitting upright, plus:
- May help relax the perineum for effective bearing down

Semisitting**

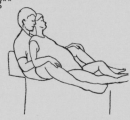

Same as sitting upright, plus:
- Makes a vaginal exam possible
- Easy position to get into on a bed or delivery table

---

* These positions are particularly helpful for slow labor or back labor.
** These positions are also useful during the birthing stage.

POSITION/MOVEMENT	UNIQUE BENEFITS
Sitting and rocking in a chair or swaying on a birth ball 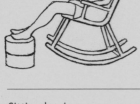	Same as sitting upright, plus: • May speed labor • Helps relax the trunk and perineum 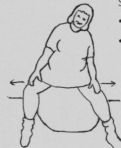
Sitting, leaning forward with support* 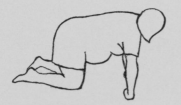	Same as sitting upright, plus: • Relieves backache • Makes it easy for the partner to give a back rub
Hands-and-knees position* **	• Helps relieve backache • Assists the rotation of a baby in OP position • Allows for pelvic rocking and other body movements • Takes pressure off hemorrhoids
Kneeling, leaning forward on a chair seat, the raised head of the bed, a birth ball, or the side of a tub* 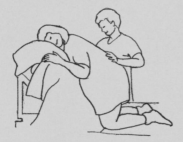	Same as hands and knees, plus: • Puts less strain on wrists and hands • Relieves back pain very effectively when done in a large tub 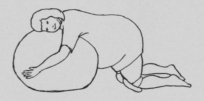

POSITION/MOVEMENT	UNIQUE BENEFITS

Open knee–chest position: Laboring person gets on hands and knees, lowers the chest, spreads the elbows, and rests their head on their hands. Make sure the knees are back far enough to raise the buttocks higher than the chest. You can support them by sitting on a chair, your feet about 9 inches (23 cm) apart. They put their head between your shins, and lean their shoulders against your shins.* This should be done for 30 to 45 minutes .

If partner's shins are uncomfortable, fold hand towels for padding.

- May be helpful in pre- or early labor
- Uses gravity to move baby's head (or buttocks) out of the pelvis, which may be desirable in early labor if the laboring person has backache or the baby is OP
- May reduce pressure on the cervix, which helps if it is swollen (also used for prolapsed cord; see page 290)

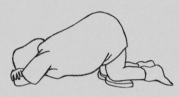
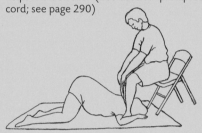

Side lying or semiprone: In the side-lying position, the laboring person lies on their side with both knees flexed and a pillow between them (a). In the semiprone position, they straighten the lower leg, roll slightly toward the front, flex the top hip and knee, and rest the top knee on one or two pillows (b) or a peanut-shaped ball (c). During the birthing stage, you can hold the birthing person's top leg up as they push (d).**

- Gives the laboring person some rest
- Makes interventions easy to perform
- Helps lower elevated blood pressure
- Safer than standing or the hands-and-knees position if pain medications are used
- May promote the progress of labor when alternated with walking
- Can slow a very rapid second stage
- Shifting between side-lying and semiprone positions helps change the baby's position.
- Works well with an epidural

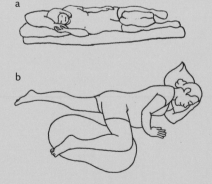
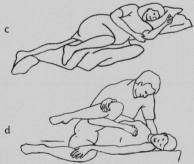

* These positions are particularly helpful for slow labor or back labor.
** These positions are also useful during the birthing stage.

POSITION/MOVEMENT	UNIQUE BENEFITS

Squatting: The laboring person squats on the floor or bed, holding on to your hands (a) or a railing or a squatting bar (b) attached to the bed. Or, if you sit with your thighs spread, they may stand between your knees (facing away from you) and lower themselves into a squat, with their arms resting on your thighs for support (c).**

- May relieve backache
- Uses gravity to help the baby descend
- May aid the baby's rotation
- Widens the pelvic outlet
- Provides the mechanical advantage of the upper trunk pressing on the uterus
- May help bring on the urge to push
- Requires less bearing-down effort
- Allows freedom to shift weight for comfort

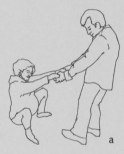 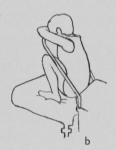 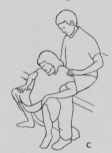

a   b   c

Lap squatting: Sit on an armless straight chair. The laboring person sits on your lap facing you, straddling your thighs. Embrace each other. When a contraction begins, spread your thighs, allowing their buttocks to sag between. Have a support person or doula stand behind you and hold the laboring person's hands for safety. After the contraction, bring your legs together and raise the laboring person onto your thighs again.**

Same as squatting, plus:

- Avoids strain on birthing person's knees and ankles
- Allows for more support with less effort for an exhausted laboring person
- Enhances feelings of well-being, as the laboring person is held close by a loved one

CAUTION: This may not be possible if the laboring person weighs more than you can support.

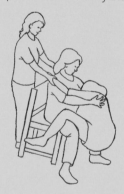

** These positions are also useful during the birthing stage.

POSITION/MOVEMENT	UNIQUE BENEFITS
Dangle with partner: Hold the laboring person under their arms as they lean with their back against you during contractions. They lower themselves so that you are bearing all their weight. Between contractions, they stand.** 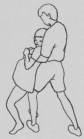	• Lengthens the laboring person's trunk, allowing more room for the baby to maneuver into position • Enhances pelvic joint mobility, allowing the baby to push the pelvic bones as needed to descend • Uses gravity to help the baby descend **CAUTION:** This position requires much strength from the partner. See following for a way to dangle while the partner sits.
Dangle: Sit on the edge of a high bed or counter, with each foot supported on a chair and your thighs spread. Standing, the laboring person backs between your legs and places their flexed arms over your thighs. During contractions, they lower themselves as you grip their chest with your thighs and they lower. You support their full weight. Between contractions, they stand.**	Same as dangle with partner, plus: • Puts much less strain on the partner 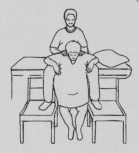
On back with legs drawn up: The laboring person lies flat on their back, raises their chin, and holds their knees apart, drawing them to their shoulders. They lower their legs between contractions. You can help them get into position with each contraction.**	• Do not use routinely • Tiring and works against gravity • May be helpful in prolonged second stage • Rotates pubic bone upward; may help if baby's head is not descending beneath the pubic bone, by moving pubic bone over the baby's head

* These positions are particularly helpful for slow labor or back labor.
** These positions are also useful during the birthing stage.

POSITION/MOVEMENT	UNIQUE BENEFITS
Hands and knees rocking forward and back: The laboring person is on hands and knees (a); they rock back, flexing knees and hips (b). They may stay in position (b) or rock forward and back throughout the contraction.	Alternating positions (a) and (b) causes movement and changes shape of pelvic joints; position (b) increases dimensions of pelvic basin. It may aid fetal head rotation during second stage. (with thanks to Susan Steffes, P.T. for this suggestion)

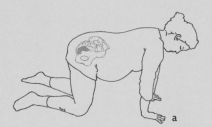
a

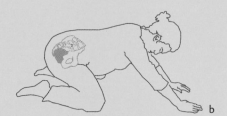
b

Comfort Aids and Devices

In addition to the self-help comfort techniques you just learned about, there are also many comforting items or devices: some are built in or available in the birth setting; others you may wish to bring with you. Use the information here to explore these items and decide which you might want to use during labor. Most items are easily found in popular stores or online. If you cannot locate some, ask your childbirth educator, midwife, or doula where to get them.

Baths and Showers (Hydrotherapy)

One of the safest and most effective forms of pain relief in labor is immersion in deep water or a warm shower. Hydrotherapy has been used for relaxation, healing, and pain relief for centuries and today is widely used in physical therapy, sports medicine, and other health

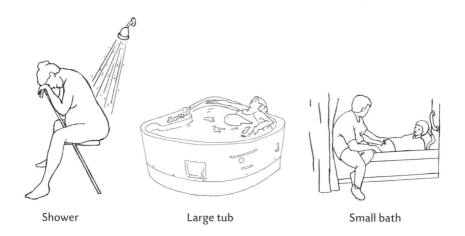

| Shower | Large tub | Small bath |

disciplines. Now, it is also widely used in childbirth. Showers are available in most hospitals, and bathtubs (some large enough for the laboring person to move around in or share with their partner) have been installed in many modern hospitals and birth centers. Some hospitals have tubs on wheels that can be moved from one birthing room to another. Lightweight tubs can be rented or purchased and set up temporarily in one's home for a home birth or possibly even in a hospital, if staff are willing and arrangements have been made in advance (see Recommended Resources, page 418).

Most people who use water in labor use it for pain relief. As you likely have experienced, soaking in a tub or lingering in the shower is soothing and relaxing. Numerous studies have shown that hydrotherapy, when used correctly during labor, is safe, reduces pain, and frequently speeds labor. It has advantages over pain medications: The laboring person can move about normally, and they remain clearheaded.

Showers and baths differ in their effects on the laboring person. While both enhance relaxation and reduce (but not eliminate) pain, the shower is simpler to use and requires fewer precautions. Water temperature is less of a safety concern with the shower than the bath (see page 178). The laboring person can use the shower early in labor, whereas the bath is better reserved until active labor. On the other hand, the shower is more tiring because one cannot easily recline, and it does not seem to have the labor-enhancing effects that immersion in deep water often has.

How Does a Bath Reduce Pain and Speed Active Labor?

When a laboring person sits in a deep, warm bath, a series of physiological changes begin immediately. These changes alter hormone production and fluid distribution throughout the body, quickly resulting in the following:

- Immediate relaxation and some pain relief from the warmth and buoyancy of the water, which can cause a drop in stress hormones

- Increased oxytocin production in the pituitary gland, located in the brain, causing stronger contractions; labor progress often speeds up without an increase in pain.

- Feelings of calm and well-being, from the increased oxytocin (**Note:** intravenous oxytocin does not have calming effects because it does not reach the brain.)

These benefits last for up to 2 hours or so, after which changes in the laboring person's circulation often lead to a slowing of contractions. To prevent this, the laboring person might get out of the water after about 1½ hours or at any time the contractions seem to space out or become less intense. Once they have been out of the water for a 30 minutes or so, they can return.

When Should a Laboring Person Get into the Bath?

As there is a time limit for benefits from the bath, the laboring person should not get in too early unless the caregiver wants to try to stop premature contractions or because they are having a long and tiring prelabor. Otherwise, the laboring person should wait until the cervix has dilated at least 5 centimeters and the contractions are clearly getting stronger and closer together (about 4 to 5 minutes apart), each lasting close to 1 minute. Getting into the bath at this point, they are likely to experience immediate and profound pain relief, along with faster dilation. Before this point they can take a long shower, which will not slow labor.

What Water Temperature Is Best?

The water temperature should not be higher than body temperature—around 98.6°F (37°C). This is very important: If the water is too warm, the laboring person's temperature goes up, which can cause a fever in the baby. Even when it is not caused by infection, any rise in temperature can cause the baby's heart rate to increase too much for safety. The laboring person should get out and cool down; be sure the temperature of the water is correct before returning to the bath. Also, labor progress may slow if the water is too hot. And, if the laboring person feels uncomfortably hot, they may lose energy (and so will you if you are in the bath together!).

Is a Bath Safe if the Membranes Have Ruptured?

Numerous research studies indicate that a bath in clean water does not increase the risk of infection if the person has ruptured membranes.

Can Staff Monitor the Baby While the Person Labors in the Water?

Yes. Most midwives who attend water births outside of hospitals have waterproof, handheld ultrasound stethoscopes (Dopplers), and some hospitals also have these. A portable telemetry fetal-monitoring unit can be used as well.

There are two types of telemetry monitors: In one, a radio transmitter is wired to sensors on the laboring person's abdomen. As long as the radio is kept out of the water, it works well. In the other, which is wireless, each sensor contains its own waterproof transmitter. In both, the transmitters send information on the baby's heartbeat and the laboring person's contractions to the nursing station or to the monitor in the labor room.

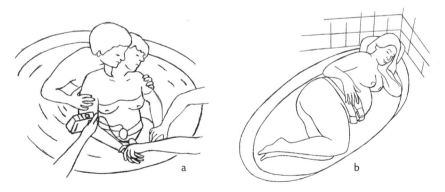

Laboring in a large bath with a partner (a) and using wireless telemetry fetal monitoring (b)

What about Modesty?

If the laboring person does not want to be naked in the water, consider an opaque sports bra or camisole and, until the birth becomes imminent, loose-fitting shorts. Or, they can use a towel to cover exposed body parts. It is unlikely they will be able to cover up completely all the time, unless they are in a conventional-size bathtub, where a towel will probably be adequate.

What if the Baby Is Born in the Water?

This is possible in a rapid labor, which is not always easy to control. If the hospital has a strong policy against birth in the water, the laboring person will need to be watched closely and will be asked to leave the bath when pushing begins. If born in the water, the baby is brought immediately to the surface and held with its head completely out of the water. The head is dried with a towel. The birthing person will be helped out of the water before the expulsion of the placenta.

Water births are everyday occurrences and are considered a safe option for healthy pregnant people in hospitals in many countries, especially Europe and Australia. Numerous studies have found water birth to be as safe as birth on land when the caregiver is confident and skilled, the person is healthy, and labor has proceeded without complications. In North America, water births take place in homes, birth centers, and only a handful of hospitals. They are attended mostly by midwives, although a few doctors also attend water births (see Recommended Resources, page 418, for more information).

The Birth Ball

Large inflated balls (also called exercise or yoga balls) made of tough polyvinyl are widely used by nonpregnant people to correct balance problems, ease back ailments, build strength and flexibility, and aid relaxation. In childbirth, we call them birth balls, and they are used by laboring people for comfort and labor progress in the following ways.

- Sitting on it and swaying during contractions, as this helps relax the trunk and pelvic floor

- Kneeling on the floor (with padding under the knees) or on a bed and leaning forward with the head, shoulders, arms, and upper chest

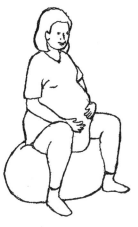
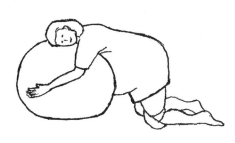

Sitting on a birth ball

Kneeling while leaning on a birth ball

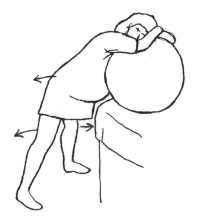

Standing, swaying with the ball

resting on the ball. This provides the same benefits as the hands-and-knees position (relief of back pain, rotation of an OP baby, and possible improvement of a baby's heart rate), but is more restful. They can also sway effortlessly.

• Standing next to a hospital birthing bed, which may be raised or lowered to a comfortable height, or a counter, the ball is placed on the bed. The laboring person may rest their head and upper body on the ball, swaying rhythmically and effortlessly, side to side, during contractions. This gives many of the same advantages as kneeling while leaning on the ball and also uses gravity to help the baby descend.

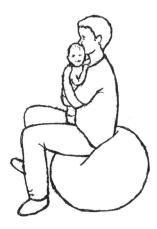

Using the ball to help soothe a crying baby

• Lastly, after the baby is born, the birth ball is a great help at home. You can almost always quickly soothe a fussy baby by sitting on the ball with the baby against your shoulder and bouncing, gently or vigorously—whatever works. This is a wonderful way to create a soothing up-and-down motion for the baby without wearing yourself out. Of course, a baby crying from hunger needs to be fed, not bounced.

Birth balls come in a variety of sizes and shapes. A person of average height (5 feet 3 inches [1.6 meters] to 5 feet 10 inches [1.8 meters]) seems to benefit most from a ball with a diameter of 65 centimeters (25½ inches) when inflated. Shorter people do well with the 55- or 65-centimeter (21½ to 25½ inches) balls, and taller people do well with the 75-centimeter (29½ inches) balls.

When seated on the ball, the pregnant person's thighs should be parallel or slightly higher than their knees. The thickness and elasticity of the vinyl vary from one brand to another and may affect whether a particular ball will actually inflate to its stated diameter. The degree of inflation can be varied to adjust the size and firmness of the ball. Some families need two sizes if the parents' heights are different.

Similar inflated devices come in other shapes, such as a peanut shape. The round balls are best for labor because they allow movement in all directions. It's a good idea to practice sitting and swaying on the ball before labor begins, so you both feel secure using the ball in labor. Partners find the ball can be a comfortable seat when the laboring person is not using it. The peanut ball is helpful as a positioning aid (see following).

Even if your hospital has birth balls, you may want to buy your own to use to soothe your baby in the months after birth. The balls are available from many sporting goods stores, department stores, or online retailers. Make sure that any ball you buy is intended to hold 500 pounds (227 kg) or more; the box usually has the weight limit printed on it. Less expensive balls may not be sturdy enough to hold an adult.

Your ball may come with a pump. If not, you can inflate it with a party balloon pump, an air mattress pump, or a service station pump. The balls bounce best when fully inflated.

Safety Precautions Using a Birth Ball

- If using the ball on a hospital room floor, place a clean blanket or sheet on the floor beneath the ball to keep it clean.

- Place a sheet, towel, or waterproof pad over the ball before the laboring person uses it in labor.

- When the laboring person lowers onto the ball, always have them hold on to something or someone stable with one hand while holding the ball still with the other hand.

- When the laboring person sits on the ball, their feet should remain planted on the floor, in front of the ball and about 2 feet (61 centimeters) apart. They should not straddle the ball.

- Stand close by, holding their hand, until it is clear they are completely safe and comfortable on the ball. This may take 1 to 2 minutes with some people; longer with others.

- When they are done and want to get off the ball, assist them.

- The ball should be cleaned between uses if different people will use it. (Hospitals use the same cleaning compound used to clean a hospital bed.)

- Keep the ball away from sharp objects and heat sources.

The Peanut Ball

Many hospitals now have peanut-shaped balls of various sizes. These are used as positioning aids. They are especially useful as pictured, to support the laboring person's upper leg when side lying or semiprone. It is

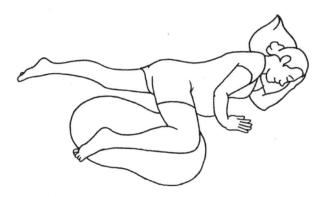

The peanut ball as an aid to positioning with an epidural, and an aid for pushing.

particularly helpful when one has an epidural, to support a position that may enhance labor progress, and also during pushing with or without an epidural, when the upper leg needs support. Otherwise, the partner is often the one to provide that support, which is hard work!

Heat and Cold

Heat and cold can be used at any time during labor and afterward to relieve a number of discomforts. For example:

- Place a hot water bottle, a hot damp towel, a warm rice-filled sock, or an electric heating pad on the laboring person's low abdomen, back, or groin to ease pain during the dilation (first) stage. (Check with the hospital before using an electric heating pad; some hospitals do not allow this.)

- Use a warm blanket to relieve trembling during the transition phase.

- Use warm compresses on the birthing person's perineum during the birthing stage to relieve pain and help them relax the birth canal. The nurse usually does this so they can keep track of the baby's progress down the birth canal. You might ask for the warm compress, as it can be very comforting.

- Use a cool damp washcloth to wipe the laboring person's neck, brow, and face between contractions.

- Use a cold wrap (see Recommended Resources, page 418), an ice bag, a rubber glove filled with crushed ice, frozen wet washcloths, or even a bag of frozen vegetables to relieve low back pain. Or, use a can of cold juice or a frozen, round plastic bottle of water to roll over their low back.

• Put frozen wet washcloths into a plastic bag and lay the bag over the anus to relieve pain from hemorrhoids or stitches after the birth.

> **CAUTION:** Be careful not to make the packs so hot or so cold that you cause burns or frost damage to the laboring person's skin. The rule is this: If you can't hold it in your own hands, don't put it on them. Let the hot pack cool, if necessary, and always put one or more layers of cloth between the skin and the hot or cold pack to protect their skin.

Other items that are useful for labor include an electric fan, rice-filled sock (to microwave for heat or freeze for cold), handheld fan, hot water bottle, cold wrap to strap on lower back, fleece blanket, massage roller, and foam kneeling pad.

Transcutaneous Electrical Nerve Stimulation (TENS)

TENS has been used successfully for years to treat postoperative and chronic pain. It is used in many countries for back pain during labor, especially early labor. Because TENS is unknown to many obstetric care-givers in the United States, you may have to suggest it yourself if you are interested in it. If needed, the laboring person's caregiver can obtain more information about TENS from a physical therapist. Many doulas are also trained in the use of TENS in labor. A doula may be able to lend you a unit and show you how to use it.

Look for a TENS unit designed specifically for use in labor. These are controlled with a single thumb switch, which the laboring person can use to control the intensity. At the moment, maternity TENS units are hard to find in the United States, but they are more readily available in Canada and can be rented or purchased from British companies through the internet (see Recommended Resources, page 418). They come with clear, simple instructions.

A TENS unit consists of four flexible 1 by 4 inch (2.5 by 10 cm) stimulating pads (electrodes) connected by wires to a small, handheld, battery-operated device that generates electrical impulses. The pads adhere to the skin alongside the lower spine. The stimulation level can

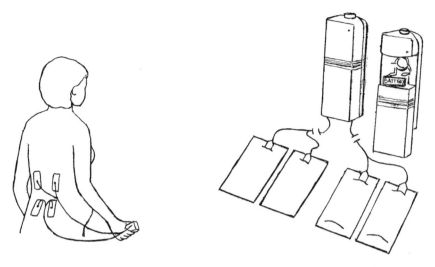

A maternity transcutaneous electrical nerve stimulation (TENS) unit in use (left) and a detailed look at the device (right)

be adjusted up or down, according to the laboring person's comfort level. When a contraction begins, the laboring person presses the thumb switch and they will feel a continuous vibration, or a tingling or prickling sensation, which will diminish their awareness of the pain. When the contraction ends, they press the button to change the stimulation to an intermittent pattern.

Many people who have used TENS during labor swear it enabled them to avoid using pain-relieving medication; others report TENS was helpful in diminishing pain, especially back pain; and still others say it did little good. It's important to start TENS use early; it is unlikely to help at all if begun in active labor. Starting it in pre- or early labor when the laboring person is having back pain may make a great difference in the ability to tolerate back pain.

It works like this: The TENS is thought to stimulate the release of endorphins (pain-relieving neurotransmitters) in the area being stimulated. If started early, the endorphin levels can build to a point where they reduce the pain. Getting started early helps ensure that, by the time the pain is significant, there will be endorphin protection.

As for safety, no adverse effects have been reported. The pads are removed if the laboring person wants to get into a shower or bath (they are reusable and can be reapplied later).

Comforting Techniques

In this section, we look at some simple techniques you can use to soothe and comfort the pregnant/laboring person, such as touch and massage, music, and pleasing scents. Practice them with the person and get their feedback to adapt them as needed.

Touch and Simple Massage

Touch conveys a kind, caring, comforting message to the laboring person. Find out what kind of touch the person finds soothing and use it during labor.

They may appreciate gentle, comforting, or reassuring touch—rubbing a painful spot, patting their back or shoulder, embracing them, holding their hand, scratching their back, or stroking their hair or cheek. With your fingertips or with your full hand, you might lightly stroke the skin on their abdomen during contractions, or the thighs, or wherever they want. Some people prefer a rhythmic rubbing or kneading of the back, legs, buttocks, shoulders, hands, or feet.

Before beginning, pour a small amount of light massage oil into one palm and rub your hands together briskly to warm them and the oil. Some people like being rubbed or stroked during early labor but stop liking it during transition. If this happens, switch to holding the laboring person's head, shoulders, hand, foot, or thigh firmly, without rubbing. A massage device—handheld or battery-operated—may also be soothing and may be handy if you are not very good at massage.

How to Give Great Mini-Massages

During labor, brief, 1- to 3-minute, massages of the shoulders, back, hands, or feet may relax and soothe the laboring person. Practice these ahead of time to learn what they like. Perhaps they will even reciprocate! Follow these general guidelines:

- Explain which massage you want to do and ask permission ("I'd like to massage your back. Is this okay with you?").

- Make sure your hands are clean and warm and that the pregnant person is comfortable.

- Use massage oil—scented, if they like, although you'll want to have some unscented oil on hand for labor, in case anyone in the room is sensitive to scents. (Ask before using it.) Place a little oil on your hands and rub them together briskly to cover them with the oil and warm it.

- Once you begin the massage, try not to remove both hands at the same time. It is unsettling to relax into a massage only to have the massager's hands vanish without warning and to reappear somewhere else.

- As you work, encourage the pregnant person to tell you where they want more or less rubbing or a lighter or firmer touch.

- When you're finished, wipe any excess oil from their skin and your hands.

Following are some of my favorite mini-massages.

Three-part shoulder mini-massage: Use this massage during or between contractions, at any phase of labor, to help the laboring person feel nurtured and to relax their shoulders (shoulders are one of the most common tension spots in people). Have the laboring person sit up or lean forward and rest their head on their arms or a pillow. Stand behind them.

1. Place your hands comfortably on their shoulders near the neck. Stroke firmly from the neck to the shoulders and over the shoulders to their upper arms. Knead their upper arms a few times and stroke firmly back toward the neck. Do this three or four times.

2. With your hands on their shoulders, squeeze and release the shoulder muscles as firmly as they like for 1 to 2 minutes.

Crisscross massage over the small of the back and/or hips: Use this massage at any phase of labor, during or between contractions, to ease back pain or help relax the lower back.

Have the laboring person kneel and lean over the birth ball or a chair seat. It will be easiest for you if they use a ball on the bed, but you can also do this with them kneeling on the floor. They may want to wear kneepads or kneel on a foam pad such as those sold for gardeners.

1. Facing the pregnant person's side, place your left hand on the narrowest part of their waist on the side farthest from you, with your fingers pointing down. Make sure your hands are not pressing on their ribs as that is uncomfortable. Place your right hand on their waist on the near side, fingers pointing up. Press their sides firmly; they should like the feeling. Keep your hands below their ribs and be sure you don't dig your fingertips into the soft flesh of their sides (it hurts!). If you have large hands, you may need to tilt them so they cover less surface area while staying within the small of their waist.

2. Using both hands, stroke firmly up, over, and across the back. (Cross one hand over the other to the original starting spots at their waist.)

3. Maintaining the same pressure, press the sides in again and repeat the crossover movement over and over as long as they want.

4. You may also move the crisscross strokes down over the hips and back up to the waist. Ask for feedback and adjust the placement and firmness as they wish.

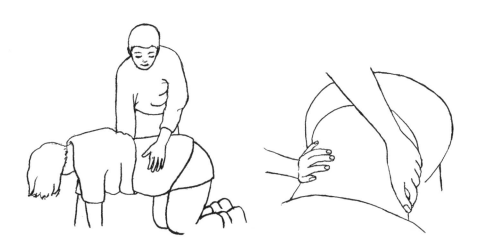

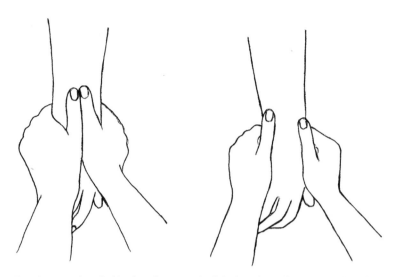

Thumbs together (left); thumbs apart (right) "breaking the ice pop" hand massage

"Breaking the ice pop" hand massage: If the laboring person has been clenching their fists or gripping your hand, the bedrail, or something else during contractions or if they seem generally tense, they are creating pressure on the palms of the hands where there are specialized nerve endings that are actually soothed by this pressure. Unfortunately, the gripping causes so much tension it loses much of its benefit. This quick massage technique will relax the hand and entire arm while providing the same pain-relieving pressure on the palm they were getting from gripping things. You can do this massage during or between contractions. Massage one hand, then the other, or have someone else do one hand while you do the other.

1. Stand or sit facing the pregnant person. Ask them to relax their arm. Take their hand, palm down, in both of yours. Grasp the hand so your thumbs touch, from their tips to their fleshy bases, on the back of the wrist and the pads of your fingers (not your nails) press into the palm. Your thumb joints should be placed at their wrist joint (see illustration).

2. Without moving your hands, increase the pressure on the palm gradually. Ask for feedback so you know when you are squeezing "hard enough" for it to feel good. You may be surprised at how much pressure they like. When they say it is enough, maintain that pressure while slowly moving your thumbs and hands

entirely off the back of their hand (see illustrations). You'll notice the skin on their hand blanches with your pressure. You are combining pressure on the palm with friction over the back of the hand. Adjust it so it feels good to them.

3. Repeat these strokes ten times or so. Does this massage remind you of how you broke apart twin ice pops when you were a child?

CAUTION: If the laboring person's hands are very swollen or if they have carpal tunnel syndrome (tingling or numbness in the hands that worsens with pressure), they will want very little pressure or not want this massage at all.

Three-part foot massage (breaking the ice pop with extras): If the laboring person complains of aching or tired feet during labor, this massage restores circulation and relieves tired aching feet caused by prolonged standing and walking.

1. Breaking the ice pop: Facing the pregnant person as they sit or lie down, ask them to relax their legs; take one foot in both your hands. Grasp it so your thumbs are together on the top of the

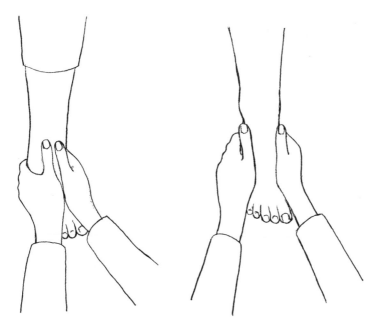

Part 1: Breaking the ice pop foot massage

foot. Press the pads of your fingers (not your nails) into the sole of the foot. Squeeze until the laboring person says it is enough. You may be surprised at how much pressure they like. Maintaining that pressure, move your thumbs and hands apart so your hands are entirely off the top of the foot. You are combining pressure on the sole of the foot with friction over the top of the foot. Do this ten times or so.

2. Squeezing the heel: Cup the heel of the person's right foot in your right hand and press the "heel" of your hand firmly into the arch. Squeeze the person's heel firmly with the pads of your fingertips several times, as if you were squeezing a tennis ball, and release it. Avoid digging in with your nails. This should feel wonderful. Repeat, using your left hand to cup the person's left heel.

3. Three-finger circle massage: If you're massaging the left foot, hold it in your left hand; if you're working on the right foot, hold it in your right hand. With the pads of the three middle fingers of the opposite hand, give a deep circle massage in the "magic spot" on the top of the foot just below the ankle bone. The spot is slightly off the center of the foot, toward the outside. They'll tell you where it feels best. Do not move your fingers on the skin; rather, move the skin over the underlying muscles and bones. Do this for 30 to 60 seconds.

Once you have completed all three steps on one foot, repeat with the other foot. Then, they will be ready to walk some more!

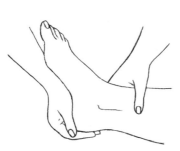

Part 2: Squeezing the heel: Press the "heel" of your hand into the arch of the person's foot; squeeze and release their heel.

Part 3: Three-finger circle massage with fingertips

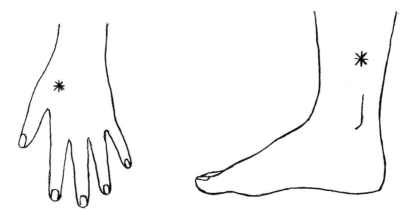

The Hoku point (left) and Spleen 6, four finger-widths above the inner ankle bone (right)

Acupressure: Acupressure or Shiatsu, has been practiced in Asia for many centuries. This healing art is derived from the ancient Chinese understanding of the principles of yin and yang. The body is made up of twelve meridians, along which vital forces flow; acupressure corrects imbalances in the flow of these vital forces that impair health and well-being. Acupressure uses the same points for stimulation as does acupuncture, but involves finger pressure instead of needles. The use of acupressure and acupuncture has grown rapidly in the West, and scientific studies of their use in labor have found beneficial effects on childbirth pain. Many people successfully combine acupressure with other methods to enhance comfort and progress in labor.

By pressing with your finger or thumb at certain acupressure points, you may be able to relieve the laboring person's pain and speed up labor. You may want to try this if they are facing induction or if the labor slows (see page 221). The two most popular points for labor are the Hoku point and Spleen 6. Both are sensitive spots that may hurt a bit when pressed. Your goal, however, is not to cause pain, so do not press hard enough to hurt.

The Hoku point is on the back of the hand, where the bones forming the bases of the thumb and index finger come together. Press steadily into the bone at the base of the index finger with your thumb for 10 to 60 seconds, three to six times, with a rest of equal length in between. You can repeat this as often as you and the birthing person want.

Spleen 6 is on the inner side of the lower leg about four finger-widths above the ankle. From slightly behind it, press your thumb into the bone

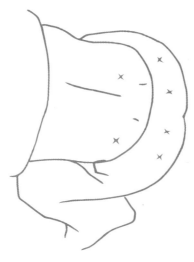

Each x marks hand placements for counterpressure

for 10 to 60 seconds at a time, three to six times, with a rest of equal length in between. You can repeat this in labor whenever you and the laboring person want. A good way to identify the best spot for the pressure is to press in several spots close together; one spot may be more sensitive than the others. That's the place to apply the pressure. Acupuncture, which uses needles to stimulate these and many other points for a variety of purposes, is described on page 214.

CAUTION: Experts advise against pressing these points on a pregnant person before the due date, as they can cause contractions and increase the risk of premature labor. Find the points on yourself, but don't use them on the pregnant person until the need arises.

Counterpressure for back pain: Try this during contractions if the laboring person has back pain. While the person in labor stands or kneels and leans forward over a bed or birth ball, hold the front of their hip with one hand to help maintain balance, and, with your fist or the heel of your other hand, press steadily and firmly in the low back or buttocks area. The "right" spot is usually off center, but it varies from person to person and at different times during the same labor. Press in several places, and they will tell you which feels best. Keep the pressure steady throughout the contraction; don't "pulse" or rub. If you release it too soon, the pain will worsen immediately. You will probably have to press hard during every contraction. Between contractions, you might massage the area or use cold or warm compresses (see page 184).

The double hip squeeze: This also helps ease back pain. In fact, this technique and counterpressure can often make the difference between tolerable and intolerable back pain.

The laboring person stands or kneels and leans forward onto a bed, birth ball, or chair seat or gets on their hands and knees. The hips should be flexed. From behind, use your fingers to locate the pelvic bones at the sides of their hips, just below the waist. From there, move your hands down the hips to the roundest part of their buttocks. Press on both sides of the buttocks with your whole, flat hands (not with just your fingertips; that will hurt). Push toward the center, pressing their hips together. Experiment to find the right places to press. When you have found the right places, press them steadily throughout each contraction. Apply as much pressure as needed.

The double hip squeeze is difficult and tiring work for one person. It is much easier with a helper. The illustration shows how two people can use this technique.

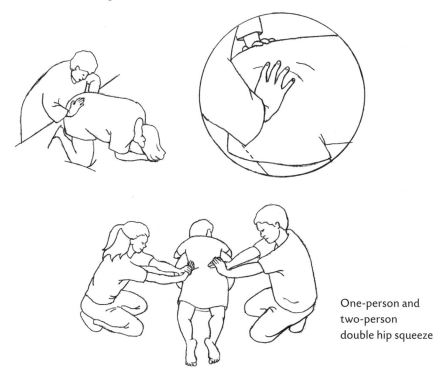

One-person and two-person double hip squeeze

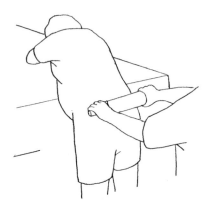

Rolling pressure over the low back: This is another helpful technique for backache. Use a rolling massager, similar to the one illustrated on page 185, a rolling pin, or a cold can of juice or soft drink (keep a six-pack in a bowl of ice so you'll always have a cold can). Rolling pins and cans of juice are usually not available in hospitals (though soft drinks are), so you may want to bring such an object with you, especially if the laboring person has a backache with contractions before you leave home. During or between contractions, roll the object, with some pressure, over the low back.

Besides the bath, shower, acupressure, massage, heat, and cold, many of the positions shown in the chart on pages 169–176 and marked with an asterisk are especially helpful for back pain, as are the techniques described under "Slow Progress in Active Labor and the Birthing Stage" in chapter 5.

Music and Sound

Many people can relax and focus better if their favorite music, relaxation narration, or environmental sounds (ocean waves, a babbling brook, a rain shower) are played during labor. Familiar and well-loved music has been found to raise levels of endorphins (the body's own pain-relieving substances). Soothing sounds may cover up some of the beeps, voices, and other sounds that are part of any modern birthing room.

You might suggest that the pregnant person select some favorite music to play during labor. Make a playlist and bring your own player. Some laboring people appreciate having two labor playlists; one with calming, soothing music and a second with music that makes them want to get up and move.

Aromatherapy or Pleasing Scents

Pleasant aromas create feelings of well-being and relaxation and cover up hospital smells. Scents such as lavender, sandalwood, citrus, and peppermint may appeal to the birthing person. You can purchase scented massage oil, sachets, bath beads, liquid soap, or cologne, or you can simply cut a lemon in half for them to sniff.

Because scent preferences are personal, ask the pregnant person whether they want them available and, if so, which ones they prefer. They may want none or pick a couple favorites to have available during labor.

Unless a trained aromatherapist prepares special mixes of essential oils for specific purposes, stick with store-bought lotions and oil mixes. Essential oils are very strong and, if too concentrated or used incorrectly, can cause burns, allergic reactions, and other side effects. Doulas are not aromatherapists and do not prepare essential oils for clients.

Check with the hospital or birth-center staff before using scented products, as some staff may have negative reactions to some essential oils. See Recommended Resources, page 418, for books on aromatherapy.

Taking Care of Yourself

Labor can be long, tiring, stressful, and demanding for the laboring person as well as the birth partner. Losing a night's sleep is never easy. Standing for long periods, skipping meals, and offering the laboring person continual encouragement are tiring, especially if you are worried or overextended. To be an effective birth partner, you will need to pace yourself, draw on the experience and wisdom of others, and look after your own basic needs. This cannot mean taking long breaks for naps or meals because the laboring person may need you and want you to stay. They will probably depend heavily on you for help through every contraction, especially if you are the only support person. There are ways you can take care of both yourself and the person in labor at the same time. Here are some suggestions to help you conserve energy and get appropriate help from others:

• Have your supplies handy. Review the list of suggested items for the birth partner's use during labor (see page 33).

• Eat and drink tasty, nourishing food and beverages regularly during labor. Choose foods without strong odors (think about how they will affect your breath) and keep them with you so you do not have to leave the room to get them.

Checklist of Comfort Measures for Labor

Check the following list of comfort measures at any time during labor when you believe a change from what you are doing may be helpful.

Relaxation/Tension Release

☐ During or between contractions
☐ Aromatherapy (lotions, oils, fruits)

Rhythmic Breathing

☐ Slow
☐ Light
☐ Horse-lips

Rhythmic Activities/Rituals

☐ Movements/vocalizing
☐ Stroking/tapping
☐ Being stroked
☐ Rhythm talk to partner

Attention Focusing

☐ Visual focus, focus on music, voice or touch
☐ Mental activity
☐ Visualization
☐ Count Breaths
☐ Chant, mantra, song, prayer

Hydrotherapy

☐ Shower
☐ Bath

Bearing Down

☐ Avoiding bearing down
☐ Spontaneous bearing down
☐ Self-directed pushing
☐ Directed pushing

Measures for Backache

☐ Counterpressure
☐ Crisscross
☐ Double hip squeeze (by 1 or 2 people)
☐ Rolling pressure
☐ TENS
☐ Cold pack
☐ Warm pack
☐ Shower
☐ Large bathtub (with room to kneel and lean over the side)
☐ Open knee-chest position
☐ Abdominal lifting
☐ Hands-and-knees
☐ Kneeling, leaning forward on ball or chair
☐ The lunge (standing or kneeling)
☐ Walking, slow dancing

Massage/Touch

- ☐ Still touch, stroking, hand holding
- ☐ Shoulders
- ☐ Crisscross
- ☐ Hand
- ☐ Foot
- ☐ Acupressure
- ☐ Rolling pressure

Warm Packs

- ☐ To lower abdomen or groin
- ☐ To perineum duirng second stage
- ☐ To low back

Cold Packs

- ☐ To low back
- ☐ To perineum after birth

Positions and Movements

- ☐ Standing, leaning forward
- ☐ Walking, slow dancing
- ☐ Hands and knees
- ☐ Kneeling, leaning forward on ball or chair
- ☐ Side lying/semiprone
- ☐ Semisitting

Positions for Pushing

- ☐ Flat on back (tilted slightly to side)
- ☐ On back, knees drawn up to shoulders
- ☐ Squatting
- ☐ Supported squat/dangle
- ☐ Lap squatting
- ☐ Hands and knees
- ☐ Semisitting
- ☐ Side lying, top leg supported

Help from Birth Partner/Doula

- ☐ Suggestions, reminders
- ☐ Encouragement, reassurance
- ☐ Compliments
- ☐ Patience, confidence in birthing person
- ☐ Immediiate response to contractions
- ☐ Undivided attention
- ☐ Aid with positions, relaxation, rhythm, rituals
- ☐ "Take-Charge" Routine
- ☐ Hugs, kisses, caresses
- ☐ Rhythm talk

- Wear comfortable clothes and have a change of clothes, a sweater, and slippers available.

- Rest by making yourself comfortable near the laboring person. Don't stand when you can sit. If the laboring person is lying down and you also need rest, lie down next to them if the bed is wide enough or sit and rest your head on the bed beside them. If there is enough time between contractions, doze. You will not have trouble waking up to help if you keep a hand on their arm or belly.

- Ask for reassurance and guidance. If you are worried about the length of labor or about the laboring person's pain, discouragement, or fatigue, ask the caregiver or nurse whether everything is all right; express your concerns. It is best, however, to do this away from the laboring person's hearing.

- Ask the nurse or caregiver for ideas for comfort measures. If you are uncertain whether you are helping the laboring person enough, ask for suggestions.

- Make arrangements to have a doula or friend or relative help you during labor.

A person in labor often needs the help of two people, one in front helping maintain rhythm and the other behind them, pressing on their back; or one running an errand or resting while the other remains.

A doula, with a broad perspective on childbirth and her experience, can apply or suggest appropriate comfort measures, help you remember some of the things you learned in childbirth class, and remind you and the laboring person of the birth plan. Also, if you have a helper, either of you can take a break during a long labor without leaving the person in labor alone.

For all these reasons, you might welcome an experienced, calm, confident support person who can remain with you through the birth.

CHAPTER 5

STRATEGIES FOR CHALLENGING VARIATIONS IN NORMAL LABOR

After 14 hours of labor, Terry started to push, but her cervix swelled because of the baby's position. She needed to stop pushing until the swelling went down, but she didn't think she could stop—her urge to push was so strong. So, she opted for an epidural that she hadn't wanted. It took away the pushing feeling, and 3 hours later it was okay to begin pushing. She watched in the mirror as she pushed. When she saw her baby's head, she said, "This is surreal!" A few more contractions and he was born and placed straight on Terry's chest. J.C. said, "Oh, oh, I can't stop crying!" to which Terry replied, "This is the only time I've ever seen you cry!"

—HEATHER, THEIR DOULA

L abor, even when perfectly normal, rarely follows a predictable textbook pattern. Variations within a range of normal are to be expected. The emotional reactions of people in labor vary, depending on the type of labor pattern they have. For example, if prelabor or early labor drags on for a long time, both you and the laboring person may be challenged by exhaustion, worry, or a loss of confidence. If, instead, labor starts suddenly with long, painful contractions that threaten to overwhelm the laboring person, their pain and panic are the birth partner's main concerns. Laboring people and their birth partners cope best with labor when they are open and flexible and when they are confident they can and will (with the help of caregivers and a support team) handle whatever comes their way.

This chapter will help you deal with situations more stressful than those encountered in the average labor, but still falling within the range of "normal." These situations require more intense and active support from you. Both you and the laboring person will need more resourcefulness, effort, decision-making, patience, and reliance on the doula's or caregiver's encouragement and advice. The special situations covered here are:

- The Take-Charge routine (for labor's toughest moments)
- On-the-spot coaching (when you have had no childbirth classes)
- Very rapid labor
- Emergency delivery
- When labor must start (labor-stimulating measures)
- Slow-to-start labor
- Slow progress in active labor and the birthing stage, with or without back pain
- When the laboring person must labor in bed
- Breech baby
- Previous disappointing or traumatic birth experience
- Incompatibility with the nurse or caregiver

Not covered in this chapter are complications in labor—situations outside the limits of normal. To learn how a caregiver detects complications and treats them with medical or surgical interventions and how you can be most helpful to the person in labor, read chapters 6, 7, 8, and 9.

The Take-Charge Routine

When labor becomes very intense, the person in labor may feel panicked or frightened and may struggle to maintain rhythm or lose it entirely. If this happens, they need calm, confident, and kind, but firm, guidance to regain and maintain a rhythm. Reserve this routine for when the laboring person:

- Is unable to maintain a rhythmic ritual in breathing, moaning, or movements

- Despairs, weeps, cries out, or says they cannot go on

- Is very tense and cannot relax

- Is in a great deal of pain

The Take-Charge routine is exactly what it sounds like. You move in close and do all you can to help the person in labor until they regain their inner strength. Usually, their despair is brief; with your help, they can pass through it and their spirits will rise. If before labor they planned to request pain medication under these circumstances, use the Take-Charge routine to help until the medication can be given. Use whatever parts of this routine seem appropriate:

- **Keep your touch firm and confident, not anxious and tense.** Your voice should remain calm and encouraging. Your facial expression should reflect confidence and optimism.

- **Stay close.** Face the person in labor or stay right by their side, your face near theirs.

- **Anchor them.** Hold their shoulders or hands—gently, confidently, firmly. Do not shake them to get their attention.

- **Get the laboring person to look at you.** If their eyes are clenched shut, you will not be able to help. Tell them to open their eyes and look at your face or your hand. This is important. Say it loudly enough so they hear you—but calmly and kindly.

- **Talk to them between contractions.** Make suggestions; for example, "With the next one, let me help you more. I want you to look at me the moment it starts. I will pace you with my hand so it won't get ahead of us. Okay? Good. You're doing so well. We're really moving now."

- **Help them regain the rhythm they had by moving your hand or head up and down in that rhythm.** You can combine this with "rhythm talk" (see next item). Pause briefly after each downbeat to keep from going too fast.

One doula said, "I wear a ring with a blue stone on my right hand. I ask the laboring person to "follow my ring" as I "conduct" them in a breathing rhythm. I love to think of the many, many women who have let my ring guide them through some tough moments. It's one reason I never take the ring off."

- **Use "rhythm talk, vocally pacing the rhythm of their breathing or moaning.** Say, "Breathe with me … BREATHE WITH ME … That's the way … just like that … Good … Keep your rhythm … STAY WITH IT … just like that … LOOK AT ME … Keep your rhythm … Good for you … It's going away … Good … Good … Now just rest, that was so good."

  You can whisper these words or say them in a calm, rhythmic, confident, and encouraging tone. If the laboring person is vocalizing, you may have to raise your voice to get their attention, but do not shout. Also, you don't actually need to breathe with the person as you say the words; you shouldn't even try if your breath is stale or the breathing makes you lightheaded. They can breathe to the rhythm of your words as well as your hand or head movements.

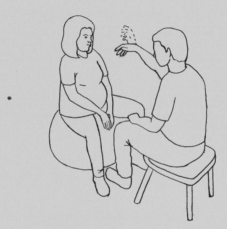

- **Repeat yourself.** The laboring person may not be able to continue doing what you say for more than a few seconds, but that's fine. Do not conclude that what you are doing is not helping. Say the same things repeatedly and help them continue.

  What if the laboring person says they can't or won't go on? Here are some guidelines:

- Between contractions, tell them you want them to **change the ritual used during contractions** because it is no longer working. Suggest a different position or breathing rhythm.

- **Don't give up on them.** This is a difficult time. You cannot help if you decide they cannot handle it. Acknowledge to both the laboring person and to yourself that it is difficult, but remind yourselves it is not impossible.

- **Ask for help and reassurance.** It can be very hard on you to see the person you love in pain. The nurse or caregiver can check the laboring person's dilation and give you advice. Perhaps the person in labor is in distress because labor is progressing very rapidly; just knowing this may help. A doula or other support person can help you, model the technique for you, suggest something new, and reassure both of you that the laboring person is okay and reacting normally. If you're having trouble with the Take-Charge routine, the doula might "take charge" while you hold the laboring person or press on their back.

- **Remember the baby.** It may seem surprising, but laboring people can get so caught up in labor they do not think much about the baby. It may help to remember why they are going through this and to recognize that the baby is working with them.

What about **pain medications**? Should you suggest them or not? This depends on:

- The laboring person's prior wishes: Did they want a nonmedicated birth? How strongly did they feel about it? (See "Pain Medications Preference Scale," pages 328–329.) Sometimes, people who ask for pain medications are really saying, "I need more help coping."

- Their rate of progress and how far they still have to go. A couple centimeters (1 inch) of dilation should be very encouraging. A complete lack of progress is very discouraging.

- How well they respond to the Take-Charge routine or the doula's help. If the person in labor cannot get back into a rhythm, even with a lot of help, and they are making little progress, they may need pain medications.

- Whether they are willing to try something else, such as a bath, a change of position, a progress check, or just coping with three more contractions to see whether things get easier

- Whether they truly want the medications or are just agreeing to the nurse's or caregiver's suggestion

- Whether they ask for medications *between* contractions. Many people ask for medications *during* a contraction, but do not mention them when the contraction ends.

- Whether they use the code word (see page 330)

Numerous people have said to their partners, "I never could have done it without you. If it hadn't been for you, I would have given up." By using the Take-Charge routine, you can indeed get the laboring person through those desperate moments when they feel they cannot go on; you can truly ease their burden by helping them with every breath. And if you both agree in advance on a code word they can use if they decide they want medications, you will know you're not forcing them to suffer.

On-the-Spot Coaching (When You Have Had No Childbirth Classes)

If the due date nears and you have not taken childbirth classes or if you took only a very short "crash" course, consider hiring a doula to help you support the birthing person and guide the two of you through labor. But what if you have no doula and labor starts early? What if you and the pregnant person have had no time to work together to learn the pain-relief techniques described in chapter 4? Here are some suggestions:

1 Don't attempt to learn everything at once during labor.

2. Use some simple breathing rhythms and a few on-the-spot comfort measures.

3. Tell the staff neither of you has had and childbirth classes.

Rhythmic Breathing

Rhythm is *everything* in labor. Once the contractions become uncomfortable, the laboring person can use rhythmic breathing or moaning through each one. They may find their own rhythm, or you can show them how to breathe in a particular rhythm. Then, breathe with them (make sure you do not have bad breath!), verbally pace them through each breath, or conduct their breathing with rhythmic hand signals. Between contractions in early labor, work together to learn *slow breathing*, which you will use first, and *light breathing*, to use later, if needed. Both breathing rhythms, described on pages 162 and 163 are simple and quick to learn.

With each exhale, encourage the laboring person to release tension. As they breathe out, you might say, "Let go right here," and touch their shoulder, brow, or any part of their body that is tense. With another contraction, help them let go in another place. (Don't just tell them, "Relax, and it won't hurt so much!" They'll know you don't understand. Be more specific, and they will be more likely to relax one area at a time.)

On-the-Spot Comfort Measures

Here are other on-the-spot comfort measures to try:

• Movement and position changes (see page 168)

• Counterpressure (see pages 194–196)

• Relaxing bath or shower (see page 176)

• Heat or cold (see page 184)

• Touch or massage (see page 187)

• Relaxation (see page 153)

• Attention focusing (see page 158)

• The Take-Charge routine (see page 202)

Most of these techniques can be used quite successfully without much preparation. In fact, you can read about them between contractions and apply them immediately.

The Very Rapid Labor

For some people, labor starts with intense, frequent, painful contractions and is over in a matter of a few hours. It seems the laboring person barely has time to adjust to being in labor before the baby is born.

Sometimes, only the first (dilation) stage is rapid. The cervix dilates so quickly that the laboring person can't catch up mentally; but then, in the second (birthing) stage, the contractions space out. If this happens, the laboring person has to cope with the difficulties of both fast and slow labors.

It is impossible to predict which people will labor in these ways, but a rapid labor seems to be more likely if:

- The pregnant person has had a rapid or quicker-than-average (less than 10-hour) labor before. A second or third labor tends to be faster than the first.

- The cervix is very soft, thin, and already partially dilated before labor begins, and the baby is low in the pregnant person's pelvis in a very favorable position.

- The bag of waters ruptures with a gush rather than a slow leak, especially if accompanied by contractions.

Few people or their birth partners are prepared for a rapid labor, especially after reading and hearing about typical labor patterns and prolonged prelabors. The pregnant person will be caught off guard if expecting that early contractions will be gentle, short, and far apart, but instead has contractions that are long, painful, and close together—almost like the contractions of the transition phase.

How Is the Laboring Person Likely to React?

You can expect any of the following reactions from the laboring person if labor begins rapidly:

- **Shock and disbelief.** They may not be able to respond constructively or even realize this is real labor.

- **Fear or panic.** They may think something is terribly wrong—that they or the baby is in danger. They may be frightened if they cannot reach you, the caregiver, or anyone else for help and may worry about getting to the hospital in time. Make alternative plans for these possibilities. Make sure you are always reachable by phone, AND have a Plan B— a friend, neighbor, or family member who agrees to be reachable (and whom you keep informed of times when you may not be immediately available). The pregnant person can call a cab or a car service (be sure you have saved numbers and a way to pay). Plan C is to call 911 and say they are in hard labor and have no way to get to the hospital.

- **Loss of confidence.** If the laboring person thinks these are the "easy" contractions of early labor, they may lose all confidence in the ability to cope with labor once it progresses.

- **Dependence on you.** They may barely be able to change positions between contractions, let alone get ready to go to the hospital. They may need your constant help to cope with the contractions.

- **Annoyance with you or the caregivers** if neither of you grasps the situation. (People tell stories of their partners going back to sleep, assuming there is a long wait ahead, and of caregivers who tell them to go to sleep, which is impossible, or to wait an hour and then call again.)

How Should You React?

- Believe what you see. If the laboring person is shaky, in pain, and having strong, fast contractions, don't assume they are overreacting to early labor. Assume this is hard labor and move right into a leadership role to help them cope.

- Don't worry about helping them relax. These contractions will not allow that.

- Use the Take-Charge routine (see page 202) if they have trouble coping with the contractions.

- Don't lose faith in them or criticize them. Give them the benefit of the doubt. Their response is telling you this labor is really hard.

- Call the caregiver, go to the hospital or birth center, or both. Drive carefully, but don't waste time.

The Emergency Delivery

What if the baby is coming and you and the birthing person are on your own—in your car or at home? You will know it is too late to go to the hospital if:

1. The birthing person says they can feel the baby coming out

2. You can see the baby's head at the vaginal opening

3. They are pushing and grunting forcibly and cannot stop

If all of this happens at home, stay where you are and call 911 for an emergency vehicle with a paramedical team. You may also call the hospital; the hospital may send an emergency team, or a nurse may stay on the phone with you to tell you what to do.

If all this happens in the car, pull over to the side of the road, put on your flasher lights, and tend to the birthing person's needs. If the weather is cold, leave the motor running and the heater on.

Basic Rules for an Emergency Delivery

Before the birth:

• Believe the laboring person if they say the baby is coming.

• Remain calm (at least pretend!).

• Get help—from paramedics, friends, neighbors, even children.

• Turn up the heat in the car or at home.

• Gather blankets, towels, or warm clothing to wrap the baby in.

• Find newspapers, a bowl, paper towels, or a plastic bag to hold the placenta.

• Reassure the person giving birth.

• Help the birthing person avoid pushing. To slow the delivery, they should pant or blow lightly with the chin up when the body starts to push.

• Help the birthing person lie down on their side or recline in a semi-sitting position. This may slow the delivery slightly and ensures a safe landing place for the baby.

• Wash your hands thoroughly, if possible, unless the birthing person needs you to stay with them or if the baby is coming out.

• Get ready to catch the baby. Have something ready to dry and cover the baby immediately (towels, blanket, your shirt, a jacket).

• Keep your hands on the baby so the baby does not fall out. If the birthing person is standing or squatting or there is no soft place for the baby to land, position your body so the baby will land on you if you don't catch the baby.

As the baby comes out:

• Help the birthing person pant, not push.

• Wipe the baby's face and head when they emerge. If the membranes cover the baby's face, tear them with your fingernail or pull them away so the baby can breathe.

• Catch and gently place the baby on the birthing person's bare chest.

As soon as the baby is out:

• Watch the baby's chest and listen to the baby's breathing. Babies normally begin breathing or crying within seconds after birth.

• Dry the baby and wipe away any mucus, blood, or vernix from the nostrils or mouth.

• If the baby doesn't begin breathing right away, rub the baby's head, back, or chest briskly or slap the soles of the feet. They might sputter and choke out some mucus or fluid from the airway.

• Place the baby, naked, on its side or stomach on the birthing person's naked abdomen and cover them both to keep the baby dry and warm. Keep the baby's face exposed so you can monitor the baby's condition.

• In the unlikely event that the baby does not breathe within 2 minutes and you know how to do infant CPR, do it now. Otherwise, get to the hospital as quickly as possible. Don't worry about tying or cutting the cord and don't wait for the placenta.

• If the placenta comes immediately, try to catch it in a bowl or wrap it in something. Then, feel for the uterus by pressing below the navel. The uterus should be hard and firm, like a large grapefruit. If you cannot feel the uterus, it is too relaxed and may bleed too much. Rub the birthing person's lower belly very firmly in a small circle (you should feel the uterus tighten as you do so) and then have them do this until the paramedics arrive or you get to the hospital.

• If the placenta comes while you are driving and the hospital is still 20 minutes or more away, it might be wise to pull over and check the birthing person's uterus as just described.

• If the birthing person is bleeding, place the baby at the breast; the baby's sucking or even nuzzling at the breast will help contract the uterus and slow the bleeding. If the baby is not ready to suck, the birthing person should roll one nipple between their fingers while massaging the uterus.

When Labor Must Start (Labor-Stimulating Measures)

Under some circumstances, the caregiver recognizes that delaying or awaiting the baby's birth for much longer carries unacceptable risks for the pregnant person or baby. The caregiver will suggest labor induction—starting labor by giving drugs, breaking the bag of waters, or other means (see "Induction or Augmentation of Labor," page 256). Rarely, the caregiver may believe that a medical induction should be done immediately (see page 258), but more often, the need is not urgent and you and the pregnant person may have a few days to try self-induction methods. If successful, they can avoid medical induction, which carries some risks and challenges (see disadvantages of induction for medical reasons, page 259).

Many doctors offer induction routinely at 39, 40, or 41 weeks, for no medical reason. This is called elective induction; see pages 256–263 for a discussion of medical and nonmedical reasons for induction and use the Key Questions for Informed Decision-Making (see page 237) to recognize whether induction is medically indicated or not. It is usually safer, especially for the first-time birthing person, to wait for labor to begin spontaneously than to have an elective medical induction or to try self-induction.

Why try self-induction methods? Probably the most compelling reason is that medical induction is considered to be indicated if the pregnant person goes two weeks beyond the due date. If they wish to avoid a medical induction and is at 41½ weeks, they may want to try to get labor to begin. Another reason could be a steadily rising blood pressure or that the baby's growth has slowed, in which case the doctor may advise induction in a few days.

Self-induction may or may not succeed. If it does not succeed, the pregnant person will end up with a medical induction anyway. Some people feel it is worth trying to get into labor on their own; others do not. The methods are easy to use and carry little risk, which persuades some to try them (but see the following sections for precautions). Chances of success depend on the pregnant person's readiness for labor (the cervix must be ripe and have begun to thin) and the techniques chosen.

Self-Induction Methods

Before using these techniques to start labor, make sure the pregnant person discusses them with the caregiver. Consult the caregiver as to whether there is any reason they should not try to start contractions, using the methods described here. If there are none, it is safe for you both to get started.

Nipple Stimulation

Stimulating the pregnant person's nipples causes the release of oxytocin, a hormone that contracts the uterus. Taking advantage of this physiological connection between breast and uterus may start labor or at least cause some contractions. Nipple stimulation probably will not work, however, if the cervix has not ripened or thinned significantly or if the pregnant person is currently breast-feeding a toddler, in which case their body has adapted to increased levels of oxytocin. The caregiver can tell them how ready the cervix is after a vaginal exam.

Either you or the pregnant person can stimulate the nipples, in one or more of the following ways, to bring on or intensify contractions:

- Lightly stroke, roll, or brush one or both nipples with the fingertips. Or, you can caress, lick, or suck the nipples. Often, within a few minutes the pregnant person will have strong contractions. The stimulation may need to be kept up intermittently for hours to keep the contractions coming.

- Massage the breasts gently with warm, moist towels for an hour at a time, three times a day.

- Use a gentle but powerful electric breast pump with double-pumping capability (which allows you to pump both breasts at once). A manual or battery-operated breast pump is less likely to work as well as one with a wall plug. Pump one breast for 30 minutes, three to five times per day, pausing when a contraction begins and resuming when it stops.

Start with one nipple or one breast. If stimulating only one does not initiate contractions in a reasonable length of time or if the contractions already occurring do not increase in frequency, length, or strength, try stimulating both breasts at once, between contractions at first, and then, if necessary, continuously. If there are no contractions after 1 to 2 hours, wait a half day before trying again or try some of the other methods.

Precautions When Using Nipple Stimulation

Many caregivers are very comfortable with their clients' use of nipple stimulation to bring on labor; others are wary because stimulating the nipples sometimes causes excessively long or strong contractions. These caregivers worry that strong contractions may stress the fetus, especially if the pregnant person is at high risk for complications. Before approving the use of nipple stimulation, the caregiver may want to check the baby's response to such stimulation by trying nipple stimulation first during electronic fetal monitoring in the hospital or office.

To help avoid excessively strong or long contractions, it is wise to time the length and assess the intensity of all contractions resulting from nipple stimulation. Stop stimulating the breasts if contractions become painful or long (more than 60 seconds).

Walking

Although effective in speeding a slow labor, walking is unlikely to get labor started. If you both want to try it anyway, take a fairly brisk walk, but don't go too far from home or the labor room. If nothing else, walking is a pleasant distraction before labor.

Acupressure and Acupuncture

Certain acupressure (Shiatsu) points can be activated to stimulate or strengthen contractions (see pages 193–194).

Acupuncture is the use of fine needles (sometimes combined with heat or electrical stimulation) to painlessly stimulate specific points along the twelve meridians along which vital forces (called chi) flow. The purpose is to remove any blockage in energy flow that may impair bodily functions. Acupuncture is becoming increasingly available for all sorts of health purposes, including pregnancy and childbirth and the need to start labor.

Acupuncture is usually arranged by the baby's parents, with the knowledge and approval of the pregnant person's caregiver. If the pregnant person is interested in trying acupuncture, check with the midwife, doctor, doula, or childbirth educator for names of licensed acupuncturists who work with childbearing people. Treatment varies depending on the acupuncturist's training and the perceived cause of the problem.

Sexual Stimulation

Sexual intercourse with orgasm is the most effective form of sexual stimulation in starting labor. Orgasm causes the release of oxytocin and contractions of the uterus, and it may also cause the release of prostaglandins, hormone-like substances that soften the cervix. Semen also contains prostaglandins.

Clitoral stimulation by hand or mouth, even without orgasm or intercourse, may also be effective in bringing on contractions.

If you choose one of these methods, make them as pleasant as possible. Try to forget your goal of starting labor and free yourselves to enjoy the sexual experience—more than once, if needed. Frequent intercourse or clitoral stimulation—several times a day—may be needed to get into labor.

Precautions When Using Sexual Stimulation

- Avoid placing anything within the vagina if the membranes have ruptured because doing so increases the risk of infection.

- Do not blow into the vagina.

- Avoid these methods if either of you has any sores that could spread or if the pregnant person has an uncomfortable vaginal condition.

Bowel Stimulation with Castor Oil and/or Verbena Oil

Sometimes, labor can be started by taking a castor oil/verbena oil cocktail. These oils are strong laxatives and also may cause powerful contractions of the bowels and diarrhea (reactions vary, but the effects can be quite unpleasant for a few hours). These oils have been used for generations to induce labor, with some success. One or both of these oils may increase the level of prostaglandins, which are produced when the bowels contract. Prostaglandins, again, cause the cervix to soften and thin.

Make sure the pregnant person checks with the caregiver before using castor oil and/or verbena oil. Some caregivers may offer their preferred recipes. If not, you might consult an herbalist or knowledgeable midwife, or search online for ways to use "castor oil and verbena to induce labor." Review your findings with your caregiver before trying this, as there are sometimes good reasons not to do it. If the caregiver sees no reason not to try it, then you might go ahead.

Contractions may come immediately after taking the first dose, but usually it takes some hours or another dose before taking effect. If it fails to get labor started, it does improve the readiness of the cervix to dilate, and then labor might start the next day through nipple stimulation or another method.

Note: You might be told that castor oil causes the baby to pass meconium (the first bowel movement) in labor. Rather than being caused by castor oil, it is likely that being postdate (at 41 or 42 weeks) is what causes this. The longer the pregnancy, the more meconium the baby has in its bowels and the more likely it is that some will be passed (see pages 64 and 369).

Enemas, previously used for starting labor, have not been found effective for this purpose, even though they do help empty the bowels.

Teas, Tinctures, Herbs, and Homeopathic Remedies

Some midwives and physicians use certain herbal teas or tinctures, such as blue and black cohosh tea and evening primrose oil, or homeopathic remedies, such as Caulophyllum, to bring on or speed up contractions. Use these teas or tinctures only with the approval of the caregiver and the guidance of an experienced herbalist or homeopath who knows about appropriate dosages and potential side effects.

The Slow-to-Start Labor

Another challenging type of labor is the one that is slow to start. In this case, contractions, sometimes painful, go on for hours or days before the cervix finally begins to dilate. We don't know exactly why this happens to some but not to others, but if the following conditions are present, it might be more likely they will have a slow-to-start labor:

• The cervix is still long (or thick), firm, and posterior when contractions begin (see "Labor Progresses in Six Ways," page 76).

• The cervix is scarred from previous surgery or injury. A scarred cervix may resist thinning and so may require more time and more intense contractions to overcome this resistance. Once thinning occurs, labor usually progresses normally.

- The uterus is contracting in an uncoordinated fashion so the contractions do not open the cervix. The reason for this is not understood, but the condition often resolves with time, rest, or medications to promote sleep or induce labor (see page 256).

- The baby's head is high in the pelvis (see page 66) or in an unfavorable position, such as OP (occiput posterior; see page 66), or other presentations, such as face, brow, or head tilted toward one shoulder (called *asynclitism*). Some babies have a hand up by their face.

- The pregnant person is very anxious and tense about labor or the baby. Increased production of stress hormones (such as adrenaline) in early labor can interfere with labor progress.

Most slow-to-start labors eventually hit their stride with time and strong contractions and proceed normally after the initial long prelabor period. Some slow-to-start labors, however, are part of a generally prolonged labor, in which all phases proceed, but at a very slow pace. When a labor begins slowly, you cannot know in advance just when it will speed up—only time will tell. Fatigue and discouragement can present a serious challenge in this type of labor, and medical interventions may be required. Your role as birth partner will be to maintain the laboring person's morale and help them pace themselves mentally and physically. If interventions are being considered by the caregiver, you can also help the laboring person be well informed about the options (see pages 237).

Strategies for a Slow-to-Start Labor

If the laboring person's long prelabor is tiring and discouraging, though not necessarily painful, the following measures will help:

- Be patient and confident. This labor will not go on forever, and your positive attitude will help keep their spirits up.

- If the laboring person is worried, remind them that *a long prelabor does not necessarily mean something is wrong* with them or the baby. The cervix simply needs more time before it thins and begins opening. The two of you need to find ways to wait without worrying.

- Call friends, family, the caregiver, or your doula for encouragement and morale boosting. Do not call anyone who will make you worry more. A doula, with their confidence, experience, and perspective, can be a great help in such labors. One doula, attending a slow-to-start labor, and, to get the parents' minds off the slow progress, suggested they all read a play together. The only play they had was Shakespeare's *The Tempest*—not an easy play to read! But the mother read her parts, and it worked as a good distraction. Before long, her labor had picked up!

- Try not to become preoccupied with the labor, analyze, or overreact to every contraction. This will only make the labor seem longer.

- Encourage the pregnant person to eat and drink high-carbohydrate, easily digested foods (for example, toast with jam, cereals, pancakes, pasta, fruit juice, coconut water, tea with sugar or honey, sorbet, or gelatin desserts).

- Create a clean, tidy environment with whatever makes the pregnant person comfortable—music, a fire in the fireplace, flowers, favorite scents, and so on.

Additionally, you can help pass the time by rotating among distracting, restful, and labor-stimulating activities. Here are some suggestions:

1. During the day, try distracting activities. Encourage the pregnant person to get out of the house. If they are willing and up to it, visit friends, go for a walk, get a massage, go to work or go to a movie, the mall, or a restaurant (you can hope you'll have to leave before you finish your meal!). You'll find that when out of the house, they will try to minimize their reactions to the contractions and, thus, avoid overreacting to them. This is easier to do when they're among other people than when alone at home.

2. At home, you can utilize these distracting activities: dance; clean; pay bills; play games; start a project such as baking bread, cookies, or a birthday cake (they might almost hope that labor doesn't start until the project is finished!); wash and put away the baby's clothes; arrange or file photos; fix and freeze meals for after the baby is born; have friends over, especially to relieve you if you are tired.

3. Help the pregnant person rest or sleep at night or nap during the day. If they are tired but cannot sleep, try the following:

- A bath: Fill the tub with warm (not hot) water; provide an inflatable bathtub pillow or folded towels for a headrest. They should plan to stay in the tub for a long time; you may have to add hot water from time to time to keep it warm enough. Rest and sleep may come more easily in a warm bath. Keep an eye on them; make sure they don't slip down with their head under the water. Remember, a bath tends to slow contractions in early labor and should be used only when the laboring person needs a rest.

- If a bath is not an option, encourage a long, warm shower. You might need to turn up the water heater.

  Caution about baths: A deep, warm bath can slow contractions, but there may be circumstances when slowing labor is not appropriate—e.g., they are overdue; the bag of waters has broken and an induction may be done if labor does not pick up on its own; or other reasons.

  Also, be careful not to exceed a water temperature of about 98°F (37°C), as the laboring person may become overheated (see page 178 for more information), which can slow labor when it is still early.

- Play soothing music.

- Give a back rub.

- Offer a relaxing beverage (warm milk, herbal tea).

- Use relaxation techniques and slow breathing during contractions (see page 162). Try labor-stimulating measures for periods of 1 to 2 hours at a time to initiate stronger, more frequent contractions. Follow the guidelines in "When Labor Must Start," page 212, noting the precautions for these procedures.

4. If the pregnant person is not only sleepless but also in pain, long baths, relaxation, massage, and slow breathing will help. See "Self-Help Comfort Measures," page 153, for ideas.

5. Try different positions and movements. The following positions and movements sometimes stimulate labor, by taking advantage of gravity, changing the shape of the laboring person's pelvis, or encouraging the baby to wiggle into a better position, while relieving backache.

- Open knee–chest position (see page 173)

- Hands and knees, with or without pelvic rocking (see page 172)

- Walking and slow dancing (see page 170)

- Abdominal lifting: While standing, the pregnant person interlocks their fingers and places them against the pubic bone under the pregnant belly. During contractions, they lift the abdomen up and slightly in, while bending their knees. This often relieves back pain while improving the position of a baby in the pelvis. You 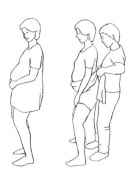 can help them by standing behind them, placing a long woven shawl, folded to about 5 inches (13 cm) wide, around their trunk and below the abdomen, and lifting the abdomen as shown in the illustration. Loosen it when the contraction is over.

The laboring person can alternate these positions and movements with rest.

If these strategies are not enough to get them through a long prelabor, the caregiver may suggest an alcoholic beverage, morphine, sleep medication, or another drug (see page 332).

If the two of you are worried that the pregnant person won't have the stamina to cope with "real" labor after this prolonged prelabor, remind yourself—and them—that they are well equipped at this time in their life to cope with a long period without sleep. Although they feel tired and discouraged, once labor begins to make progress, their energy level and spirits will likely rise, allowing them to continue without distress. If not, they may benefit from pain medications that allow them to rest.

CAUTION: Rarely, the abdominal lift makes the baby uncomfortable, causing the baby to wiggle more, indicating it's uncomfortable—so stop doing it. If you have a nurse or midwife with you, it is a good idea to ask them to listen to the baby's heartbeat during a contraction while doing the abdominal lift. These precautions are taken because it is possible, though very rare, that the umbilical cord could be in a place where it can be pressed by the shawl. If so, the abdominal lift should not be done.

Slow Progress in Active Labor and the Birthing Stage—with or without Back Pain

Sometimes, labor begins with good progress but it slows once the person gets into active labor (after 5 or 6 centimeters). We usually expect progress to speed up around this time. The delay may be temporary, or progress may continue to be slow until the birth. This delay is sometimes associated with back pain, sometimes not.

One in three people have back pain during active labor—or back labor. One possible cause is a poor fit between the baby's head and the pregnant person's pelvis. The actual size of the baby's head is less often a problem than its position in the pelvis. The most favorable head position is occiput anterior, or OA (where the back of the baby's head is toward the pregnant person's front), with the baby's chin tucked to their chest. When, instead, the back of the baby's head is toward the pregnant person's back (OP, occiput posterior), or is tightly positioned sideways (OT, occiput transverse), or tipped back or to one side, then a larger diameter of the baby's head is pressing down into the pelvis. If the baby's hand is placed next to their face as they enter the pelvis, it can also cause back pain and so can variations in the pregnant person's pelvic and spinal anatomy. All these factors, and others, may cause a delay in labor as well as back pain. Reducing this pain and repositioning the baby are the major goals when supporting the laboring person.

As for comfort measures for backache during labor, relaxation and breathing are usually not enough to cope with the pain. Try one or more of the following comfort measures, described in chapter 4: counterpressure, crisscross massage, the double hip squeeze, rolling pressure over the low back, heat and cold, baths and showers, and transcutaneous electrical nerve stimulation (TENS).

Problems that cause both back pain and a delay in active labor usually resolve spontaneously, but this is likely to happen more quickly if the laboring person is active and trying ways to help the baby change position.

Encouraging the Baby to Change Position

It is not always easy to identify the baby's position in the pelvis; even the most experienced nurses, midwives, and doctors have trouble doing this sometimes. However, you do not need to know the baby's position before trying some of the measures described in this and the preceding chapter.

If there is a delay in active labor, whether or not the laboring person has back pain, assume there is a need to change the baby's position.

Help the laboring person use the following positions and movements to encourage the baby to change position. Some of these techniques may also relieve back pain:

• Pelvic rocking (see page 176)

• Slow dancing (see page 170)

• Abdominal lifting (see page 220)

• The lunge (see page 170), during contractions. Have them lunge, using rhythmic patterns, in each direction and then continue with the most comfortable direction for five or six contractions. Help them keep their balance and keep the chair from sliding. The lunge is not easy to do, but it may very well correct the problem.

• Side lying, where the laboring person lies on their side with both hips and knees flexed and a pillow between the knees. If the nurse or midwife is quite sure the baby's back is toward the left side of the laboring person's back (left occiput posterior, or LOP), they lay on their left side; if they believes the baby is ROP, the laboring person lies on the right side. If you are not sure of the baby's position, have them turn from one side to the other every 20 to 30 minutes.

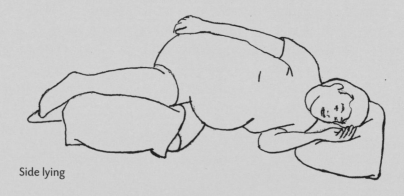

Side lying

- Lying semiprone: If the nurse or midwife thinks the baby's back is toward the left side of the birthing person's back (LOP), they lie in the right semiprone position—on their right side with the lower leg out straight. The upper hip and knee are flexed, resting the upper knee on a doubled-up pillow or peanut ball (see page 183), and they roll toward their front.

   If the baby's back is toward the right side of their back, they lie the same way on their left side. Unless you are sure of the baby's position, have the birthing person change sides every 20 to 30 minutes.

   Note: The semiprone position is quite different in its gravity effects than the side-lying position, so instructions regarding which side to lie on are different for the two positions.

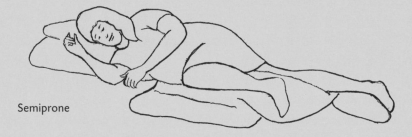

Semiprone

- Kneeling and leaning forward: The birthing person rests their upper body on a chair or a birth ball (see page 180). Some special hospital beds, called birthing beds, can be adjusted to support this position.

- Standing and walking: These take advantage of gravity in encouraging the baby to descend. In addition, the alignment of the baby within the pelvis is thought to be most favorable when the birthing person is upright. Walking also allows some movement within the pelvic joints, which may encourage the baby's rotation.

Promoting the Baby's Descent in the Birthing Stage

If there is a delay in descent during the birthing stage, it is important that the birthing person change position. They can try shifting from semisitting to side lying to squatting to sitting on the toilet. They can try unconventional positions such as the dangle, lap squatting, and lying on their back while lifting their head and drawing their knees up toward their armpits. All these positions are described and illustrated on pages 169–176.

Note: The positions that require getting out of bed are next to impossible if the birthing person has been given an epidural (see pages 171 and 173 for positions to use with an epidural).

Also, the dangle and lap squatting require practice ahead of time and may not be acceptable to the hospital staff. If you think these positions are ones you both might want to try, discuss this with the caregiver ahead of time. Also rehearse them ahead of time to be sure you are comfortable with them.

Occasionally, a baby will not reposition, despite the birthing person's efforts—especially if the baby is large. If so, the baby may be born facing forward ("sunny-side up"). Otherwise, medical or surgical interventions are likely needed to deliver the baby. Possibilities include pain medications (usually an epidural); intravenous oxytocin to strengthen the contractions (see page 258); delivery with forceps or a vacuum extractor (see pages 266–269); or, if nothing else works, a cesarean delivery (see pages 346–352). It's wise to read about these procedures ahead of time.

You can help the birthing person deal with a delay in labor by:

• Being very empathetic

• Maintaining patience and optimism

• Helping them change position so the baby can change position and descend

• Using the techniques described in chapter 4 to relieve any back pain, and, if necessary,

• Ask the Key Questions for Informed Decision-Making (see page 237)

The caregiver's role in this situation is described on pages 287–289 in chapter 7.

When the Birthing Person Must Labor in Bed

Sometimes, a person must remain in bed for labor and birth. These are the most common reasons:

• **High blood pressure:** One's blood pressure tends to drop when lying on the left side.

- **Pain medications:** If one is sleepy or groggy or if half the body is numb with an epidural, they are able to move in bed but cannot safely get out of bed.

- **Use of equipment that attaches to machines:** Intravenous lines, electronic fetal monitors, bladder catheters (thin tubes), and other devices all tend to make it difficult or impossible to move out of bed.

- **Hospital customs:** Unfortunately, in many hospitals, even people with normal labors are routinely discouraged from leaving their beds. There is no medical reason for such a practice.

Being restricted to bed may not distress the birthing person, especially if they are tired, are comfortable in bed, or this was expected. Some, though, find that lying down is most uncomfortable in labor. Some become very restless and are unable to stay down. A person who planned to use movement and positioning for comfort or to help the labor progress will be disappointed and should ask to get out of bed.

Sometimes, restricting a person to bed slows the labor and increases the pain from contractions. It also prevents the laboring person from doing many of the things that speed labor and increase comfort.

Here are some things you can do if the laboring person does not have an epidural and is confined to bed:

1. Find out the reason: The two of you may be able to persuade the caregiver to change the orders if there is no compelling medical reason to remain in bed. If bed rest is medically necessary, you will both be better able to accept it and cooperate if you understand the reason.

2. Find out how strict the order is: The laboring person may be told not to leave the bed or not to turn from their left side at all. They may be allowed up for short periods or to go to the bathroom or to take a bath, which could be as effective for lowering blood pressure as lying on the left side. These options make a positive difference.

3. Ask about alternatives: The laboring person may be able to use a telemetry unit (see page 250) for electronic fetal monitoring and an IV pole on wheels. These allow getting out of bed and walking. Even if connected to many machines and containers, they may be able to stand or to sit in a rocker beside the bed.

4. Help the laboring person focus on the many pain-coping techniques and comfort measures that can be used while in bed, without dwelling too much on what cannot be done. Try relaxation (see page 153), rhythmic breathing (see page 161), attention focusing (see page 158), spontaneous rituals (see page 151), counterpressure and other techniques for relieving back pain (see pages 194–196), massage and acupressure (see pages 187–194), heat and cold (see page 184), transcutaneous electrical nerve stimulation (TENS; see page 185), hypnosis (learned ahead of time, see page 155), or the Take-Charge routine (see page 202).

Although remaining in bed may add to the laboring person's stress, with your help, they can handle this challenge. The key is to understand and accept the reasons for remaining in bed, to focus on the comfort techniques that can be used, and not to give up.

A Breech Baby

In late pregnancy, about 1 in 30 babies is in a breech presentation—with head up and buttocks, feet, or both, down at the cervix. Many breech babies turn spontaneously to a head-down position in late pregnancy, but as the birth approaches, they are less likely to do so because, as they grow, there is less space for large movements such as a somersault.

There are three types of breech presentation: the *frank* breech, with the buttocks down at the cervix; the *complete* breech, with the knees bent so both buttocks and feet are down at the cervix; and the *footling* breech, with one or both feet down at the cervix.

Although many breech babies can be born safely, the breech presentation presents some unique problems, particularly if the baby is premature or very large. Other difficulties are due to the head being born last. Sometimes, there is a delay in the birth of the head because it is the largest part of the baby. Sometimes, the baby inhales amniotic fluid and vaginal secretions, which can interfere with breathing after birth. Also, when the head is still inside and the baby's body is outside, the umbilical cord might be pinched while the baby still depends on it for oxygen.

This does not mean that no breech babies can safely be delivered vaginally. In fact, there are excellent outcomes of vaginal breech births when the following favorable conditions exist: a healthy birthing person who desires a vaginal birth; an average-size baby in a frank breech presentation, with a tucked chin; a skilled caregiver; and a well-equipped hospital with adequate staffing day and night.

Unfortunately, because many hospitals, especially in rural areas and developing countries, could not meet the need for adequate care and facilities, vaginal breech births were almost completely discontinued in the early 2000s in favor of planned cesarean deliveries of all breeches.

Today, there are few doctors with the necessary skills because obstetric training programs stopped teaching how to assist at breech births. Ironically, however, we now have the ability to select those breeches that are safe candidates for vaginal birth, and the standard of care is now supportive of vaginal breech births. Older doctors (who formerly did vaginal breech births) and training programs are slowly reviving the practice.

Helping the Baby Move to a Head-Down Position

Today, if the baby is breech near the due date, the odds are still high that a cesarean will be scheduled before that time. Some people ask to have their cesareans after labor has started spontaneously, to reduce the odds that their babies will be born prematurely. This option of planning a cesarean after labor begins is not favored by many caregivers because the labor might progress quickly before the parents arrive at the hospital, meaning there is insufficient time for a smooth and unrushed cesarean, especially if all operating rooms are occupied. Scheduling a cesarean before labor is usually preferred in North America to reduce problems of overcrowding in the operating suite. Of course, it is impossible to control the timing of all cesareans, but they try to avoid the non-emergency cesareans as much as possible. If you and the birthing person are interested in awaiting labor before having a cesarean birth, discuss the possibility with your caregiver.

If the pregnant person wants a vaginal birth, the best bet is to try to turn the baby to a head-down position before labor. Between 32 and 35 weeks' gestation, the pregnant person can try to turn the baby by using one or more of the following techniques. Of these techniques, however, only moxibustion has shown some success in scientific studies. Still, these techniques seem generally harmless and may help in some cases.

• Breech-tilt: Three times a day, when their stomach is not full and the baby is active, the pregnant person should either get into the open

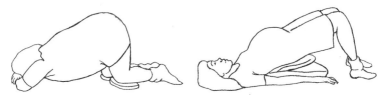

The breech-tilt position, done two ways

knee–chest position (see page 173) or lie on the floor or bed on their back with knees bent and feet flat. While they lift their hips 12 to 18 inches (30 to 45 cm), slide firm cushions beneath the hips to support the tilted position. They remain in this position for 10 to 15 minutes (less if it is uncomfortable), while consciously releasing tension in the abdomen and trunk and visualizing the baby's head pressing "down" against the top of the uterus and the baby trying to get their head "up" again. *Do not use this position if the pregnant person finds it very uncomfortable.*

• Musical or vocal stimulation (recorded music or your voice): Place stereo headphones low on the pregnant person's abdomen and play rhythmic music at a normal volume. Some people believe babies particularly like baroque or classical music. The idea is that the baby may try to move their head closer, to hear the music better. You might combine this technique with the breech-tilt position. You might also try lying with your head on the pregnant person's lap, facing their abdomen, and call the baby, at a normal voice level, to come down to hear you better. Who knows—the baby just may flip to hear your familiar voice better.

　We have no scientific studies regarding the success of the technique, but it is simple, safe, and fun for many parents—and, who knows, it may work!

• Moxibustion is an acupuncture technique where a smoldering stick or a paste of dried herb (mugwort) is held about ¼ inch (6 mm) away from the lower outside corner of the nail of each small toe for 15 to 20 minutes, two or three times per day. Many acupuncturists teach people and their partners how to do this treatment themselves. It is thought to work by increasing the baby's physical activity. If moxibustion appeals to either of you, ask your midwife or doctor, childbirth educator, doula, yoga instructor, or search the internet for a referral to an experienced acupuncturist. Be sure your caregiver is aware that you want to do this or the Webster technique (a chiropractic technique designed to gently assist the baby into a head-down position).

• Breech version, done by many midwives and obstetricians. See following for more information.

Breech Version

If the baby is still breech at 36 to 38 weeks' gestation, the most common plan for delivery in the United States is planned cesarean. However, the pregnant person and caregiver together may decide to try an *external version*, a procedure for turning a breech baby. Versions have been done for generations in many cultures. This is how they are done today in a medical setting:

1. In the doctor's office or hospital, usually with their partner or a doula to help with relaxation and distraction during the procedure (see sidebar following), the pregnant person has an ultrasound scan to confirm the breech presentation and assess the baby's size, the location of the placenta and umbilical cord, the amount of amniotic fluid, and other conditions. An electronic fetal monitor is used to perform a nonstress test to assess the baby's well-being (see page 242).

2. The pregnant person may be given an injection of terbutaline, which relaxes the uterus. Some doctors also give an epidural to relax abdominal muscles and prevent pain from the procedure. Most doctors don't do this, however, because it is too complex, time consuming, and expensive for such a brief procedure. Studies have shown that an epidural increases the chances of a successful version, when compared to no support or assistance in coping with the stress of the procedure. Support from a partner or doula who knows how to help may also increase the success.

3. The birthing person lies on their back and relaxes.

4. The care provider rubs a lubricant on their abdomen and, with the guidance of ultrasound, presses on the abdomen to lift the baby out of the pelvis and gradually turn the baby so the head is down. If unsuccessful at first, the doctor may try once or twice more, but usually not more than that.

5. The pregnant person remains as relaxed as possible; the procedure is sometimes quite uncomfortable. You can help by guiding them in light rhythmic breathing, using eye contact, and

"conducting," with your hand or head movements, as in the Take-Charge routine (see page 202).

6. The baby is checked with ultrasound throughout the procedure. If at any time the baby appears not to be tolerating the procedure, the doctor stops.

7. After the procedure, the pregnant person undergoes another non-stress test to see that the baby has tolerated the procedure well.

After the initial preparation, the version procedure takes only 5 to 15 minutes. Although breech version as practiced today has many built-in safeguards, it also has some slight risks, including fetal distress and bleeding by the pregnant person. These complications are usually identified before they are serious; to be safest, however, most caregivers notify the hospital's labor-and-delivery unit that they are doing a breech version, so if a serious problem arise, a cesarean can be performed at once.

Versions are successful 50 to 60 percent of the time, and can be more successful when used with spinal anesthesia to aid relaxation. Most people who undergo versions give birth vaginally to healthy babies. (Some have cesareans for unrelated reasons that arise during labor; see page 343.)

How a Partner or Doula Helps During a Version

Beforehand, learn how the procedure is done, including such things as how long the actual procedure takes, and plan to use some comfort techniques during the procedure. Rehearse relaxation (page 153), rhythmic light breathing (page 163), and the Take-Charge routine (page 202) in advance with the birthing person. Discuss that it will be uncomfortable for a few minutes and that it is do-able if you work together. Be sure the pregnant person knows to let you or the doctor know if they need a pause to catch their breath. The more relaxed the pregnant person can be and the more tolerant they are of the pressure on the abdomen, the more likely the procedure is to be successful.

During the procedure, maintain eye contact, give them a rhythm with hand signals, head movements, and encouraging words (in the rhythm of their breathing): That's good. . . just like that, . . . stay with me, . . . so good . . ." A kind, confident facial expression and tone of voice are very helpful. Such coaching through this procedure might make all the difference.

When a version is unsuccessful, a cesarean delivery is usually planned. If this happens, see pages 353–355 for ways to make the cesarean birth special.

A Previous Disappointing or Traumatic Birth Experience

Many people who have gone through labor have doubts about whether they can "do it again." For those whose previous birth experiences were normal and satisfying, confidence and optimism tend to outweigh apprehension or doubt. But, for the person who had an unexpected and scary cesarean birth; a difficult, exhausting, frightening, or traumatic labor; a premature, sick, disabled, or stillborn baby; or a labor in which they felt unsupported or helpless, the memories of these difficulties may remain.

You may also have sadness and self-doubt from such an experience. As you both anticipate the upcoming labor and birth, you may be haunted by various doubts and anxieties. The pregnant person may not feel confident about coping with childbirth again or may be anxious about their own safety, especially if the previous labor ended with a cesarean or a difficult forceps or vacuum delivery; or they may be worried about the baby, especially if the last baby did not survive or was very ill. You may feel guilty that you did not do enough to prevent the disappointment, and you may want to be more helpful with the upcoming birth.

The pregnant person will benefit from special preparation for labor and additional understanding and support during labor. The following suggestions should help you provide these:

- Look for books about giving birth after a previous cesarean, recovery from a traumatic birth experience, or pregnancy after the loss of a baby (see Recommended Resources, page 418), for both of you both to read.

- Look for a support group or a class that helps people and their partners prepare for labor after a previous disappointing birth experience. ICAN (International Cesarean Awareness Network) support groups, VBAC (vaginal birth after cesarean) classes, postpartum depression groups, and Pregnancy After Loss meetings may be available in your area. These programs help the pregnant person realize they are not the only people troubled by a previous difficult birth and that they *can* cope. They also teach the birth partner how to be especially helpful during labor. Ask your caregiver, doula, or childbirth educator for the names of instructors or leaders of these classes and groups.

- Browse websites and join email groups that focus on support after difficult or traumatic childbirths (see Recommended Resources, page 418).

- Consider a doula. As an onsite guide who knows the stress you are under, the doula can advise and assist you to make this birth more satisfying than the previous one.

- If either or both of you are very troubled, consider requesting counseling from a seasoned doula or childbirth educator or a psychotherapist with an understanding of birth-related disappointment or trauma.

- Consider the unlikely possibility that the pregnant person's upcoming labor might be similar to the preceding one. Which controllable factors can be different this time? For example, a change of caregivers or the birth location? If the last labor stalled for 7 hours, would earlier intervention be called for if it happens again? If the pregnant person had an induction or cesarean that they felt was unwarranted, do they want more of a say in the decision and a clearer explanation of the reasons, if the caregiver felt such an intervention were needed this time? Do they want a different plan for the use of pain medication? By facing the possibility that a similar labor could occur and knowing it will be handled differently, much of the fear may be diminished and a better experience can be anticipated.

- Encourage the pregnant person to discuss their distress and wishes with the caregiver and note the previous experience and worries in the birth plan.

Anticipate the pregnant person's unique emotional needs. Besides the typical emotional responses to labor (see chapters 2 and 3), there are additional emotional hurdles the laboring person may have to overcome during labor. They are described here, along with suggestions for how to help:

- **Early labor:** As the pregnant person gets into labor, they may suddenly lose heart. This is the "moment of truth," and they may be flooded with self-doubt. Encourage them to talk about their feelings and remind them that such feelings are normal under the circumstances. This will help them carry on and avoid overreacting to the contractions out of fear. Review chapter 2, "Getting into Labor," and "The Slow-to-Start Labor," page 216, for ideas about helping the laboring person accept, rather than dread, labor.

- **Flashbacks to the previous labor.** At times, the laboring person may not be able to escape the feeling that this labor is "just like last time." You can help by acknowledging any similarities, by discussing their feelings, and, most important, by reminding them this is not "last time," but a completely new labor to deal with.

- **Reaching the point during labor at which they a cesarean or other difficulty occurred:** Some people feel a great deal of apprehension before they reach this critical point and are relieved only after it passes. Try to help the laboring person with distraction and stress-reduction measures (see chapter 4) and then rejoice together when the critical point has passed.

A great potential for healing and growth exists when a person confronts their difficult memories and deals constructively with them. With preparation beforehand and sensitive, capable support during labor—from you, a doula, and a caring, understanding staff—the pregnant person's experience of birth is almost certain to be far more satisfying and fulfilling than the previous experience was.

Incompatibility with the Nurse or Caregiver

One shortcoming of the North American system of maternity care is that the pregnant person is usually cared for by people they have never met or only scarcely know. If their own doctor is not on call when labor starts, they are assisted by a substitute doctor who may be a complete stranger. Spending time getting to know the pregnant person is one feature of the midwifery model of care, but some busy midwives' practices have the same shortcomings as doctors'.

Most of the time, no serious problems arise in the birth room; the laboring person, the partner, the caregiver, and nurses get along quite well. What do you do, though, if one or both of you is uncomfortable with the nurse or caregiver? Differences in attitudes toward childbirth, in personality, or in perceptions of each other's roles sometimes become obvious during labor. Discomfort or friction may arise. This *never* works in the laboring person's best interests. They need to be surrounded by kind people who they believe will encourage and support them.

If, before labor, you or the pregnant person anticipates problems, prepare and discuss a birth plan with the caregiver (see page xx). Also, consider hiring a doula to work with the two of you, ahead of time and during labor, to help smooth relations with the staff and help you and the pregnant person advocate for yourselves.

Usually, problems with staff are not serious and can easily be resolved. Following are some suggestions for avoiding, minimizing, or resolving conflicts:

- Do not be the cause of any friction yourself. By your attitude and your behavior, show you are friendly, respectful, and polite, that you expect to work well with the staff, and you appreciate their experience and the contributions they can make to the laboring person's comfort and well-being. If you appear suspicious, frightened, or hostile, the staff might react defensively.

- Communicate any of the laboring person's special concerns—for example, a desire for natural childbirth, a fear of needles or blood, and so forth.

- Have a copy of the birth plan for the nurse to read. If there is time, discuss the birth plan with the nurse or caregiver and ask for help in following the plan as closely as possible. If a staff member has any concerns about the plan, it is better to discuss, than to ignore, them. Differences can usually be resolved.

- Call the nurse or caregiver by name.

If there are differences *between you or the pregnant person and the nurse,* try one or more of the following tactics:

- Deal with the nurse politely. Say, for example, "I cannot talk with you during contractions because I need to help [pregnant person] breathe and relax," or "I think there is a misunderstanding. Our doctor said it is fine for [the pregnant person] to walk around and use the shower. Would you please check with the doctor?"

- Talk to the head nurse. In a calm and objective way, explain any differences you and your assigned nurse have and ask the head nurse to assign another nurse or help mediate the problem.

- Talk directly to the caregiver (by phone, if necessary). If there is an apparent misunderstanding over the nurse's management of labor, ask the caregiver to resolve it.

If the problem is with the doctor or midwife (especially if this is someone unknown to both of you), discuss it directly. If this doesn't solve the problem, ask the nurse to intervene on the laboring person's behalf and advocate for their needs. Or, if the problem involves a clinical decision, ask for a thorough explanation, using the Key Questions for Informed Decision-Making (see page 237), or ask for a second opinion.

How can a doula help you? The doula has no authority to intervene with the staff on your behalf. They cannot be your voice or the laboring person's. They are, however, likely to recognize when a particular action or intervention may lead to a significant departure from your birth plan. They can cue you to ask the Key Questions for Informed Decision-Making (see page 237) or suggest you ask for more time before agreeing to an intervention you had hoped to avoid. This helps ensure you and the laboring person participate in decisions and are not rushed.

Sometimes, the best interests of the laboring person are served by avoiding conflict rather than by resolving it. In other words, to avoid a stressful confrontation, you may have to accept a less-than-ideal arrangement and work with it.

If you are in the unlikely position of being stuck with a nurse or caregiver with whom you are incompatible and who will not yield, accept the situation for the moment and focus your energies on helping the laboring person cope. You may feel powerless and frustrated, but you cannot stop labor while the problem is settled. And trying to resolve a disagreement in the midst of labor might make the labor harder and more stressful for the laboring person. After the baby is born, you can pursue the matter, by discussing the situation with the caregiver, a counselor, or both and writing a letter to those responsible for patient care. Although this effort will probably not benefit you, the birthing person, or the baby, your efforts may help prevent similar difficulties for another laboring person in the future.

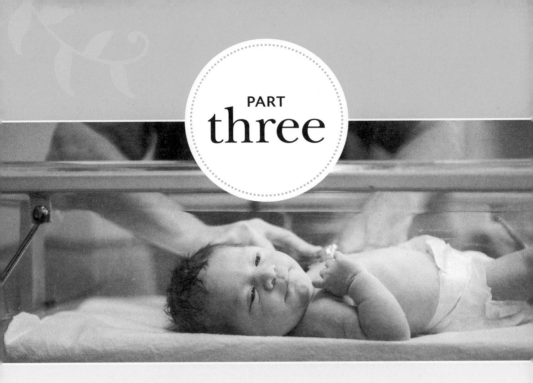

PART

three

THE MEDICAL SIDE OF CHILDBIRTH

THE CAREGIVER'S PRIMARY ROLE IN CHILDBIRTH is to safeguard the health of the laboring person and baby. Throughout pregnancy, the caregiver relies on a wide assortment of tests, technologies, and procedures to detect and treat problems before they become serious. Similar tests, technologies, and procedures (often referred to as "interventions") are available during childbirth.

Caregivers differ regarding what constitutes routine basic care during childbirth. Some caregivers feel birth is so unpredictable it is safest to use many medical procedures in every labor, whether needed or not. Others believe childbirth is essentially a normal physiological process and use medical or surgical interventions only when problems are suspected or detected. Pregnant people differ over the same issues. Some are fearful and feel more secure with a highly medical approach, while others perceive birth as normal and are wary of excessive interventions. They place more trust in their bodies and inner resources than in technology.

Research has shown that, for a healthy person, labor proceeds normally and without hazard most of the time and that careful observation is all that is necessary to detect problems in time to take medical action.

One way to *avoid* problems is to be cautious about using optional procedures and medications; these can sometimes *cause* problems. For example, any procedure that restricts the laboring person's freedom to move might slow labor or increase pain, thus making further interventions more likely and actually increase the risk of developing other problems. For these reasons, technology, medications, and procedures are appropriate and necessary only when problems already exist or are very likely to occur.

Key Questions for Informed Decision-Making

Tests and interventions always involve tradeoffs. The laboring person needs to know what they give up and what they gain before deciding whether to accept a nonemergency intervention. When considering interventions, discuss the following questions with each other and with the caregiver.

When a *test* is suggested, ask:

- What is the reason for the test?

- What questions will it answer?

- How is the test done?

- How accurate or reliable are the results? What is the margin of error? In other words, might the test miss a problem that exists or indicate a problem that does not exist?

- If the test detects a problem, what happens next (for example, further testing or immediate treatment)?

- If the test does not detect a problem, what happens next (for example, a repeat test in a day or two, other tests, or no further concern about the problem)?

- What will this test cost the pregnant person, if anything?

When a *treatment or intervention* is suggested, ask:

• What is the problem and how serious is it?

• How urgent is the need to begin treatment?

• What is the treatment and how is it done?

• How likely is it to solve the problem?

• If the treatment fails, what are the next steps?

• Are there any side effects to the treatment?

• Are there any alternatives (including waiting, doing nothing, or other treatments)?

If an alternative is suggested, again, ask how it is done, how likely it is to work, what its side effects are, and what happens if the alternative treatment fails.

In most situations, there is plenty of time to discuss these questions. When you, the pregnant person, and your caregiver exchange information, questions, and concerns and come to a decision together, it is called "shared decision-making." This approach builds trust and satisfaction because it is based on mutual respect, flexibility, and consideration for each other's points of view.

In the rare case of a true emergency, however, there may not be time for such discussion. The caregiver should tell you how serious and urgent the situation is. If it is urgent, you must trust the caregiver and help the laboring person accept the interventions. A full explanation may have to wait until the emergency is over. In this case, simply ask, "Will this intervention improve the odds of a healthy birthing parent and healthy baby?" If the answer is yes, agree to it, no questions asked. Explanations and discussion may have to come later.

Chapters 6 through 9 discuss the tests, technologies, interventions (including cesarean birth), and medications commonly used in childbirth, along with the problems they are designed to detect and treat.

CHAPTER 6

TESTS, TECHNOLOGIES, INTERVENTIONS, AND PROCEDURES

She was now a full-on tube-o-saurus—the IV and Pitocin tube in her vein, the epidural tube in her back, the urine catheter, baby heartbeat and contraction monitors up inside her, and a mask to super-oxygenate her blood so the baby could get more oxygen. The nurse checked her cervix and said she was now at 4 centimeters—she had been at 3 centimeters 6 hours earlier. I said, "All that crap for 1 centimeter?"

—KEVIN, FIRST-TIME FATHER

During the last month of pregnancy, pregnant people usually see their caregivers once a week. This is a time when problems that can affect labor may surface for the first time, and their detection now, may help the caregiver plan how best to care for the laboring person during labor. Following are descriptions of some common late-pregnancy tests and why and how they are done. This information cannot substitute for discussing the key questions (see page 237) with the caregiver but may provide background on which to base your questions. Omitted here are routine tests given in early pregnancy or at every prenatal checkup.

Late-Pregnancy Tests

During the final weeks or months of pregnancy, the caregiver watches closely for conditions in either the pregnant person or the baby that might affect the outcome of the birth. Results of the tests described here guide the caregiver in planning the clinical management of the birth.

Group B Strep (GBS) Screening

This tests the pregnant person for the presence of particular bacteria, called Group B streptococci. Offered at 35 to 37 weeks of pregnancy, the test involves culturing a sample of secretions from the vagina and/or rectum. Results are usually available in about 2 days. Reliable rapid screening tests that give results in less than 1 hour may soon be available.

One in four pregnant people is a carrier of GBS, which means the bacteria are present in their bodily fluids but they show no signs of infection. Approximately 1 in 200 babies born to these people acquires a GBS infection, which can cause serious illnesses in the newborn, such as pneumonia, sepsis (infection in the blood), and meningitis. GBS infections in newborns can be almost entirely prevented by giving intravenous antibiotics to every laboring person who tests positive for Group B strep, after the membranes rupture or when they go into labor. The antibiotics, which reach the baby via the placenta, lower the risk of newborn infection to 1 in 2,000 to 4,000. The antibiotics also lower the pregnant person's risk of developing an active GBS infection, which may cause fever, uterine or urinary tract infection, and abdominal pain.

If a GBS carrier gives birth before receiving sufficient antibiotics, the baby is observed for symptoms of infection, tested for Group B strep, or both. The tests used vary among caregivers. Some rely on a blood culture only; others also culture the baby's urine and spinal fluid. Some caregivers treat all these babies with intravenous antibiotics and observe them closely for signs of infection for 2 to 3 days, until the tests are complete. Others watch the babies closely and treat only if the baby shows signs of infection before the test results come back. If Group B strep bacteria are present in the cultures, the intravenous (IV) antibiotic treatment continues for many days, during which the baby must remain in the hospital where the IV can be monitored and the baby can be watched for signs of infection.

The main disadvantage of GBS screening is that, if the pregnant person is a carrier, they not only must take intravenous antibiotics, but will probably also have labor induced if the membranes rupture without contractions. Several doses of antibiotics may be given during the waiting period. A common practice is to give a maximum of four doses and to plan induction if the pregnant person does not go into labor within 24 hours. Some caregivers are more patient than others under these circumstances, as are some pregnant people. Either choice—large amounts of antibiotics or induction—has disadvantages (see page 256).

Many people are happy to learn the antibiotics, although given intravenously, are administered only every 4 to 6 hours, depending on the antibiotic. Between doses, the IV line can be plugged and disconnected. People planning an out-of-hospital birth do not have to switch to a hospital birth because of Group B strep, but they do have to visit their midwife every 4 to 6 hours for the antibiotics.

Most researchers agree there is need for better scientific research to determine the true value and potential harms of antibiotics in labor. Alternative treatments to prevent newborn infection, such as the use of probiotics, homeopathics, vaginal flushes, and others, have not been found effective, but also have not been adequately studied.

Ultrasonography

This complex technology involves the transmission of high-frequency (ultrasound) sound waves through a handheld probe into the uterus from outside the pregnant person's abdomen or within the vagina. This produces a detailed picture of the baby (brain, heart, other organs, facial features, limbs, genitals—everything), placenta, umbilical cord, cervix, and other structures. The picture appears on a video screen that you both can see along with the technician. Although no fetal abnormalities have been linked to ultrasound, it is recommended that exposure to this powerful technology be limited to the minimum time that is medically necessary.

Ultrasonography is used for numerous purposes throughout pregnancy. In late pregnancy, it is used mostly to identify the baby's presentation when a breech or other difficult presentation is suspected, to estimate the baby's growth and weight, and to measure the volume of amniotic fluid. A decrease in fluid may indicate the placenta is no longer functioning very well; an increase may indicate a problem with the pregnant person's fluid regulation or the baby's kidneys. Unfortunately, the margin of error with these estimates can be considerable. For example, if somewhat dehydrated when a pregnant person has an ultrasound measurement of amniotic fluid volume, it is likely to be lower than if they were well hydrated. There's a lesson here: be sure they are well hydrated if having such a test.

Ultrasonography is done this way: The pregnant person lies in a dimly lit room, and the ultrasonographer lubricates the abdomen and slides the probe over the belly. Photographs are taken and measurements made at different depths of the pregnant person's and baby's tissues. The whole scan may take up to 30 minutes.

Then, a radiologist analyzes the ultrasonographer's report for the doctor or midwife, who makes recommendations based on the findings—for example, continuing the pregnancy without concern, administering more tests, inducing labor, delivering the baby by cesarean, or trying a breech version.

If during labor the baby is suspected to be malpositioned, a brief ultrasound scan may be done to determine the baby's position (see page 66).

Nonstress Test

This test assesses the baby's well-being by measuring heart rate changes that occur when the baby moves in the uterus. The nonstress test is recommended when the pregnant person notices the baby's movements slowing in frequency (see "How to Count Fetal Movements," page 43), when the caregiver feels the baby's growth may be less than expected, or when the pregnant person is overdue or has high blood pressure, diabetes, or another medical condition.

Using an external electronic fetal monitor (see page 249), the pregnant person presses a button when the baby moves. If the baby's heart rate speeds up, this is a good sign; the heart rate is said to be "reactive." If the rate stays the same or slows—if it is "nonreactive"—this may indicate the baby may be stressed, and further tests or corrective action may be necessary.

The nonstress test is not wholly accurate. When the test indicates the baby is doing well, it is usually correct. When it indicates the baby is not doing well, however, the results are often wrong. Combining a measurement of amniotic fluid volume with the nonstress test seems to give a more accurate picture of a baby's well-being.

Essential Observations During Labor

What constitutes basic care during labor when the laboring person is in good general health, has experienced a normal pregnancy, and the baby is in a favorable position within the uterus? By making certain simple observations regularly during the labor, the skilled caregiver or nurse can accurately assess whether both pregnant parent and baby are fine or whether closer observation or treatment is needed.

Basic care includes the following essential observations of the laboring person, labor progress, the amniotic fluid (the water in the bag of waters), the fetus, and the newborn.

The caregiver or nurse makes these observations of the **laboring person:**

- Behavior, activity, and emotional state during and between contractions and after the birth

- Basic body functions: eating, drinking, urination, bowel movements

- Contractions: frequency, intensity, and duration

- Tone of the uterus between contractions

- Location and nature of labor pain (abdomen, back, or both and whether the pain is continuous or intermittent)

- Rating the laboring person's pain (on a scale of 0 to 10). Most hospitals, by policy, assess every patient's level of pain and offer pain medication if the pain is increasing or distressing to the patient.

- Vaginal secretions

- Progress of labor (determined by the pattern of contractions, the patient's behavior, and occasional vaginal exams)

- Vital signs: temperature, pulse, and respiration

- Blood pressure

- Tone of the uterus after childbirth

- Amount of bleeding after childbirth

When the bag of waters breaks, the caregiver or nurse makes these observations of the **amniotic fluid:**

- Color: If the fluid is clear, the baby has probably not been stressed. A brown or green color indicates a fetal bowel movement (meconium), which means the baby has been stressed.

- Amount (leak or gush): Sudden loss of a large amount of fluid (a gush) increases the likelihood of pressure on the umbilical cord during contractions, which could cause stress to the baby.

- Odor: A foul smell indicates infection.

The caregiver or nurse makes these observations of the **fetus:**

- Heartbeat, monitored by frequent listening with an ultrasound device (handheld or embedded in a belt around the abdomen) or a stethoscope

- Size (approximate weight)

The simple observations listed previously are made frequently by a caregiver or nurse who is with the laboring person nearly continuously. They give a very good idea of both the baby's and laboring person's condition. As long as they indicate normal conditions, these observations are all that is truly needed. If they indicate problems with the laboring person, the labor, or the baby, then additional interventions (described in the next pages) are used to correct the problems.

Immediately after birth, the caregiver or nurse makes these observations of the **newborn.** They are a quick assessment of the newborn's well-being:

- Apgar score at 1, 5, and, perhaps, 10 minutes after birth

- Baby's temperature, respiration, and pulse

Apgar Score (assessed at 1, 5, and, sometimes, 10 minutes)

SIGN	0 points	1 point	2 points
Heart rate	absent	below 100 per minute	more than 100 per minute
Breathing	absent	slow, irregular	good, crying
Muscle tone	limp	arms and legs close to body	active, moving
Reflex irritability	no response to mild pinch	grimace	struggle, cough, or sneeze
Color	blue-gray	body usual skin color; fingers and toes blue	all pink or ruddy

- Baby's general behavior and state of alertness
- Baby's physical appearance

A score of 7 to 10 at 1 and 5 minutes of age is considered good health. Below 7 indicates the baby needs attention, such as suctioning their mouth and nose; giving oxygen or other aid to breathing; rubbing and stroking the baby's skin; or having the parents speak or sing to the baby. Lower scores indicate the need for more skilled medical care.

Conditions Influencing the Use of Intervention During Labor

Beyond the essential observations already discussed, other tests, procedures, and medications are used if potential problems are discovered. They include the use of highly specialized equipment, a variety of drugs, and surgery. How and when they are used depends on a number of considerations:

- **Medical condition of the pregnant parent:** As already noted, there is less need for intervention when the pregnant parent experiences a healthy pregnancy, labor is progressing well, and all vital signs are normal.

- **Apparent well-being of the fetus:** If the fetus is fully developed and mature, of normal size, and apparently unstressed, most interventions are not needed.

- **Training and philosophy of the caregiver:** Some caregivers routinely use more interventions than others, preferring to prevent problems before they arise. Although this results in unnecessary treatment, these caregivers feel that overtreatment is harmless and that without it, they might miss problems. Better safe than sorry, they believe. Other caregivers are comfortable watching the laboring person, baby, and labor progress and using interventions only if a problem arises; they believe unnecessary treatment can cause problems. The scientific literature supports the latter approach.

- **Usual practices or policies of the institution and nursing staff:** These practices or policies are determined by current standards of care, nurses' training, the size and competence of the staff, customs in the hospital, legal concerns, financial considerations, and other factors. There is much variation in usual practices among hospitals—even in the same geographical area. In one hospital, for example, laboring people may be encouraged to be out of bed and moving about or using the bath in labor. In another hospital nearby, they may be discouraged from doing these same things. Rates of labor induction, epidural analgesia, and cesarean delivery also vary widely among hospitals.

- **Preferences of the pregnant person:** Within each institution and within each caregiver's practice, there is room for choice. Make sure the caregiver knows the pregnant person's preferences (see "Prepare and Review the Birth Plan," page 45); help ensure their preferences are considered in all decisions made.

Common Obstetric Interventions

Following are descriptions of many common obstetric procedures and their purposes, disadvantages, and possible alternatives. These are usually unnecessary when labor is normal, but may become necessary if problems arise. Chapter 7 discusses the circumstances under which these procedures are necessary for medical reasons.

As the birth partner, you may be the liaison between the laboring person and the hospital staff. A doula can advise you in this role. It is important for you to be familiar with common obstetric interventions so you can inform the staff about the laboring person's preferences, help them make decisions about optional procedures, and help handle any additional discomfort—emotional or physical—arising from the interventions. It is also important that you both understand any circumstances that require interventions for safety.

Intravenous (IV) Fluids

An intravenous drip is a plastic bag of liquids that includes water and electrolytes, dextrose, or medications. The bag hangs from a pole attached to the bed or a pole on wheels; the latter allows the person in labor to walk. A tube extending from the bag is inserted into a vein in the laboring person's hand or arm. The liquid drips into the vein.

Intravenous fluids may be given to provide the laboring person with liquids, calories, or both, instead of taking them by mouth; to administer medications; with an epidural, to increase blood volume to help protect against a drop in blood pressure; or to keep a vein open, just in case they require medications quickly later on.

Many caregivers give intravenous fluids to all patients in labor because they do not want the laboring person to eat or drink anything. They feel an empty stomach is best. Their reason dates from the time when most people gave birth while unconscious under general anesthesia. It was dangerous to have a full stomach while under general anesthesia because they might vomit and breathe in the vomited material. General anesthesia is now rarely used for childbirth and, when it is, better techniques help protect the patient from this complication. Still, many caregivers today continue the out-of-date and unnecessary policy of withholding food and drink and giving every patient IV fluids.

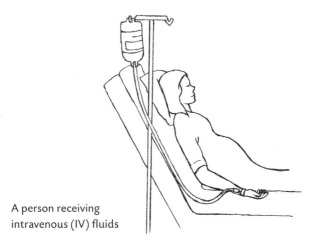

A person receiving intravenous (IV) fluids

Some caregivers have a less positive attitude toward intravenous fluids. They believe intravenous fluids are problematic and they encourage laboring people to drink sufficient fluids to satisfy their thirst. Intravenous fluids are reserved for times when they are "medically indicated"—that is, when necessary or desirable because of the medical condition of the laboring person or baby, such as when:

• Labor is very long.

• The laboring person has continuous nausea and vomiting.

- They will receive epidural, spinal, or general anesthesia (see pages 315–326).

- They need certain IV medications—to stop preterm labor, induce or augment labor, control blood pressure, reduce pain, or for another reason.

- They have a condition that might require immediate medical action.

Disadvantages of Giving IV Fluids:

- Large amounts of IV fluids cause fluid retention in the laboring person, especially in the legs and breasts. It may take days for this to disappear, and the increase in breast engorgement makes breast-feeding more difficult during the first week. Rarely, excessive fluids accumulate in the laboring person's lungs (called pulmonary edema).

- An IV line is inconvenient and somewhat stressful for the laboring person, who must make sure it is out of the way when rolling over or getting out of bed.

- IV lines sometimes "infiltrate"—that is, poke through, the vein. The fluids then go directly into the laboring person's tissue, causing pain and swelling. If the fluids contain medications, they do no good, as they do not get into the bloodstream.

IV fluids are unnecessary if the laboring person drinks enough liquid and does not need IV medications. The best policy is usually to encourage them to drink when thirsty or to offer liquids after every contraction or two for them to take or not, as desired.

You and the laboring person can discuss the following alternatives to an IV with the caregiver:

- After every contraction or two, offer the laboring person fluids to drink, such as water, fruit juice, coconut water, or sports beverages (with added electrolytes), or frozen juice bars to eat. If they decline, there is no need to urge them to drink large amounts. Usually, the laboring person's thirst is a good guide.

- Keep a vein open so the caregiver can give intravenous medications quickly if needed. The caregiver or nurse places a short, flexible tube in a vein in the laboring person's arm above the wrist, but then plugs it instead of connecting it to an intravenous line. This procedure (called a heparin lock or saline flush) allows the laboring person more freedom to move around than does an intravenous line.

Electronic Fetal Monitoring (EFM)

There are three methods of electronic fetal monitoring (EFM): external, internal, and portable external.

With external monitoring, the nurse or caregiver places two stretchy belts around the laboring person's abdomen. One belt, placed low on the abdomen, holds an ultrasound device that detects the fetal heartbeat. The other, placed higher, holds a device (a tocodynamometer) that detects contractions.

With internal fetal monitoring, a thin spiral wire electrode is attached to the skin of the baby's scalp to detect the fetal heart rate electronically, and a fluid-filled tube (intrauterine pressure catheter) is placed within the laboring person's uterus to measure the intensity of the contractions. When the uterus contracts, fluid is squeezed out of the tube, and a gauge precisely measures the strength of the contraction.

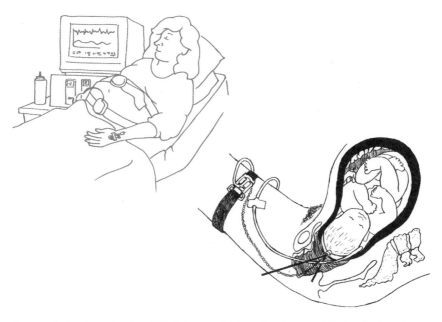

Electronic fetal monitoring (EFM): external (above) and internal (below); they also have a saline flush in place above the left wrist.

The information about contractions and the baby's heart rate response to them is transmitted either by wires to a bedside display or wirelessly to a screen at the nurses' station. The readings can also be printed out continuously.

With *portable electronic fetal monitoring* (telemetry), the laboring person may wear a radio transmitter around their neck, which connects by short wires to the sensors in the belts (instead of wires connected to the bedside console). Or, they may use a newer wireless version. In these, radio transmitters are located within each sensor, and the sensors are waterproof, so the laboring person can be monitored in the water. Either type allows the laboring person to move about freely (within about 200 feet, or 61 meters, of the nurses' station) while information is radioed back to a central monitor and the monitor in the labor room. External monitoring is easier to apply, less invasive, and much more widely used than internal monitoring, but the latter is more accurate and reserved for times when external monitoring is not tracking the fetal heartbeat or the contractions accurately enough (as with a laboring person who is also obese, contractions of questionable intensity, and other situations).

Purposes of EFM During Labor

EFM detects, displays, and records the baby's heart rate response to contractions. A permanent record of the length, frequency, and (with internal monitoring) intensity of the contractions, along with the fetal heart rate, is produced.

EFM is **medically indicated** during labor when:

• Labor is prolonged and the caregiver is considering speeding progress by administering synthetic oxytocin (see page 258). The length and frequency of the contractions can be assessed with the external tocodynamometer. If the caregiver needs an accurate measurement of the intensity of the contractions, the intrauterine pressure catheter is used.

• A nurse or a midwife cannot be with the laboring person continuously or frequently.

• The laboring person receives synthetic oxytocin or other medications that may make the contractions too intense for the fetus.

- There are doubts during labor about the fetus's well-being (because of prematurity, small size, meconium-stained amniotic fluid, or possible lack of oxygen).

- The laboring person is considered to be at high risk for complications.

Disadvantages of EFM are:

- The laboring person's movements are restricted, although they can change position in bed and sometimes even stand by the bed or sit in a chair. Portable monitoring allows for more movement, including walking around, and wireless monitoring is possible while in a bath or shower. Internal monitoring is less restrictive but more invasive than external monitoring.

- Sometimes, more attention is paid to the machine than the laboring person. As the birth partner, do not allow yourself to fall into this trap. The laboring person needs your attention, not the machine.

- Interpretation of the monitor printouts (tracings) is extremely complex, and experts even disagree about what different heart rate patterns really mean and when intervention is necessary.

- Internal monitoring requires breaking both the bag of waters and the skin of the fetal scalp. These procedures slightly increase the risk of infection to the laboring person and baby, especially if the laboring person has an infection or sore in the vagina. Also, breaking the bag of waters may cause additional stress to the fetus by removing the cushion of fluid that protects the head and cord.

- EFM measures only the fetal pulse, but it cannot detect whether the fetus is experiencing a shortage of oxygen. When cesareans are done solely because of EFM tracings, the babies often show no signs of having been oxygen deprived. For this reason, attempts to confirm the findings of EFM are sometimes used (see "Fetal Scalp Stimulation Test," page 253).

Alternatives to consider: Before labor, you and the pregnant person can discuss the following alternatives to EFM and state your preferences in your birth plan.

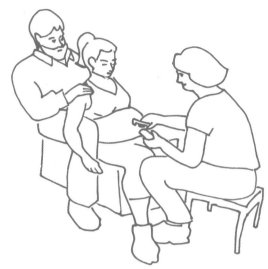

Auscultation of fetal heart tones with an ultrasound stethoscope (doppler)

- Have a nurse or midwife listen frequently to fetal heart tones with an ultrasound stethoscope or a fetal stethoscope, for 1 to 2 minutes at a time during and after a contraction. Many studies have compared this method of monitoring with continuous EFM, and all have found that listening to heart tones intermittently results in equally healthy babies and fewer cesareans. This method, called *auscultation*, requires the nurse or midwife to be trained and experienced and be available for about 5 minutes out of every 15 during active labor and continuously during the birthing stage. Auscultation is the method used in home or out-of-hospital birth centers.

- Use external EFM intermittently for 10 to 15 minutes each hour, removing it the rest of the time. This enables the laboring person to move around when not being monitored. Some caregivers are comfortable doing this in early labor, but prefer continuous monitoring in active labor and beyond.

- Use a portable (telemetry) EFM unit (see page 250). Find out whether the hospital has portable telemetry units available.

- Use a handheld waterproof ultrasound stethoscope or the waterproof telemetry units for listening to the baby when the laboring person is in the bath. These are not available in all hospitals. Ask the caregiver about them.

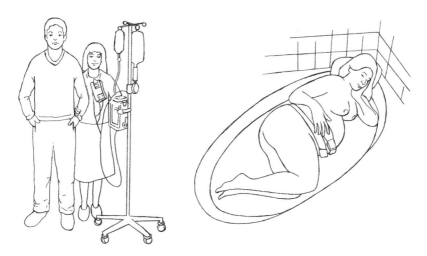

Portable telemetry units: wired (left) and wireless (right), with woman in the bath

Fetal Scalp Stimulation Test

The caregiver performs this simple test by pressing or scratching the baby's scalp during a vaginal exam. If the baby is in good condition, the heart rate will speed up with such stimulation. If the baby is distressed (that is, short of oxygen), the heart rate will not speed up. The results of this test have been found to correlate well with the actual condition of the fetus.

This test is performed to check whether the baby is still tolerating labor even though the EFM tracings or audible heart sounds raise concerns. The test is medically indicated at any time fetal heart tones are unclear (the medical terms for this are "nonreassuring" or "indeterminate," meaning there is concern about the baby's well-being) and certainly before a cesarean is performed for fetal intolerance of labor (which is considered to be diagnostic of oxygen deprivation). This simple test can be performed any number of times during labor.

Alternatives to consider: Instead of performing the fetal scalp stimulation test, you can simply rely on EFM alone or on frequent listening to the fetal heart rate, which may result in overcalling fetal intolerance of labor.

You and the laboring person can ask for the fetal scalp stimulation test whenever fetal distress is suspected. Discuss it with the caregiver in advance and state your preference for it in the birth plan.

Artificial Rupture of the Membranes (AROM)

To rupture the membranes, or break the bag of waters, the caregiver inserts a thin instrument (amnihook) into the vagina and through the cervix and makes a hole in the sac holding the amniotic fluid, which then comes streaming out. The procedure is no more painful than a vaginal exam. Sometimes, following AROM, the laboring person's contractions suddenly increase in intensity; this is usually the goal of the procedure.

In the past, laboring people were warned against taking baths after their membranes were ruptured, but scientific trials have found that bathing in a clean tub after AROM does not increase the chance of infection in either the laboring person or the baby.

AROM is done:

• To speed labor. If timed correctly and the baby is well positioned, AROM shortens labor by an average of 40 minutes. If the baby is malpositioned, however, the procedure may actually lengthen labor. Rupturing the membranes removes the cushion of fluid around the baby's head, causing the malpositioned head to wedge more firmly into the pelvis, which lessens the chances that the baby's position will improve. It cannot always be predicted which labors will be shortened by AROM and which will not. The gamble may be worth taking if labor progress is poor as other interventions to speed labor are more complex and potentially risky.

• To induce labor with other methods, such as prostaglandins or oxytocin (see pages 257–258). AROM alone is not likely to induce labor unless the cervix is very soft and thin.

• To check the amniotic fluid for a fetal bowel movement (meconium, which signals fetal stress), for infection, for bleeding, or for other signs of problems

• To apply the electrode and catheter for internal EFM (see page 249)

When is AROM medically indicated? This question is controversial. The frequency with which caregivers use AROM, especially in early labor, varies widely. Some believe it is innocuous and use it for most of their patients in labor. Others believe its advantages rarely outweigh its disadvantages; they reserve it for situations in which they feel they must intervene. Otherwise, they prefer to leave the membranes intact.

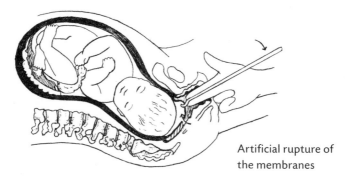

Artificial rupture of the membranes

Disadvantages of AROM are:

- No effect. Frequently, it does not start or speed labor.

- Chances of infection for the laboring person or baby increase with time after the bag of waters is broken and with the number of vaginal exams performed.

- Removing the protective cushion of fluid from around the baby's head may increase pressure on the head during contractions and cause indeterminate or nonreassuring fetal heart rate changes.

- If the baby's head is malpositioned, removing the thin fluid layer surrounding the head may take away any wiggle room, thereby decreasing the chance of the head repositioning.

- AROM increases the risk that the umbilical cord will be compressed during contractions. This compression could cause fetal heart rate changes that indicate a shortage of oxygen for the baby.

- If the baby's head (or buttocks, if the baby is breech) is high when AROM is done, the danger of a prolapsed cord (see page 290) increases.

Alternatives to consider:

- The caregiver can refrain from breaking the bag of waters to speed labor and suggest that the laboring person try self-help methods to stimulate contractions (see pages 212–217).

- Or, they can use other methods to check fetal well-being (see "Electronic Fetal Monitoring," page 249 and "Fetal Scalp Stimulation Test," page 253) or to induce labor.

Amnioinfusion

In this painless procedure, saline solution (salty water) is sent into the uterus via a plastic tube, the same kind used in internal EFM to assess the intensity of contractions (see page 249). Amnioinfusion is done after the bag of waters has broken to replace the fluid lost if the baby's umbilical cord is being compressed during contractions.

The added fluid helps cushion the cord and may protect against fetal distress. The procedure is also helpful if the baby has passed meconium in the uterus. The fluid dilutes the meconium to protect against problems that would occur if the baby were to inhale thick meconium during birth. Although the injected fluid gradually runs out of the uterus, the procedure can be repeated as necessary to maintain sufficient volume. This simple technique, which is extremely low cost, sometimes makes it possible to safely avoid a cesarean for fetal intolerance of labor.

Disadvantages of amnioinfusion are:

• It is invasive and can increase the chance of uterine infection.

• The laboring person must remain flat in bed during and after the procedure or the fluid will run out quickly.

Alternatives to consider:

• The caregiver can go straight to a cesarean if and when fetal distress warrants quick delivery.

Induction or Augmentation of Labor

Sometimes, labor is induced (started artificially) and at other times, a labor that has slowed is augmented (speeded up). There are several ways labor can be induced or augmented:

1. Self-help methods (see pages 212–217)

2. "Stripping" the membranes to begin labor induction. The caregiver inserts a finger in the vagina through the cervix and circles the finger around inside to separate the membranes from the lower segment of the uterus. This is usually uncomfortable or painful for the pregnant person—it feels like a vigorous vaginal exam—and sometimes results in inadvertent rupture of the

membranes. Stripping the membranes usually does not actually start labor, but it may hasten ripening and thinning of the cervix to make it more ready for dilation (see "Labor Progresses in Six Ways," page 74). The procedure cannot be done if the cervix is hard to reach because it is very posterior (pointing toward the pregnant person's back) instead of anterior (in the center of the vagina) or if it is tightly closed.

3. Artificial rupture of the membranes (AROM, see page 254). This sometimes speeds or augments labor when timed correctly.

4. Prostaglandin gels, suppositories, or tablets. Prostaglandins are hormone-like substances produced by the body. They can also be manufactured. Like the prostaglandins a pregnant person produces, synthetic prostaglandins promote the softening, thinning, and, sometimes, dilation of the cervix. They are used when labor must be induced before the cervix has naturally softened or thinned. Prostaglandins come in these forms:

• A water-soluble gel containing prostaglandin (dinoprostone or Prepidil), applied to the inside or the outside of the cervix through a syringe. More may be applied after 6 hours or so.

• A tampon-like device containing prostaglandin (Cervidil), placed in the vagina behind the cervix, where it gradually releases prostaglandin over about 12 hours

• A tiny tablet containing another synthetic prostaglandin, misoprostol (Cytotec), either placed in the vagina behind the cervix or given by mouth. Tablets are given by mouth when a pregnant person's membranes have ruptured because placing anything in the vagina increases the risk of infection. A second tablet may be administered after 4 to 6 hours. Cytotec should be given in low doses (25 micrograms vaginally or 50 micrograms orally) and usually acts gradually, as Prepidil and Cervidil do. Higher doses can cause sudden, very intense, contractions and fetal distress. This is less likely to happen with the other prostaglandin agents.

These agents are only used in the hospital and require careful observation of the pregnant person and fetus for unwanted side effects. Dosages and treatment schedules vary depending on the caregiver's preferences, the pregnant person's preferences, and the state of the cervix. Lower doses are generally safer but act more slowly.

5. Intravenous administration of a synthetic form of the hormone oxytocin (also called Pitocin) can start or speed up labor. Pitocin is mixed with intravenous fluids in a continuous drip. By regulating the dose, the caregiver can usually control the intensity and frequency of the contractions quite well. Electronic fetal monitoring is required, along with a nurse's close observation, to detect and correct excessively strong or long contractions. Attempts to start labor with Pitocin often fail when the cervix is firm and thick. If prostaglandin is used before Pitocin, this problem is often avoided.

If an induction is done for medical reasons and fails, cesarean delivery is the only remaining option. If an induction is done without a medical reason (that is, for convenience) and fails, the pregnant person may be sent home to await spontaneous labor, but this rarely happens today. Usually, the baby is delivered by cesarean.

Induction or augmentation of labor is **medically indicated** when:

• Pregnancy is prolonged. Caregivers disagree about when pregnancy has gone on too long. Some offer induction at 39, 40, or 41 weeks, but there is scientific evidence that, statistically, if there is no medical problem, the risks to the baby of inducing before 42 weeks exceed the risks of waiting. However, waiting beyond 42 or 43 weeks increases the risk of stillbirth. *In 2016, the American College of Obstetricians and Gynecologists recommended that, without a medical reason, induction of labor should be postponed until 42 weeks of pregnancy.*

• Medical problems are such that continuing the pregnancy might harm the pregnant person or the baby (for example, when the pregnant person has high blood pressure or diabetes).

• The baby is not thriving in the uterus.

• The bag of waters has been broken for a long time and labor has not started spontaneously or the pregnant person has tested positive for Group B strep (see page 240).

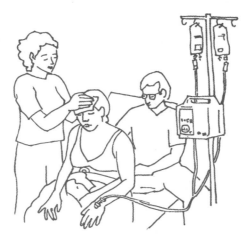

A pregnant person having labor induced with Pitocin. Contractions and fetal heart rate are monitored electronically.

- The pregnant person who has frequent herpes outbreaks is free of herpes sore in the genital area. Being induced is a way to avoid a cesarean (which is done if a pregnant person has a herpes sore in or near the vagina when going into labor; see page 280).

- The pregnant person is having a prolonged prelabor and the cervix is firm, in which case the use of prostaglandins may be appropriate (see "Prelabor," page 85 and "The Slow-to-Start Labor," page 216).

- Contractions in the active phase slow and decrease in intensity, causing a delay in progress. In this case, augmentation with intravenous Pitocin may be appropriate.

Disadvantages of induction for medical reasons include:

- Medical induction usually includes more interventions for safety than does spontaneous onset of labor; such interventions include continuous electronic fetal monitoring, IV fluids, and others.

- Because the pregnant person is hospitalized before the first contraction—possibly hours before—they can become tired and hungry, perhaps discouraged, and even begin to perceive that their labor is very long and something is wrong.

Sometimes, labor is induced out of fear that the baby is becoming too big. The reasoning is, inducing labor before the baby grows too much will make the birth easier and prevent complications and, possibly, a cesarean. Although this seems to make sense, studies have shown that:

- It is not possible to assess an unborn baby's size accurately. Estimates are often wrong by 10 percent or more, even when ultrasound is used.

- When babies are thought to be large, cesareans are actually more likely if labor is induced than if labor begins spontaneously, and induction, in these cases, produces no improvements in the babies' health and well-being.

- Although the odds of a difficult labor increase when the baby's weight exceeds 8½ pounds (3.9 kilograms), inducing labor does not prevent a difficult labor or a cesarean birth.

- Most cases of shoulder dystocia (in which a baby becomes stuck after the head is out) happen in average-size babies; this problem cannot be predicted. When this serious complication occurs, doctors and midwives use well-practiced techniques to resolve it.

Nonmedical reasons for induction: While it is difficult to quantify exactly, many inductions are elective; that is, not for medical safety but for reasons such as:

- Convenience—for the pregnant person, caregiver, or both. An elective induction may be scheduled to occur when the caregiver is on call or when the pregnant person has household help.

- Routine procedure, whenever a pregnant person reaches week 39 or 40. Many caregivers see no reason not to induce labor at this point, and they are not concerned about the possibility of prematurity or the increased likelihood of a cesarean (see disadvantages, following).

- The pregnant person's discomfort. Swelling, backache, itching, or fatigue makes some women want to end their pregnancies as soon as safety allows.

- Avoiding the stress of going to the hospital in labor, especially if the pregnant person lives far from the hospital or has had a previous rapid labor.

It can be very appealing to be able to plan when the baby will be born. As the birth partner, you might appreciate knowing the date and being able to plan your schedule accordingly. However, inductions are more successful if done when the cervix has already ripened (softened and thinned) considerably.

Disadvantages of elective induction: Because induction is not an innocuous procedure, you and the pregnant person should carefully consider the benefits and risks of an elective induction before making a decision. There are many potential disadvantages:

1. Inductions sometimes proceed very slowly, especially if the pregnant person's cervix has not undergone some of the predilation changes (see "Labor Progresses in Six Ways," page 74). A day or more may pass before the baby is born, and, in some cases, the induction procedures are carried out during the day and stopped at night to allow the pregnant person to eat and get some rest. The reason for allowing plenty of time for the process is to try to avoid a cesarean; however, a slow induction can be exhausting and demoralizing for both the pregnant person and birth partner. (If the bag of waters has broken, the caregiver usually intervenes with a cesarean earlier.) Some caregivers are reluctant to put the pregnant person through a long induction or to wait several days for the birth, and so they decide on a cesarean after 12 hours or so, although labor may not have even begun in this much time. You may wonder if the induction for no medical reason is worth these risks.

2. The timing of an elective induction may not be best for the baby, who might benefit from another few days or weeks in the uterus. Most babies continue to mature and develop greater strength and other capabilities until labor begins spontaneously. Normally, the baby, when mature enough, starts the labor process, by secreting the hormones that initiate labor. If the pregnant person's due date is uncertain and labor is induced, the baby might be premature. In fact, elective induction has been identified as one large and preventable contributor to the high rate of prematurity (10 percent) in the United States.

3. Prostaglandins used to ripen the cervix sometimes cause nausea and rapid changes in the pregnant person's blood pressure.

4. The chances of a cesarean are greater in a first-time pregnant person who has an elective induction compared to a first-time pregnant person whose labor begins spontaneously.

5. Sometimes, even though the induction date is planned, the hospital is too busy or lacking an available bed when the day comes. The pregnant person may be told not to come in or may even be turned away on arrival. They may be asked to call the hospital every few hours until a bed becomes available. This can be frustrating and worrisome, especially if they have not been warned in advance that this could happen or if they think the induction was suggested for medical reasons.

6. Induced labors may cause contractions that are too long or too strong for the baby (or the pregnant person) to tolerate. Sometimes, the staff, in the desire for a fast labor, may begin with contractions that are much stronger than natural contractions and that could harm the baby. To detect such a problem, the pregnant person must have continuous electronic fetal monitoring (see page 249). To protect against this happening, you can ask the staff to start and increase the contractions gradually— more like a natural labor.

   If the laboring person's contractions are too strong for the baby to tolerate well, the nurse takes measures to stop them. If the laboring person is receiving intravenous Pitocin, the nurse can turn it off or turn it down; the contractions, usually, quickly subside. If the laboring person has had prostaglandin placed in the vagina, the nurse either removes the insert (Cervidil) or washes out the gel (Prepidil) or the tablet (Cytotec). If the pregnant person has swallowed a Cytotec tablet, another drug, such as Terbutaline, may be given to slow the contractions.

7. Use of pain medications early in the dilation process is more likely with induction, for several reasons:

   • The laboring person may be restricted from using comfort measures, such as changing positions, walking, and massage, by the intravenous line and the electronic fetal monitor's belts and cords.

   • Fatigue and discouragement over a slow onset of labor may lower the laboring person's motivation to deal with the contractions. They also may feel hungry, as they may not be allowed to eat before or while the Pitocin is being given.

(A request to eat lightly is a good item for the birth plan, though some hospitals routinely deny food in labor.)

- As said earlier, with induced labor, Pitocin may be given in high enough doses to cause stronger and more frequent contractions than those that usually occur in noninduced labors. Contractions in early labor (before 4 or 5 centimeters) may be more difficult to handle than if labor began spontaneously.

- If the pregnant person is hospitalized before contractions start, the labor seems much longer and slower than if labor begins at home where they can keep busy with normal activities. They might become concerned that labor is going too slowly and lose confidence in the ability to handle it.

Although medically indicated induction has some of the same disadvantages, knowing there is good reason for the induction makes these disadvantages more acceptable.

Alternatives to consider: If there is *no medical reason* for induction, you and the pregnant person can:

- Wait for spontaneous labor. If the pregnant person asks about postponing an elective induction, the caregiver may be willing to wait for labor to start on its own, at least until they are 1 to 2 weeks past the due date—as long as there is careful surveillance of the pregnant person's and baby's well-being.

- Try the nonmedical methods for stimulating labor contractions described on pages 212–217, "When Labor Must Start"

Episiotomy

An episiotomy is a surgical cut, made with scissors, from the vagina toward the anus shortly before delivery. Anesthesia may be given before the procedure, but, even if done without anesthesia, the birthing person is hardly aware of it. Strange as it may seem, rather than feeling pain, there is relief from the stretching and burning sensation when the episiotomy is performed. Local anesthesia is given after the birth to relieve pain that occurs when the episiotomy is stitched. The incision usually heals within 1 to 2 weeks, although pain at the site may linger, during physical exertion and intercourse, for weeks or, rarely, months. If there is still pain after a few weeks, consult the caregiver.

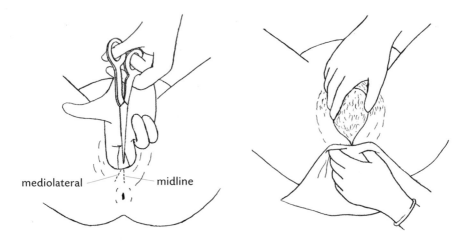

Episiotomy. The midline incision is most common in the United States.

Once routine, episiotomies are rarely performed by midwives; physicians also do far fewer now than in the early and mid-1990s. The main reason for doing an episiotomy was to avoid a tear in the perineum (the area between the vagina and the anus) or in the front of the vagina. Episiotomies became less common when scientific evidence showed that this rationale was unsupportable (see disadvantages, below).

Purposes of episiotomy are:

- To speed delivery by 5 to 10 minutes, if the baby appears severely compromised

- To reduce pressure on the baby's head, if the baby is premature or has other problems

- To enlarge a very tight vaginal opening, when necessary, to allow delivery. It is very rare that the vagina will not stretch adequately.

- To allow easier placement of forceps

Disadvantages of episiotomy: An episiotomy will *definitely* damage the birthing person's perineum—they will have a cut, stitches, a healing period, and some discomfort or pain. If no episiotomy is done, however, there is about a 30 to 60 percent chance that the birthing person's perineum will have a tear. Research indicates that spontaneous tears are almost always smaller, require fewer stitches, and are quicker to heal than the average episiotomy.

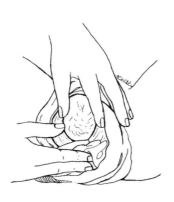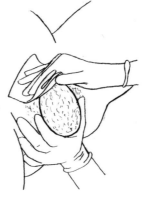

Normal delivery without episiotomy, with the birthing person on their side.
Left: The caregiver uses warm compresses to promote relaxation and circulation and gently supports the perineum. Right: With the birthing person rolled toward their side, the caregiver provides slight counterpressure as the baby's head emerges.

In addition, episiotomies sometimes *extend*—that is, after the cut is made, the pressure of the baby's head can enlarge the incision. This happens in approximately 1 person in 20. Spontaneous tears are rarely (fewer than 1 in 100) as large as extended episiotomies. In other words, the chance of a serious tear is greater *with* an episiotomy than without.

Alternatives to consider: The caregiver can simply forego an episiotomy, even if it appears that the birthing person may tear. They may incur no injury, one or several small tears, or, rarely, a tear as large as an average episiotomy (rarely larger).

The caregiver can protect the perineum from tearing seriously—for example, by placing warm compresses on the perineum, controlling the birth of the head and shoulders, suggesting positions that facilitate the baby's descent, and allowing spontaneous rather than directed bearing down (see "The Crowning and Birth Phase," page 127, and "Spontaneous Bearing Down," page 165).

You and the birthing person can improve the chance of an intact perineum after birth by doing prenatal perineal massage (see page 40).

Whether or not a birthing person ends up with a perineal tear or an episiotomy, exercising the pelvic floor muscles after birth seems to be very important to the recovery of pelvic floor tone; see page 38 for a discussion of the Kegel exercises.

Vacuum Extraction

Vacuum extraction is sometimes used during the birthing (second) stage of labor, only after the birthing person has pushed for a long time without progress. A plastic suction cup (about 3 inches, or 7.5 cm, in diameter) is placed in the vagina on the baby's head. The suction cup is connected to a handle and a pump that creates a safe level of suction. The caregiver pulls on the device attached to the baby's head while the uterus contracts and the birthing person pushes. Once the baby's head is out, the suction cup is removed and the birthing person pushes the baby out. An important safety measure is that the suction cup comes off if the caregiver pulls too hard, thus protecting the baby's head. If the vacuum doesn't succeed, a cesarean becomes necessary.

Vacuum extraction is done to assist or hasten delivery after the baby's head is in the birth canal. This procedure is **medically indicated** if:

- The birthing (second) stage of labor is prolonged because fatigue or anesthesia has made it difficult for the birthing person to push effectively.

- The birthing stage is prolonged because the baby's head is angled so it doesn't fit through the pelvis, and the birthing person's efforts need assistance.

- There is last-minute fetal distress.

Compared with forceps (see following), vacuum extraction less often requires an episiotomy, may cause less damage to the birthing person's vagina, and appears to be about equally safe for the baby.

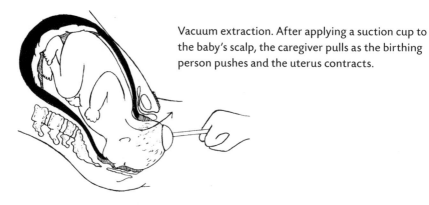

Vacuum extraction. After applying a suction cup to the baby's scalp, the caregiver pulls as the birthing person pushes and the uterus contracts.

Disadvantages of vacuum extraction are:

- Vacuum extraction frequently causes a fluid-filled lump and a bruise or abrasion on the baby's head where the suction cup was. It may take days or weeks for the lump to disappear.

- Serious injury to the baby's head is possible, though very unlikely when the vacuum extractor is used according to safety guidelines set by the Food and Drug Administration (FDA) and the obstetric profession.

- If the suction cup pops off during use, both the birth partner and the birthing person may be alarmed. Remember, it pops off to protect the baby from excessive strain.

Alternatives to consider:

- The birthing person can bear down (push) in different positions, such as squatting or standing (see "Positions and Movements for Labor and Birth," pages 169–176).

- Forceps can be used for delivery (see "Forceps Delivery," following).

- A cesarean delivery can be performed (see chapter 9).

Forceps Delivery

Forceps are used late in the birthing stage to deliver the baby more quickly. Two steel instruments, like spoons or salad tongs, are placed, one at a time, within the vagina on either side of the baby's head. They are then locked together into position so the forceps cannot squeeze the baby's head, no matter how hard the doctor grips the handles. This protects the baby's head from undue pressure. The doctor pulls during contractions while the birthing person pushes. Sometimes, forceps are used to rotate the baby's head.

A forceps delivery is **medically indicated** when birth is delayed because the birthing person is not able to push effectively; there is a decrease in uterine contractions; or the baby is large or poorly positioned.

Forceps are also medically indicated if the baby is distressed when low in the birth canal. If the baby is too high in the birth canal for the safe use of forceps, a cesarean delivery (see chapter 9) is a safer choice than forceps.

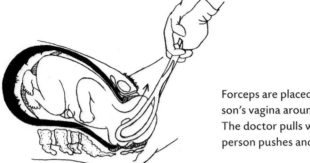

Forceps are placed in the birthing person's vagina around the baby's head. The doctor pulls while the birthing person pushes and the uterus contracts.

If a forceps delivery appears difficult, the attempt is abandoned, and a cesarean is performed.

Disadvantages of forceps delivery are:

• A forceps delivery usually requires an episiotomy and anesthesia.

• Forceps may bruise the baby's face or the side of the head.

• Though rare, forceps may injure the baby's head or neck, especially if used with excessive force and contrary to the professional guidelines for the safe use of forceps.

• Forceps may injure the birthing person's vagina.

Alternatives to consider:

• The birthing person can use directed pushing in positions that enlarge the pelvis, such as squatting with or without support, the dangle, rocking forward and back on hands and knees, or lying flat on their back and pulling the knees up toward the shoulders (see "Positions and Movements for Labor and Birth," pages 169–176 and "Directed Pushing," page 167).

• The caregiver can monitor the baby and birthing person; if both are doing well, they can give the labor more time.

• The caregiver can use vacuum extraction (see page 266). The choice between forceps and vacuum extraction is best made by the doctor, according to training and expertise.

• The caregiver can attempt a forceps delivery once or twice, but, if it appears the baby is not moving, the caregiver can remove the forceps and prepare for a cesarean.

- The doctor can perform a cesarean delivery. This is the only alternative if vacuum extraction does not work and a forceps delivery is not appropriate.

In summary, the purpose of medical interventions is to improve birth outcomes for the birthing person and baby. Most interventions carry some risks or disadvantages along with benefits. Therefore, they should be used only when needed.

Except in emergency circumstances, there is usually more than one way to accomplish the intended purpose of any proposed intervention. For this reason, you and the birthing person will want to be prepared to make informed choices about what options might be used and when.

CHAPTER 7

COMPLICATIONS IN LATE PREGNANCY, LABOR, OR AFTERWARD

The labor went really well. I was so proud of Bess. As she held our sweet little Todd, though, her bleeding got worse. She lost a lot of blood. We're so thankful the doctor took care of it quickly, and that both Bess and Todd are fine. But I'm pregnant now, and that scary time haunts me.

—MAUREEN, FIRST-TIME CO-MOTHER

This chapter discusses a number of complications that may arise before, during, or after labor, how they are treated, and how you can help the laboring person if they occur. More serious than the difficulties discussed in chapter 5, these complications require hospitalization and medical assistance for a good outcome. They fall into four major categories: problems with the laboring person; problems with the labor; problems with the fetus; and problems with the newborn.

As you can imagine, the laboring person will be upset, worried, shocked, stunned, frightened, anxious, or even suspicious if serious problems arise—and so will you. You both may have difficulty accepting that there is a problem, especially if they feel normal, as is often the case with gestational diabetes, high blood pressure, or threatened preterm labor (when contractions often feel quite mild; see page 70). It is hard to cope with much more than labor itself, and they may rely on you to assume the responsibility for decision–making.

If the situation is serious and a quick decision must be made, the single most important question to ask the caregiver is: Will this (procedure, medicine, or treatment) improve our chances for a healthy birthing person and baby after the birth?

If the answer is yes, give up some priorities. If no, you have time to consider options, using the Key Questions for Informed Decision-Making (page 237).

As the birth partner, you can help in the following ways:

- Learn what is happening, why it is a problem, how serious it is, and the rationale for and the expected results of any corrective action to be taken. Ask the caregiver the key questions (page 237), adding the most important question just noted. Help the pregnant person understand the answers.

- Remain assertive and cooperative with the caregiver. Inform the staff of the laboring person's wishes and learn any alternative ways of handling the problem. Use the birth plan (see page 45) as your guide.

- Recognize the need to accept the caregiver's judgment without discussion if there is a true emergency—when time is of the utmost importance.

- Help the pregnant person adjust to the need for a change in management. If the birth plan reflects the understanding that complications sometimes arise unexpectedly, they will realize a departure from some previous preferences is warranted to ensure a good outcome for both the baby and themselves. A doula can help you both ask the right questions, adjust to the change in management, and maintain perspective.

- Remain with the laboring person throughout. When things go wrong, they need your help and support more than ever.

- Afterwards, allow them time to recover emotionally. You will also need time to recover.

Complications for the Pregnant Person

This section includes explanations of complications and why they are problematic; descriptions of the ways each might be managed; how the pregnant person may react; and how you can help. If complications arise, this information may be useful as the two of you discuss them with your caregiver.

Priorities for Childbirth

Every parent-to-be cares about their baby's birth and how it will go. Preferences vary among expectant parents, and some place a higher priority on some things than other people would. For example, whether the baby is born vaginally or by cesarean; whether the labor is induced or starts on its own; whether the laboring person prefers medications over self-help and nonmedical ways to manage the pain; and many more. Some priorities are more important than others—a healthy birthing person and a healthy baby trump all others. Please remember that while all your priorities are important, you must be ready and willing to give up some, if safety or well-being is at stake.

Most people agree with the following priorities for their birth and the baby. They want:

• A healthy full-term pregnancy

• Spontaneous onset of labor

• A normal labor pattern without need for interventions

• Use or nonuse of medications as planned (and no undesirable side effects if medications are used)

• Spontaneous vaginal birth in the desired location

• Successful breast-feeding

• Healthy birthing person and a healthy baby after the birth

Unfortunately, childbirth is not always controllable or predictable, and some of these outcomes do not materialize. This can be surprising and disappointing for parents and caregivers. For example, premature labor sometimes occurs unexpectedly. Sometimes, risk factors develop during pregnancy or during labor in the pregnant person or fetus, making induction, medications, forceps, a vacuum extractor, or even cesarean delivery necessary. If pain medications are planned, a very fast labor or an anesthesiologist who has other laboring people waiting for anesthesia may mean the laboring person does not get medication when desired. If an unmedicated labor is planned but labor is very long or complicated, pain medications may become necessary. Challenges in breast-feeding, such as weight loss in the baby or insurmountable problems for the new parent, may mean the baby needs formula.

Sometimes, the pregnant person or couples cannot have all their other priorities met because their most important priority—**a healthy birthing person and healthy baby after the birth**—requires accepting some interventions they hadn't previously wanted.

Premature Labor

Labor is premature if it begins before 37 weeks of pregnancy (see "Signs of Labor," page 67, for an explanation of signs of premature labor). If a pregnant person suspects they are having premature labor, call their caregiver for a diagnosis and advice. Early treatment sometimes stops premature labor. Babies born prematurely are at greater risk for a number of medical problems, such as breathing difficulties, jaundice, infection, difficulty maintaining body temperature, and feeding problems.

Management of premature labor depends on the baby's gestational age, well-being, and stage of development. Measures may include the following:

- Vaginal exam to determine how much the cervix has dilated

- Assessment of contractions (how long, strong, and frequent they are)

- Attempts to stop labor using bed rest and medications such as terbutaline, ritodrine, indomethacin, naproxen, nifedipine, or others. Treatment is more likely to be effective if the cervix has not dilated beyond 2 centimeters.

- Amniocentesis and testing of the amniotic fluid to indicate whether the baby's lungs are mature, that is, capable of breathing without difficulty after birth. This helps the caregiver determine how aggressively to try to stop the labor.

- Medications (corticosteroids) given to the pregnant person via injection to hasten the maturation of the baby's lungs and prevent respiratory distress syndrome, if birth cannot be postponed and the baby's lungs are immature

- Electronic fetal monitoring to detect contractions and track the fetal heart rate responses to contractions

- Assessment for infections that sometimes cause premature labor (including, among other organisms, Group B strep, described on page 240). The pregnant person is treated with antibiotics if there are signs of infection.

- If delivery cannot be postponed, transport of the pregnant person to a hospital with an intensive-care nursery, especially if the baby will be born very early (at less than 33 weeks' gestation)

- Summoning of a pediatrician or neonatologist to care for the baby immediately after the delivery

- If delivery is successfully postponed, the pregnant person may be sent home on medication and asked to reduce activity or remain on bed rest until 36 weeks or so.

How the Pregnant Person May React

Both you and the pregnant person will be eager to do everything possible to help the baby get a healthy start in life. The pregnant person may feel guilt and self-blame that, in some way, they caused the contractions or if reduced activity or bed rest prevents them from doing their share of running the household. They may feel concerned about adding pressure on you. They may worry how a lengthy period of bed rest will affect their strength and fitness (if so, the caregivers may be able to recommend a physical therapist who can visit your home and teach some safe in-bed exercises). The pregnant person may become very bored lying around all the time.

How You Can Help

Do not add to their feelings of guilt. Take on added responsibilities cheerfully; consider them your contribution to your baby's and the pregnant person's health and well-being. Ease your burden by getting household help, if possible. Encourage the pregnant person to shop for the baby by catalog or online. They might communicate with others on bed rest via the internet, too (see Recommended Resources, page 418).

This is also a good time for them to read books and watch videos on baby care and feeding. Their childbirth educator or public library may have such videos available. YouTube and other websites also are good sources.

High Blood Pressure

About 5 percent of pregnant people have chronic high blood pressure, or hypertension, that begins either before or soon after becoming pregnant. This condition needs to be monitored carefully throughout pregnancy. Medications may be necessary, and they may need occasional adjustment.

Five to 8 percent of pregnant people develop high blood pressure (over 140/90 in two consecutive readings) after 20 weeks of pregnancy. They are said to have gestational hypertension (GH), also called pregnancy-induced hypertension (PIH), which is usually mild. Mild GH may be accompanied by swelling in the legs, hands, and face and protein in the urine. The caregiver monitors it carefully. The condition usually goes away after birth, but sometimes it becomes more severe during labor.

More severe GH, or chronic hypertension, can be scary. In addition to the swelling and protein in their urine, the pregnant person may have blurring or spots in their vision, upper abdominal pain, headaches, increased reflexes (that is, when the knee is tapped, the foot jerks more than usual), and liver and kidney problems (the last are detected by a blood test). The function of the placenta may be impaired, and this may slow the baby's growth. If the GH is very severe, the pregnant person may experience convulsions. Very rarely, women die from this condition. The complications arising from severe GH are referred to by the terms *preeclampsia*, *eclampsia*, *toxemia*, and *HELLP syndrome* (HELLP stands for hemolysis [breakdown of red blood cells], elevated liver enzymes, and low platelets, which interfere with the body's ability to clot blood).

Management of High Blood Pressure During Pregnancy

Measures may include:

- Reduction or modification of activity (reducing exercise, quitting work, or reducing work hours) or bed rest. The number of hours of bed rest each day depends on the severity of the GH and the caregiver's belief in the value of bed rest. Opinions vary a lot, while research findings on the benefit of total versus partial bed rest indicate that complete bed rest is rarely necessary.

- Medications to lower blood pressure, magnesium sulfate to prevent convulsions, or both. Hospitalization may be required. Some medications used to control chronic hypertension are unsafe for the unborn baby, so the caregiver may switch the pregnant person to another that is safer.

- Close monitoring of the pregnant person's blood pressure and other signs of worsening GH (through blood and urine tests, checking reflexes, tests of fetal growth and well-being, and weight checks)

- Induction of labor, or even a cesarean, if the condition worsens

Management of High Blood Pressure During Labor

Measures may include:

- Restriction to left-sided bed rest. Some caregivers allow a warm shower or bath from time to time during labor, as these also lower blood pressure.

- Continuous electronic fetal monitoring and intravenous fluids

- Frequent blood-pressure checks

- Medications to lower blood pressure and magnesium sulfate to prevent convulsions, if the condition is severe

- Intravenous Pitocin (see page 258), if magnesium sulfate is used, as the latter drug slows labor. Pitocin also may be used to induce labor.

How the Pregnant Person May React

During pregnancy, the pregnant person may feel:

- Disbelief, because many people with mild, or even moderate, GH feel fine. They may not want to comply with orders to quit work or reduce activity or stay in bed. They may feel the doctor is overreacting.

- Relief, if they can quit or cut down at work, especially if it has become tiring or stressful

- Worried, when they learn some of the possible serious consequences for themselves and the baby if the condition cannot be controlled

During labor, the pregnant person may feel:

- Disappointment over the required interventions, especially induction of labor (see page 256), restriction to bed, and electronic fetal monitoring (see page 249).

- Discomfort from the effects of medications, especially magnesium sulfate, which may make them twitch, sweat, and feel hot, flushed, and nervous. Blood pressure medications may also have uncomfortable side effects: headaches, nausea, drowsiness, shortness of breath, and trouble urinating.

How You Can Help

Empathize with the pregnant person and help them focus on what they must do—for their welfare and the baby's. Discuss the comfort measures they can use (see "When the Birthing Person Must Labor in Bed," page 224). Severe GH is a serious condition and requires cooperation from both of you. Remain informed of their condition, the baby's well-being, and treatments.

Gestational Diabetes Mellitus (GDM)

Gestational diabetes mellitus (GDM), also called glucose intolerance or simply gestational diabetes, first appears during pregnancy and is a potentially serious disorder regarding how the pregnant body adjusts to the increased glucose load that normally occurs in pregnancy to support fetal growth. The result is extra-high blood glucose levels in the pregnant person, which can increase the chances of urinary tract infections, preterm labor, a large baby, and stillbirth. The newborn is also at added risk (see page 278). Early detection and appropriate treatment help prevent these problems.

For that reason, pregnant people are offered a two-step test to detect gestational diabetes. At 26 to 28 weeks, most pregnant people take the diabetes screening test, which involves drinking a sugary beverage and having blood drawn to assess it for blood sugar. This simple, inexpensive test identifies most who have low blood glucose and do not have GDM. Those whose blood glucose levels are high on the screening test then take the diagnostic test, which is the more accurate 3-hour glucose tolerance test; they have their blood drawn before drinking the same sugary beverage and then have blood drawn three more times over the next 3 hours. If blood sugar is still high at these readings, they have gestational diabetes. However, most who have high blood glucose on the screening test do *not* have high readings in the 3-hour glucose tolerance test and thus do not have GDM.

The mainstay of treatment is a very healthy, individualized, and tightly controlled low-sugar and low-carbohydrate diet combined with regular exercise. This may be all that is necessary to keep blood sugar levels normal. If not, the pregnant person may also need to take insulin.

Management of Gestational Diabetes During Pregnancy

Besides diet and exercise, the caregiver may recommend these measures:

- Frequent blood sugar testing with a special glucose meter by the pregnant person at home; high readings are reported to the caregiver.

- Consultations with a dietitian for guidance and support in the special diet

- Fetal movement counting (see page 43)

- Close monitoring of fetal growth and well-being with ultrasound, nonstress tests, and other tests

- Self-administered insulin injections, if necessary, to control blood sugar levels

Concerns for the Baby

Especially if the pregnant person's blood sugar is not well controlled, the baby's organ systems are at increased risk for uneven development because of inadequate insulin production. Effects may include:

- Large size (because of excess glucose that crosses the placenta to the baby) and associated increased risk of difficult birth

- Low blood sugar at birth due to the sudden drop in glucose from the pregnant person that occurs at birth

- Prolonged jaundice, possibly due to liver immaturity at birth

- Respiratory problems, due to developmental immaturity of the lungs, despite the baby's large size

Gestational diabetes is managed with the goal of preventing these complications. A neonatologist or pediatrician is usually present at the birth to observe and care for the newborn. The prognosis for the baby is very good when the pregnant person's diabetes is well controlled.

Management of Gestational Diabetes During Labor and Afterward

Measures may include:

- Induction of labor at 38 or 39 weeks, or earlier if blood sugar is not well controlled

- Greater likelihood of a cesarean, especially if the baby seems to be very large

- Frequent checks of the pregnant person's blood sugar during labor

- Intravenous administration of glucose or insulin, depending on whether the pregnant person's blood sugar is high from too little insulin or low from too much. Insulin levels are sometimes challenging to control.

- Frequent checks of the newborn's blood sugar until levels are normal

- Management of low blood sugar in the postpartum person or baby after birth

- Treatment of respiratory problems, jaundice, and other problems in the baby that result from gestational diabetes

- Subsequent checks of the postpartum person's blood sugar because people who have had gestational diabetes are at increased risk of developing type 2 diabetes at a later age

How the Pregnant Person May React

During labor, the pregnant person may feel:

- Disbelief they are ill, especially if feeling fine

- Disappointment over the added interventions

- Worry about the baby

- Helpless or unable to understand the complexities of the treatment

How You Can Help

• Learn about gestational diabetes and any options the pregnant person may have (see Recommended Resources, page 418).

• Encourage the pregnant person to ask the Key Questions for Informed Decision-Making (see page 237).

• Help them understand and adjust to the demands of their diet and blood sugar testing regimen and to the necessary interventions they will experience during labor.

• Emphasize the things they can do to help themselves in labor, rather than dwelling on all the things they cannot do.

Herpes Lesion

If the pregnant person has or has ever had genital herpes, which causes sores to appear in the genital area, they should report this to the caregiver. If the virus is active when labor begins, the baby could contract the virus during vaginal birth. Though rare, herpes in the newborn is very serious; it frequently causes brain damage and death. If the herpes has been present for a long time, the risk that a sore during labor could give the baby herpes is about 1 to 3 percent; the risk is much higher if the pregnant person has recently acquired herpes.

In an effort to prevent herpes outbreaks in late pregnancy, many caregivers offer antiviral medication (such as acyclovir or valacyclovir) during the last weeks of pregnancy to all pregnant people who have ever had herpes sores. Such treatment has resulted in a great decrease in the number of newborns who acquire the disease. A person who has not had an outbreak in years may reasonably refuse the medication, but a person who has had one or more recent outbreaks may be wise to accept it.

Complementary measures that may reduce the incidence of symptoms include reducing stress and maintaining a balanced diet. If one has a herpes outbreak at or near term, the caregiver will recommend taking acyclovir, which can shorten the duration and severity of the outbreak (and perhaps protect the baby). These drugs are not associated with birth defects or other adverse effects in the baby. The caregiver may also offer to induce labor at a time when no sore is present.

Management During Labor for the Pregnant Person with a History of Herpes

At the hospital, the caregiver may:

- Carefully inspect the genital area for the presence of a sore

- Culture the pregnant person's vaginal secretions for asymptomatic presence of the virus

- Perform a cesarean to prevent the baby from coming into contact with a sore, if one is present

    If no sore is visible but the culture indicates the herpes virus was present, the baby will be treated with acyclovir. Or, the baby may be tested for herpes and treated only if the test indicates the baby is infected.

How the Pregnant Person May React

The pregnant person will probably be disappointed, shocked, angry, or depressed when learning they have an active herpes lesion, especially if it was unexpected. Expect them to need time, support, and, perhaps, counseling afterward to deal with the disappointment over any changes in plans for the birth or any problems in the baby caused by the herpes.

How You Can Help

- Give the pregnant person an opportunity to express their anger or disappointment.

- Give them time to adjust to the need for medications.

- Try not to become defensive if you were the source of the herpes. Your defensiveness will prolong their anger and postpone their adjustment to the cesarean.

- Explore ways to make the cesarean more satisfying (see page 353).

Excessive Bleeding During Labor

Most bleeding during labor comes from the site of the placenta, when it begins to separate from the uterine wall. The amount of visible bleeding and the seriousness of the problem depend on where and how extensive the separation is and whether the bleeding is concealed, that is, blood does not flow out. If the placenta is very low in the uterus and covers the cervix fully or partially (this condition is called placenta previa), blood comes out of the vagina. If the placenta is high in the uterus when it begins to separate (this condition is called placental abruption), the uterus may become very firm between contractions and the laboring person is in constant pain (rather than the intermittent pain that normally comes with contractions). In either case, both pregnant person and baby are in danger; *potentially, this is an acute emergency.*

Left: placenta previa; right: placental abruption

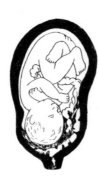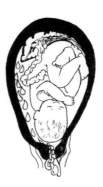

Management of Bleeding During Labor

This complication is managed in the following ways:

- If severe bleeding begins early in labor or before labor begins, a cesarean delivery is probable. The pregnant person may receive a general anesthetic if blood loss is rapid; the anesthetic quickly puts the pregnant person to sleep for the surgery. If there is time, a spinal block, which allows the pregnant person to remain conscious, is used.

- If severe bleeding begins late in labor or if bleeding begins in early labor but is not severe and the baby is not in distress, the doctor or midwife may monitor the baby's heart rate continuously. If the baby's heart rate remains normal, a vaginal birth may be possible.

How the Pregnant Person May React

During labor, the pregnant person may:

- Be caught off guard

- Be frightened for their health and the baby's health over abnormal bleeding, leaving other priorities irrelevant

- Feel very nervous about waiting and preoccupied with the baby's condition

- Wonder whether the caregiver is overreacting

How You Can Help

- Remain well informed about the severity of the bleeding and the baby's condition. Share the information with the pregnant person.

- Continue supporting the laboring person during contractions and remind them to deal with each contraction as it comes, not fret about what may happen.

- Be prepared to comply with changes in management and help the pregnant person comply, if the baby shows signs of distress.

Excessive Bleeding After Birth (Postpartum Hemorrhage)

Some bleeding immediately after birth is normal; it comes from the area in the uterus where the placenta was attached. The uterus usually contracts vigorously after birth, causing the bleeding to subside. You may be surprised, though, at how much blood there seems to be even under normal circumstances. Losing as much as 2 cups (475 ml) of blood is considered normal.

Postpartum hemorrhage, or excessive bleeding immediately after birth, usually occurs for one of three reasons: relaxation of the uterus, a retained placenta or fragments of placenta, or lacerations in the vagina or cervix. The loss of blood may cause the just-birthed person's blood pressure to drop; the skin may become clammy, and they may feel faint. To remedy the low blood pressure, they will be asked to lie flat, with their head low, and they will be given intravenous fluids, possibly containing a drug to raise the blood pressure.

For a few weeks after someone gives birth, they experience a dwindling discharge, called *lochia*. This fluid is composed of blood and some of the tissue that lined the uterus during pregnancy. Lochia is like a longer-than-usual menstrual period.

Management of Bleeding After Birth

If the uterus relaxes after the birth, it leaves the blood vessels open at the placental site. When the uterus is made to contract, it will squeeze these vessels closed and the bleeding will stop.

As a preventive measure, many caregivers routinely inject synthetic oxytocin (Pitocin), or administer it through an IV, as the baby is being born or immediately afterward, without waiting to see how much blood loss there is. Research has found that, under usual conditions in the hospital, this practice has lowered the incidence of postpartum hemorrhage significantly.

After birth, the caregiver may vigorously massage the low abdomen to make the uterus contract. The massage can be painful for the person who gave birth, but it is the quickest way to get the uterus to contract.

If there is excessive bleeding, with or without the preventive administration of Pitocin, the caregiver may inject Pitocin or Methergine into the birthing person's thigh or have you or the nurse stimulate the laboring person's nipples to increase the body's secretion of oxytocin.

If the placenta or parts of it are retained, there may be excessive blood loss. The caregiver manually removes the placenta or the placental fragments. This is very painful, so intravenous narcotics or an inhaled anesthetic gas may be given first. If, however, the procedure will be quick, the birthing person may be given the option of going without pain medication to save time. If manual removal fails, surgery is required to clean out the uterus and close off the large blood vessels or, in rare but very serious, life-threatening cases, to remove the uterus.

If there are lacerations in the vagina or cervix, the lacerations are sutured.

If the birthing person has lost a significant amount of blood, they may receive transfusions of blood or other fluids to restore the blood volume.

How the Birthing Person May React

The birthing person may:

• Fail to realize, at first, how serious the blood loss is

• Feel weak or faint if a large amount of blood is lost

• Become frightened if bleeding continues and urgent measures are taken to stop it

The Breech Presentation

See page 226 for a discussion of managing the breech presentation.

Complications with Labor Progress

The caregiver or nurse regularly observes and records the progress of labor. They perform vaginal exams to determine changes in the cervix and in the position and station of the fetus. They also observe the quality of the contractions (frequency, duration, and intensity) and the laboring person's reactions to them. Two situations that may signal problems are very rapid progress and slow progress.

Very Rapid Progress

When contractions are exceptionally efficient or unusually powerful or when the cervix is exceptionally yielding, labor may progress rapidly. Although not usually considered a complication, a fast labor may present clinical challenges and be extremely painful and frightening for the laboring person.

Main Concerns of the Caregiver

These are:

• Getting the laboring person to the hospital or birth center in time (or, in the case of a home birth, getting the caregiver to the home in time) to care for them adequately

• How well the fetus tolerates the powerful, frequent contractions

• Possible damage to the birthing person's perineum during a rapid birth

• The newborn's adjustment afterward. Breathing problems and head trauma may be more likely as a result of this kind of birth.

Management of Very Rapid Labor

This involves:

• Supporting and reassuring the birthing person

• Placing the birthing person on their side or on hands and knees (gravity-neutral positions) to avoid speeding labor

• Monitoring the fetal heart to assess the baby's response to the contractions and, possibly, using interventions (changing the laboring person's position, giving oxygen) to improve oxygenation

• Attempting to control the speed of delivery by coaching the birthing person not to bear down and by applying manual pressure against the rapidly emerging head

How You Can Help

See "The Very Rapid Labor," pages 207.

Arrest of Active Labor (Dystocia)

By the time the cervix dilates to 6 centimeters, the cervix is usually quite thin and ready to open more easily. So, even if it has taken many hours, or even a day or two, to reach this point (see "The Slow-to-Start Labor," page 216), dilation now usually speeds up. Sometimes, though, it does not. Dilation may be very slow (this is called *protracted labor*) or it may seem to stop for 2 or more hours (this is called *arrested labor*).

The reasons for a delay in the active phase are more likely to be serious than are the reasons for a slow prelabor or a slow latent phase. It is not always possible to determine why labor is delayed, nor is it possible to know just how serious the delay is until time has passed.

Slow progress is not necessarily a problem, but an arrest of labor is a concern for the caregiver as well as the parents. The caregiver begins to worry that the laboring person is becoming exhausted, especially if they have tried everything and there is no end in sight. At some point, the caregiver begins to think the labor should be sped up. This is when the laboring person crosses the line from having a difficult labor, as described in chapter 5, to having a complicated labor—one requiring medical intervention.

Causes of Arrest in Active Labor

The delay may be due to one cause or a combination of causes, such as:

- Poor fit between the baby's head and the laboring person's pelvis: This condition is sometimes called cephalopelvic disproportion, or CPD. *Cephalo* means head, and in the case of CPD, the baby's head will not fit through the pelvis, despite the measures suggested on page 221 in chapter 5. The head may not fit because it is simply too large for the pelvis or more likely because it is positioned in a way that doesn't fit (occiput posterior, see page 66), chin tipped up, to the side, or back.

- Inadequate contractions: They lose intensity, slow down, or become shorter in duration. Or, they do progress, but remain too weak, too infrequent, or both.

- Exhaustion, dehydration, excessive fear, or tension in the laboring person

Management of Delay in Labor

The caregiver tries to determine the cause or causes of the delay by assessing the laboring person's contractions, cervix, size and position of the baby, and the laboring person's physical and emotional state.

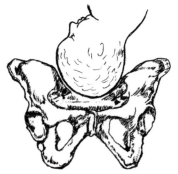

A poor fit between the baby's head and the pregnant person's pelvis

Many things can be done to speed a prolonged labor and to support the laboring person undergoing it. You both can do some of these things (see pages 221–224); others must be done by the nurses and caregiver.

During the prolonged labor, the **caregiver** may:

- Monitor the fetal heart rate more often, or continuously, to help determine whether the baby is tolerating the delay

- Offer the laboring person a narcotic or an epidural to reduce pain and help them relax, especially if they are exhausted. With an epidural or, to a lesser extent, a narcotic, they may be able to sleep, and progress may resume.

- Start intravenous fluids in the hope that improved hydration and some calories might reenergize the uterus

- Rupture the membranes in hopes of speeding labor (see page 254)

- Use intravenous oxytocin (Pitocin) to stimulate contractions if they appear to be decreasing or inadequate to change the cervix or the baby's position (see page 258)

- Use an intrauterine pressure catheter (internal electronic fetal monitoring) to find out just how strong the contractions are or whether Pitocin improves them

- Use forceps or a vacuum extractor (see pages 266–269) if the delay occurs in the birthing (second) stage

- Recommend a cesarean delivery if there is no progress even with the passage of considerable time and after efforts have been made to correct the problem (see chapter 9)

How the Laboring Person May React

The laboring person may:

- Be willing to try suggested measures to improve progress

- Feel exhausted and discouraged if nothing seems to work

- Want a break and ask for an epidural, even if they originally wanted to avoid one (see page 330 for discussion of the code word)

- Need acknowledgment of their great efforts and validation that this labor is unusually difficult

- Fear something is wrong with their body or the fetus

- Be ready for Pitocin, a cesarean, or anything that will end the labor and bring the baby

How You Can Help

You can help the laboring person during an arrest of labor in these ways:

- Confer with the doula or nurse on suggestions to help the laboring person

- If the laboring person hasn't tried them yet, suggest the measures discussed in chapter 5 (see "Slow Progress in Active Labor and the Birthing Stage," pages 221–224 and "Nipple Stimulation," pages 213–215). They may not have thought of a bath, changing positions, or labor-stimulating measures.

- If tired and discouraged, the laboring person may be reluctant to do things to make the contractions more intense. Consider their prior preferences regarding the use of pain medications (see pages 327–329). An epidural under these circumstances may allow them to sleep while the contractions intensify and (hopefully) progress to vaginal birth.

- Be attentive and understanding of the laboring person's emotional state during an exhausting labor. If they feel ignored when they express discouragement, they may later feel they were alone or unheard by you or others (see "A Previous Disappointing or Traumatic Birth Experience," page 231).

- Take care of your own needs. Eat, rest, and refresh yourself by washing your face and brushing your teeth, but do not leave the laboring person unless someone else (a doula, friend, or relative) is with them to help.

How a Doula Helps

A doula can be a huge help during a long or exhausting labor. When you and the laboring person are tired and discouraged, the doula, who has been in such situations before, knows that labors such as this can change at any time. If the baby is malpositioned, for example, they have witnessed situations where other babies did change position and labor progress improved. This experience helps the doula remain patient, hopeful, and able to give you and the laboring person incentive to keep going with movements, position changes, and comfort measures and not give up too soon.

Of course, a doula is realistic and would not push the laboring person beyond where they are willing to go. The doula knows some labors will not be correctable and can help you and the laboring person recognize this while also recognizing you did everything you could. When you and the laboring person look back on the labor, you can both feel very good about the role you played in the difficult labor.

Complications with the Fetus

The ability of the fetus to tolerate labor varies. Usually, labor benefits the baby by facilitating alertness, respiration, temperature regulation, and suckling. Sometimes, however, conditions that existed prior to labor interfere with the fetus's or newborn's well-being. The laboring person's caregiver watches for signs that the fetus is not tolerating labor well and that interventions may be needed.

Prolapsed Cord

On very rare occasions, the umbilical cord prolapses—that is, slips below the baby into or through the cervix. This can occur before or during labor, and it is a *true obstetric emergency* that can result in the baby's death if not promptly and correctly managed. The danger is this: If the cord prolapses, it can be pinched by the baby's head at the cervix. This obstructs blood flow through the cord and deprives the baby of oxygen. The baby can survive only a few minutes without oxygen.

Signs to Recognize

A prolapsed cord is rare under any circumstances, but is most likely to happen if two conditions are present—the baby is in a breech presentation (buttocks or feet down) or the head is high or off the cervix *and* the bag of waters suddenly breaks with a gush, either spontaneously or because the caregiver ruptured it. With this combination, the cord may slip down around the baby's head or buttocks as the fluid escapes; then the baby, who has been "floating," presses on the cord, slowing or stopping blood flow to the placenta and oxygen to the baby.

A cord prolapse is extremely unlikely when the baby is already low in the pelvis and the head or buttocks are already pressing against the cervix.

Management of a Prolapsed Cord

The caregiver gets the laboring person into the open knee–chest position and places a hand in the vagina to hold the baby off the cord. A cesarean section is performed as soon as possible. With this rapid action, the baby will likely be born in good health.

CAUTION:

In late pregnancy, at each appointment, the pregnant person should ask the caregiver whether the baby is high and floating, low in the pelvis, or pressed against the cervix. A vaginal exam is not needed to determine this. The caregiver can palpate the abdomen to feel the location of the baby's head.

The pregnant person should also ask, "If my bag of waters breaks with a gush with my baby at this level, should I be concerned about a prolapsed cord?" If the caregiver says yes, and the bag of waters later does break with a gush of fluid, you both should take the following measures just in case the cord has prolapsed:

- Call the caregiver and hospital. If you or someone else can't drive the pregnant person to the hospital immediately, call 911 and say that the pregnant person's bag of waters has broken. To ensure a rapid response, indicate there may be a prolapsed cord (even though chances are small).

- With your help, the pregnant person should get onto their hands and knees and then drop their chest down to the floor or bed. This open knee–chest position uses gravity to move the baby away from the cervix and off the cord.

- Go immediately to the hospital. Before the pregnant person stands to walk to the car, move the car close to the door of the house, move the front seat forward, and open the back door of the car for them.

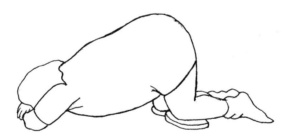

- The pregnant person should ride in the back seat, or in the ambulance, in the open knee–chest position, with their buttocks high. Drive carefully, but wasting no time, to the hospital emergency entrance. Leave the laboring person in the car in the open knee–chest position. Go in and tell the person on duty that the pregnant person's bag of waters broke and you think they may have a prolapsed cord. The pregnant person should remain in the open knee–chest position on a stretcher until a doctor or nurse can listen to the fetal heart rate. If the heart rate is normal, as it most likely will be, you can all relax and rejoice. If, however, the cord had prolapsed, this could save the baby's life.

How the Pregnant Person May React

They may:

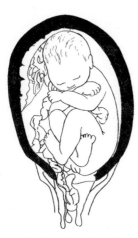

Prolapsed cord with a breech baby

- Feel excited that the bag of waters has broken because this is a sign of labor

- Feel reluctant to get into the open knee–chest position for the ride to the hospital, thinking they are being overly dramatic

- Be willing to go straight to the hospital but insist on sitting up for the ride

- Feel frightened that the baby may be in danger and willing to do whatever will improve the odds for the baby

- Feel they know just what to do because they have asked the caregiver whether the baby was high or low in the pelvis and whether they should be concerned about a prolapsed cord if the bag of waters should break with a gush before labor

How You Can Help

As scary as all this is, the odds of a prolapsed cord, even if the baby is high or breech *and* the bag of waters breaks with a gush are low—perhaps 1 in 100. In the event of a cord prolapse, however, your and the pregnant person's actions will be most important; time and their position are the crucial factors in the baby's well-being. Cooperate with the hospital staff in whatever way possible.

Fetal Heart Rate Problems

Although a healthy baby has a remarkable ability to compensate for temporary oxygen deficits during labor, brain damage can occur if oxygen deprivation is severe and continues too long or if the baby has another problem that reduces the ability to compensate.

Fetal distress means the unborn baby is receiving less oxygen than normal and is showing signs of having to adjust physiologically. The terms *indeterminate* or *nonreassuring fetal heart tones* and *fetal intolerance of labor* are preferred today by physicians over the term *fetal distress* because they are more precise in quantifying the severity of the condition. Indeterminate heart tones are not as concerning as intolerance of labor. It means the heart tones are not clearly normal or abnormal. They will watch closely for any change that could clarify the situation. You may hear any of these terms used by the staff to express concern for the baby's well-being.

Diagnosing Fetal Distress

At present, the two main indicators of fetal distress are the fetal heart rate and the presence of meconium in the amniotic fluid. They are assessed in the following ways:

- **Auscultation:** A nurse or midwife listens to the fetal heart rate with a fetal stethoscope or an ultrasound fetoscope at frequent intervals during labor (see page 252). This requires the nurse or midwife to remain by the bedside much of the time.

- **Characteristics of the amniotic fluid:** If the bag of waters breaks spontaneously or is broken by the caregiver (see page 71), the amniotic fluid is examined for the presence of meconium, which might indicate fetal distress.

- **Electronic fetal monitoring (EFM; see page 249):** This traces the fetal heart rate, as well as the strength of the laboring person's contractions. The nurse or midwife observes the monitor tracings in the laboring person's room or, possibly, at the nurses' station.

Remember, if EFM indicates fetal distress, this does not necessarily mean the baby is in trouble. It may only mean the baby is compensating for a temporary oxygen deficiency by slowing the heart rate to spare oxygen use. In other words, the baby may either be in trouble or adjusting well to the decrease in oxygen.

To evaluate whether the baby really is in trouble, the caregiver may want to check the fetus's present condition with the simple fetal scalp stimulation test (see page 253) to determine if the baby is still doing well.

Management of Fetal Distress

If monitoring indicates the fetus may be in distress, the nurse or caregiver may do any or all of the following:

- Try to correct the fetal distress by having the laboring person breathe extra oxygen through a mask. The oxygen is carried via the bloodstream to the placenta and through the cord to the baby.

- Have the laboring person change position to relieve pressure on the umbilical cord, which may be causing the fetal distress

- Discontinue any drugs that might be causing the distress, such as high doses of Pitocin, which can cause contractions that are too long or too strong, or narcotics, which may affect the fetal heart rate. During such contractions, oxygen flow through the placenta may be reduced.

- Give a drug to slow contractions (see page 332)

- Call for further testing: a change from external to internal monitoring (the latter is more accurate) or the fetal scalp stimulation test

- If the fetal distress appears to be severe, immediately deliver the baby vaginally, with forceps or vacuum extraction (possibly with an episiotomy), or by cesarean. The choice of delivery method depends on how close the laboring person is to giving birth.

The truth is, there is no technology that can give a clear and accurate indication of how well a baby is doing at the moment or is likely to be doing in the next hours. In a risky situation, most caregivers (and parents) are less inclined to be patient and "wait and see" whether the baby will remain stable and healthy. They are more inclined to act quickly before the condition becomes an emergency.

How the Laboring Person May React

The laboring person is likely to react in these ways:

- Fright and shock when told the baby shows signs of fetal distress

- Accept the caregiver's decisions—no questions—under these circumstances

- After delivery, especially if it was sudden and frightening, the birthing person may have very mixed feelings: relief and joy that the baby is all right, confusion about all that happened, and regrets or doubts about the cesarean and their own behavior or decisions.

How You Can Help

- Keep abreast of what is going on and what staff are thinking.

- Ask questions, but do not keep the caregiver from doing what is necessary if the baby seems to be in danger.

- Ask for the quickly performed fetal scalp stimulation test to confirm the diagnosis of fetal distress.

- Follow the suggestions near the beginning of this chapter, pages 270–271, keeping in mind that, if the situation is urgent, there will not be time for discussion.

How a Doula Helps

The doula can help the two of you remain calm, ask the right questions so you can still make informed decisions, and adjust to the change in the birth plan while preserving your remaining priorities. The doula can be very helpful in a time of crisis so you don't feel alone or confused.

Complications in the Placental Stage

Immediately after the birth of the baby, the uterus normally continues to contract, separating the placenta from the uterine wall and expelling it. This is usually completed in 30 minutes or fewer, with blood loss of about 2 cups (475 ml). Sometimes, this critical transition does not proceed smoothly; here are some reasons.

Excessive Postpartum Bleeding

Excessive bleeding during this time causes symptoms of shock in the birthing person (rapid pulse, paleness, faintness, trembling, chills, or sweating). This may be caused by poor uterine tone (uterine atony) or the uterus has stopped contracting, which is necessary to stop the bleeding.

Management of Excessive Bleeding

The care provider may give Pitocin via IV or intramuscular injection, massage the uterus to encourage contractions, or have the birthing person nurse the baby or stroke the nipples to stimulate the release of oxytocin. In rare circumstances, the bleeding isn't controlled with these methods and a blood transfusion may be necessary.

Retained Placenta

The lack of muscle tone in the uterus may prevent the birth of the placenta. Sometimes, pieces of the placenta or membranes are left behind after most of the placenta has been expelled. These fragments can also prevent the uterus from contracting fully and cause excessive bleeding.

Management of Retained Placenta

The care provider may use their hand to remove the placenta or any fragments left behind. Vigorous uterine massage and additional use of Pitocin may also be necessary. Sometimes, the care provider and birthing person will transfer to the operating room where there is better lighting and more tools available to remove the placenta or fragments. Rarely, a D & C (dilation and curettage) operation may be needed under anesthesia to remove the fragments. You may be expected to stay out of the operating room, but, if the birthing person is awake and you would like to be there, request that you accompany them. It is worth a try.

It is very helpful if the caregiver speaks reassuringly to both of you about what is happening and what they are doing to help.

Lacerations

Sometimes, as the baby comes down the birth canal and exits the vagina, some tearing of tissues can occur and result in bleeding.

Management of Lacerations

The caregiver sometimes packs the vagina with sterile gauze to stop the bleeding and under local anesthetic, repairs the tears with dissoluble suture.

How The Birthing Person May React

The birthing person may not be fully aware of the seriousness of the complication and may be surprised at the actions of the staff. If they have symptoms of shock from the bleeding or fear for their own well-being, they will probably be frightened, especially if you are also frightened. They will benefit from reassurance and some explanation of what is happening, especially if the caregiver will talk with them.

How You Can Help

Stay beside the birthing person; talk to them; and help them keep calm by breathing slowly and fully and focusing on the baby, if the baby is near or with them. Ask the caregiver or nurse to explain what is happening. If possible, encourage the birthing person to hold the baby skin to skin (with your help) and keep talking to the baby. Encourage the baby to suckle at the breast. If you are worried, sit near the birthing person and do not show your fear. Focus on the birthing person and baby at this time.

How a Doula Helps

This is a frightening time and the doula's calm presence can make a positive difference. These actions can be very helpful: making the parents as comfortable and safe as possible; attending to their physical well-being; watching for symptoms of shock or panic and being ready to comfort and steady them if they are very upset or worried. Doulas put their own feelings aside, so they can assist the parents. Later, the doula will need to debrief with colleagues or mentors.

Complications with the Newborn

The newborn baby is assessed immediately after birth. If all is normal, the baby is usually placed in the birthing person's arms for cuddling and suckling. If there are problems, the baby may need to go to the nursery for special care.

If the baby has problems, take part in the decision-making about appropriate care. The Key Questions for Informed Decision-Making (see page 237) will help. The birthing person may be unable to think clearly right after the birth because of the excitement and the effects of drugs, exhaustion, or problems of their own. Provided you are legal next of kin, it may fall upon you to agree to the course of treatment. (If you have no legal or biological tie to the baby—if you are, for example, a co-parent in a state where your relationship to the birthing person is not recognized or a relative or friend—make arrangements ahead of time whereby you may make decisions about the baby if the biological parent cannot.)

If the baby must remain in the special-care nursery for several days or more, you may need to be the baby's advocate, despite your distress. When a baby is hospitalized, many caregivers (for example, pediatricians, neonatologists, other physician specialists, nurses, laboratory personnel, X-ray and ultrasound technicians, respiratory or physical therapists, and social workers) are usually involved. They come and go, each providing care and information according to their roles and responsibilities. Keeping track of everything can be most confusing and may seem next to impossible. Parents and their partners often feel help-less, depressed, confused, and either distrustful of the baby's caregivers or resigned to accepting whatever they say. Good communication and record keeping are ways to prevent these feelings of helplessness.

Remain with the baby as much as possible. The baby needs a loving person close by, to hold them (if the condition permits), to stroke and talk and sing to them, and to keep track of what is going on.

When you need to leave, ask a relative or friend to stay with the baby, at least some of the time you are gone. The point is to remain informed as the various professionals participate in the baby's care.

- Keep a written log of each visit by staff, including the professional's name and specialty, date, time, purpose of the visit, and a summary of any communication regarding the baby's condition, plans for test-ing, medications, and so on.

- Keep all the records in one notebook, not on scraps of paper; this will make it easier for you to locate the items you want to ask about. Sometimes, there are differences in advice and contradictory infor-mation. Your notes will be most helpful as you work to keep everything straight.

- Write down your questions so you do not forget to ask them.

- Above all, know who is coordinating the baby's care and how to reach that doctor or, when off duty, a substitute.

The birthing person should remain with the baby as much as possi-ble. Make sure they have a comfortable chair or bed and access to nourishing food. If the baby cannot breast-feed, the birthing person should be given a breast pump and instructions for using it. Pumped breast milk can usually be fed by bottle; if the baby cannot yet take a bottle, a stomach tube is used. Even if the birthing person is not plan-ning to breast-feed, the pediatrician may ask them to provide their own colostrum or milk until the baby can take formula well, as breast milk helps protect the baby from infection during this vulnerable time. For-mula cannot do this.

Detailed descriptions of all possible newborn problems are beyond the scope of this book, but following are some fairly common problems that might arise shortly after birth.

Kangaroo Care

Studies show that being held skin to skin on a parent's chest and covered with a blanket keeps a baby warmer than a heated baby bed. The baby benefits not only from the parent's warmth but also from their movements, soothing voice, touch, and even heartbeat sounds. Both parent and baby are more content when they spend some hours each day in this *kangaroo care*.

Babies who have been "kangarooed" gain weight faster, suckle better, cry less, and are discharged from the hospital sooner. Kangaroo care has been done even with babies receiving oxygen or tube feedings or who are very premature or sick. Ask the baby's caregiver or nurse about kangaroo care and see Recommended Resources (page 418) for more information on this subject.

Breathing Problems

A newborn may have difficulty breathing because of fluid in the lungs, meconium aspiration (see "Suctioning the Baby's Nose and Mouth," page 368), lingering narcotic drugs that were given to the birthing person during labor (see chapter 8), infection, immature lungs, or congenital abnormalities. A baby who is slow to breathe on their own, or who breathes very fast and grunts as they breathe, may need medications, intravenous feeding, an incubator, deep suctioning, resuscitation, mechanical assistance with breathing, extra oxygen, or other help.

Low Body Temperature

A baby whose body temperature drops below normal uses oxygen and energy to bring that temperature up. It is important to keep the baby warm (see "Kangaroo Care," above, and "Warming Unit," page 374).

Infection

A newborn sometimes acquires an infection while in the uterus or soon after birth. Depending on the organism causing it, the infection may be serious (see "Group B Strep Screening," page 240, or genital herpes, page 280). Prompt diagnosis and treatment with antibiotics or other medications, along with special care in the nursery (intravenous feeding, an incubator, and close observation), are needed.

Because infection in a newborn can become very serious very quickly, painful interventions may be necessary. These may include tests of various body fluids, obtained by heel sticks; spinal taps; bladder taps; scalp-vein intravenous lines; nasogastric tubes; and many other complex procedures. You and the birthing person will find all this confusing and frightening. Keep informed so you understand what is done and why and follow your baby's progress.

Birth Trauma or Injury

Some babies are injured during the birth process, especially if the birth is difficult. A very rapid birth or a prolonged or difficult forceps, vacuum, or cesarean delivery can cause bruises, a broken collarbone, cuts, or nerve damage. Although wise management reduces the chances of such injuries, they can occur even with the most skilled caregivers.

For some vulnerable babies (for example, premature babies, babies with birth defects, and babies with genetic or other preexisting problems), even the normal birth process is too much. Some very large babies also suffer, if great effort by the caregiver is required to deliver them. Vulnerable babies can usually, but not always, be identified before labor, and plans can be made in advance for their special care.

Sometimes, even with the best of care, a baby is unexpectedly born with serious problems requiring emergency treatment or long-term care. This possibility haunts parents and professionals alike and motivates attempts to develop better diagnostic and treatment methods.

Drug Effects

Improvements in pain medications and other drugs used during labor, and in the ways these drugs are given, have reduced the severity of side effects. Still, if babies are born with drugs in their system, the drug may subtly or noticeably affect their behavior. Depending on the drug and the amount used, they may show some degree of sleepiness, poor suckling and breathing, lack of muscle tone, irritability, jitteriness, jaundice, or sluggishness of some reflex behaviors, or other atypical signs. When the drug wears off, they behave more normally. Sometimes, other drugs, such as narcotic antagonists, can be given—these counteract some narcotic effects and hasten the baby's recovery.

Low Blood Sugar

Low blood sugar is rather common in:

• Babies of diabetic birthing persons

• Very large, small, or premature babies

• Babies whose birthing parent received large amounts of intravenous dextrose or glucose solution during labor

• Babies born after prolonged labors

• Babies born under other rare conditions, such as sepsis (infection), delayed feeding, or Rh incompatibility

Symptoms of low blood sugar in the baby include jitteriness, irritability, breathing problems, temperature problems, and others. The diagnosis of low blood sugar is made by drawing blood from the baby's heel and analyzing it. Treatment usually consists of giving the baby some glucose water or formula and rechecking blood sugar levels. The problem usually resolves itself quickly (see chapter 10, page 273).

Jaundice

If the baby's skin or the whites of their eyes become yellowish, the baby is jaundiced. Usually harmless, physiologic jaundice is caused by elevated levels of bilirubin, a yellow pigment that results when red blood cells break down after birth as part of their normal life cycle. Physiologic jaundice is mild and goes away on its own, usually in a few days, but extra-high levels of bilirubin in some vulnerable babies may cause brain damage. Premature babies, babies who had particular difficulties during birth, and those with blood types incompatible with the gestational parent's are more vulnerable to brain damage from high bilirubin levels.

Jaundice is diagnosed by measuring bilirubin in the baby's blood, a sample of which is taken with a heel stick. Further tests of blood type, liver function, and bowel function help determine the cause of jaundice.

Jaundice is treated with phototherapy, which consists of exposing the baby's skin to special bright light almost constantly for a few days. Light breaks down (photooxidizes) bilirubin as it circulates through the blood vessels in the baby's skin and lowers total bilirubin levels. Portable phototherapy units are available for treatment at home. These are blankets or sleeping bags containing fiber-optic light filaments that can be wrapped around the baby to expose large areas of skin to the light. Treatment usually lasts for a few days after which the jaundice begins to recede. Prolonged exposure to indirect sunlight (through a window) helps, but less reliably than artificial light. Frequent nursing (more than eight times per day) also helps relieve jaundice.

If bilirubin levels are very high or if the baby is premature, jaundice is more serious, and a complete exchange transfusion of the baby's blood may be done. This is very rare today.

Prematurity or Low Birth Weight

The premature infant (born before 37 weeks' gestation) or the low-birth-weight infant (weighing less than 5 pounds, or 2.5 kg) is more susceptible to all the newborn problems described here than is the full-term, average-size baby. Premature babies are therefore watched more closely and receive more aggressive treatment. As they approach average size and weight, their vulnerability to problems decreases. See Recommended Resources (page 418) for more on prematurity.

Death of a Baby

Rarely, a baby dies during or around the time of birth. Words cannot describe the shock and grief felt by the parents and their loved ones. Of course, nothing can bring the baby back to life, but memories can be created that will have great meaning as time passes.

As difficult as it is to think through the possibility that your baby could die, it is a good idea to learn about the kinds of things that can be done to bring some positive meaning to such a tragedy. Please see pages 49–50 for some suggestions. Decision-making is very difficult when one is grieving intensely, but parents may later feel regret it if they did not say goodbye in the way they would have chosen. See Recommended Resources (page 418) for more helpful information.

Many hospitals have sensitive and compassionate staff members who do all they can to create a meaningful opportunity for parents to be alone with their baby. Staff members may also provide referrals for support groups and grief counseling. Please make a plan and then put it aside, with the peace of mind that you have it in case you need it. Now, focus on a healthy outcome and a beautiful baby.

After It Is All Over

Any complication during labor or the early postpartum period, whether in the birthing parent or baby, presents a challenge to your family, the caregiver, the nurses, and the doula.

Each complication requires quick acceptance of a change in plans and expectations, often without a complete understanding of the situation. You do what must be done, even if in a state of shock. Afterward, as you, the parents, look back over the events, the feelings hit. Even if both birthing parent and baby have come through alive and healthy, the emotional impact can be great. Unanswered questions and feelings of guilt, anger, or disappointment may arise, especially if everything happened too quickly for either or both of you to grasp, or if you, the birthing parent, or the baby was treated unkindly or disrespectfully.

It may take time, especially for birthing parents, to come to terms with unrealized expectations. They will benefit from your patience and acceptance of what is, in reality, a grieving process. Your doula may be able to help with some of the practical matters, such as phone calls, lining up friends and family to help, and be a listening ear as you relive the experience with someone who was there. For both of you, a conference with the caregiver may fill gaps in your understanding of the events and answer your questions. Sometimes, consulting with a childbirth educator, trauma counselor, or psychotherapist helps either or both parents sort out feelings and gain a healthy perspective on a physically or emotionally traumatic birth experience. Please see page 353, "Your Role During and After a Cesarean Birth," for further discussion of emotional reactions following a difficult birth.

In the end, with the birth in the past, let us hope that the birthing person recognizes the courage and grace they displayed as they dealt with the unexpected challenges posed by a complicated labor.

CHAPTER 8

MEDICATIONS FOR PAIN DURING LABOR

We both thought it would be great to make it through without an epidural, but labor went on and on and the pain got worse, and she (and I) got really tired. Every contraction was like this huge ordeal. She asked for an epidural. It went in smoothly and her pain was gone. She didn't even know when she was having a contraction! We both slept. It was almost hard to believe she was in labor.

—JOHN, FIRST-TIME FATHER

She had wanted an unmedicated birth this time, but she also knew she couldn't count on it because of all the unknowns of labor. I didn't know why it mattered so much to her. In labor, though, I really got into it. We were a real team. I loved working with her. But, after a long time, with no end in sight, we ran out of gas. The epidural really helped. She feels she used it just the way she planned and feels great about the birth.

ANDY, SECOND-TIME FATHER

Next to the health of birthing persons and their babies, the major concern of everyone—birthing person, caregiver and nurses, you, and the support team—is the birthing person's comfort during labor. Although the pain of labor is usually very intense, it does not have to be overwhelming (see the discussion of pain and suffering on page 144). There is much the laboring person can do to keep the pain manageable; they can learn and rehearse many effective comfort measures in advance, from childbirth classes and this book (see chapter 4) other books, films, and the internet. As you know, however, the laboring person will need help from you, your doula or other supporters, and the staff in using these comfort measures. Labor is simply too demanding for most people to manage without advance preparation and help at the time.

In hospital births, drugs are also used to relieve labor pain (only nondrug remedies are used in home and birth-center births). To a great extent, drugs for pain are optional—the laboring person can decide whether and when to use them. Because they are readily available in a variety of forms and because they can have profound effects besides pain relief, they require precautions and extra procedures for safety. The laboring person should learn from the doctor, midwife, or childbirth classes about the pain-relief methods available and think about how they feel about using them during labor. You should also think about these things. Are your feelings about the use of pain medications compatible with the laboring person's? What if you favor natural childbirth without drugs, but the pregnant person wants to use them? Can you agree? Plan to support them in accomplishing what they want.

It may seem somewhat foolish to plan whether or not to use pain medications in advance because the level of pain and reactions to it are all unknown. Although this is true, the birthing person does know some things that may help them decide: For example, do they prefer to feel as little pain or other sensations as possible? Or, do they want to experience the labor and deal with the pain using nondrug approaches as much as possible? Using the information in this chapter, you and the birthing person can make a plan that will guide you both as you encounter the pain of labor together. There is not a right or wrong way to deal with the pain of labor. The laboring person should be supported as much as possible with their choice.

Management of Normal Labor without Pain Medications

The pain of normal labor, though severe, can be successfully managed without suffering and without pain medications if these four conditions are met:

1. The birthing person wants to avoid pain medications. In this case, they should decide whether they want to avoid pain medications and how strongly they feel about this (see pages 327–329). One's motivation is key.

2. The birthing person knows about the birth process and ways to relieve pain without medications. If the desire is to avoid pain medications, you both need to know the comfort measures described in chapter 4. It helps to rehearse these together and adapt them as needed. They will also cope better with access to such aids as a bath, shower, rocking chair, birth ball, hot packs, cold packs, a squatting bar (as pictured on page 174), and music (see page 196).

3. The birthing person has emotional support and assistance. They need competent, caring support from you—someone who loves them, knows them well, who wants to share the birth, and who wants to help them follow their wishes. The continuous help of a doula improves the odds of using less pain medication or avoiding it altogether, if that is the plan.

   The doula accomplishes this with encouragement, reassurance, information, and guidance in the use of techniques that lessen pain and help labor progress. Their experience and confidence rub off on both of you and help you know if what they are going through is normal. (Of course, if a pregnant person plans to use pain medications, the doula helps get them. If the laboring person plans to avoid pain medications, but labor is very difficult, they may decide to use them, and the doula helps get them.)

   The laboring person also needs the support of the professional staff. A person in labor is vulnerable to both positive and negative suggestions, especially from the experts—nurses, midwives, and physicians. If they believe in the laboring person and provide encouragement, the laboring person is more likely to carry on; being pitied or ignored by the staff will discourage the laboring person from using the comfort measures they learned, and they are more likely to give up.

4. The birthing person has a reasonably normal labor. This is key and is at least partly a matter of luck. The labor must not require painful interventions and must not thoroughly exhaust and

discourage the laboring person. This does not mean labor has to be short or painless. If the first three conditions are present, a person can handle more challenges without pain medications, but you both and your doula must realize and accept that, in some labors, pain medications and painful interventions are required.

If the laboring person prefers to cope without medications, prepare yourself for an active and satisfying support role.

What You Both Need to Know About Pain Medications

To make an informed decision about pain medications, you and the birthing person need information. Do not wait until the birthing person is in labor to get this information. When they are in pain and asking for medication, it is too late to learn all about the drugs.

- What is the drug? How does it work? How effective is it in relieving pain? What other effects does it have—on the birthing person, the progress of labor, the fetus, and newborn?

- What precautions or added interventions are needed to ensure safety?

- How does one support the birthing person who has taken pain medications?

Remember, although various drugs are available, effective, and widely used in labor, they involve tradeoffs: The birthing person gets pain relief, but they or the fetus may experience unwanted side effects—directly, from the drug itself, or indirectly, through potential problems such as restriction of the laboring person's activity or the need for other interventions.

Long-term detrimental effects on the baby of drugs used judiciously in labor have not been established. There may be no harm, or, in some cases, there may be subtle long-term effects. This is a subject of great debate in the medical literature, and it is unlikely to be settled in the near future.

For these reasons, I advocate planning to use nondrug methods of pain relief, at least for part of labor (see chapter 4), and seeking a birth place that has the amenities (bathtub, shower, squatting bar, birthing bed, places to walk, rocking chair) that enhance a laboring person's comfort. You may bring your own music, hot or cold packs, and birth ball (see page 180) if the hospital or birth center doesn't have them. If you're planning a home birth, you probably have furniture to lean on and hold on to for squatting and pillows to support the birthing person in various positions in bed.

By using nondrug pain-relief methods for at least part of the labor, the birthing person can comfortably postpone the use of pain medications. In this way, they reduce the total amount of medications received and lessen the likelihood of undesirable effects and the need for additional interventions.

Many birthing persons find these nondrug methods sufficient to keep their pain at a level at which they can cope throughout the labor. Afterwards, the absence of mental or physical side effects of the drugs on the birthing person and baby and the ability to get up and move freely immediately after the birth contribute to a feeling that these rewards are worth the pain.

Preparing to deal with labor pain using nondrug methods is time consuming, however, and going through labor without drugs can be a challenge. And, if labor is exhausting or complicated, the benefits of pain medications will outweigh potential risks. Many birthing people do not have the time or inclination to master the nondrug approaches and so plan to rely on the epidural to take away most pain in labor or wait to see whether they need it. About 70 percent of American women (and more in urban areas) use an epidural today.

As you both learn more about pain medication, you will be able to help the birthing person make informed choices. To begin our discussion of pain medications, here are several definitions.

- **Analgesia:** reduces pain; analgesics are drugs that relieve pain.

- **Anesthesia:** loss of sensation, including pain sensation; anesthetics are drugs that take away feeling.

- **Systemic:** taken up by the bloodstream, affecting the entire body and reaching the baby in concentrations similar to those reaching the birthing person

- **Neuraxial:** affecting areas of the body supplied by specific nerves coming from the spinal cord (the neuraxis is the brain and spinal cord)

- **Neuraxial analgesic:** pain medication injected near spinal nerve roots to block or decrease awareness of pain in the area supplied by those nerves; neuraxial analgesics are used in epidural and spinal blocks.

- **Block:** medication that interrupts the transmission of pain impulses, creating numbness

- **Local:** affecting specific tissues—such as the cervix, vagina, and perineum; a local anesthetic blocks the feeling provided by nerve endings in these tissues.

- **General anesthesia:** complete loss of consciousness caused by a systemic medication, a *general anesthetic*

When pain medications are used, several factors influence the area where pain is relieved and the severity of side effects:

- Choice of medication—a narcotic or narcotic-like drug, a sedative, a tranquilizer, a gas, an injected anesthetic, or an amnesiac (a drug that causes loss of memory of events taking place while the drug is in effect)

- Total dose—the concentration of the drug, the volume of each dose, and the number of doses; if medication is given continuously, the total amount of drug given

- Route of administration—injection into a muscle, a vein, the cervix, or the vaginal wall; inhalation into the lungs; injection into the epidural or spinal (intrathecal) space; or swallowing

- Individual characteristics of the birthing person—weight, sensitivity to medications, blood-clotting ability, anatomic variations, physical condition, the number of weeks of pregnancy (gestation), and overall health

How Pain Is Relieved by Medications

Medications reduce pain by altering some part of the nervous system, the system that makes it possible to recognize, interpret, and react to pain.

Labor pain originates with pressure, stretching, or compression involving tissues in the uterus, vagina, or pelvic joints. Contractions of the uterus, dilation of the cervix, and the baby's movement through the pelvis create the pain. Nerve endings in these tissues are stimulated to send pain impulses over nerve fibers to the spinal cord and brain.

The transmission of the pain signals can be modified anywhere along this pathway—in the nerve endings, in the nerve roots (situated where the nerves leave the spine), in the spinal cord, or in the brain.

This is how various pain medications work:

• Local anesthetics block nerve endings in the injected areas from sending the pain impulses over the nerve fibers to the spine and brain.

• Epidural and spinal (neuraxial) medications are either injected directly into the spinal fluid or injected just outside the spine (into the epidural space). They block transmission of pain signals from the nerve fibers where they enter the spinal cord.

• Systemic medications (such as narcotics) act in the brain to reduce recognition of pain or reactions to it.

The rest of this chapter presents specific information about the various medications used during labor. You and the pregnant person may use these pages as background for your discussions with the caregiver, for seeking further information, and for making decisions.

The drugs are grouped in the text according to general characteristics (subtle differences among the drugs in each group are not described here). For more details, consult the table "Pain Medications and Their Effects" (see pages 332–339), which lists all the medications and techniques and important information on each. The chart "When Are Pain Medications Used?" on page 331 indicates at which stages of labor the various pain-relief methods are most safely used and when the drugs' effects will ideally have worn off. When you have both read the chapter, you will be ready to use the "Pain Medications Preference Scale," on pages 328–329, as a tool in your decision-making.

Systemic Drugs

Drugs that affect the whole body—the entire system—are called systemic drugs. *Systemic analgesics* (pain-relieving drugs) use the bloodstream to transport the medication to the brain, where the drug exerts its pain-relieving effect. Systemic drugs can be given in several forms: as pills, as gases to inhale, as injections into the skin or muscle, or as part of an intravenous (IV) solution that drips continuously into a vein.

Systemic drugs give short-term relief (30 minutes to 2 hours, depending on the specific drug and dose). Another dose might be given after this period, or the birthing person might have an epidural. While under the effect of a systemic drug, the birthing person feels groggy and dozes between contractions.

Systemic drugs circulate not only to the birthing person's brain but also throughout their body; they also cross the placenta to the baby. Because their effects on the baby after birth may be profound, these drugs must be given early enough in labor to allow time for them to wear off (let the birthing person's liver metabolize and excrete the drug) before birth. If a systemic drug has not worn off sufficiently by the time of birth, another drug, such as a narcotic antagonist, is given to counteract the unwanted effects of the original drug.

Even when the timing is appropriate, some of a drug (or its metabolic by-products) almost certainly remains in the baby's bloodstream after birth and may subtly alter their behavior and reflexes for a few days following. How severely medication affects the baby depends on the baby's health and maturity, the choice of drug, the dosage, and when it is given during labor. If the baby is in good health and the amount of medication is small and there is a long time between when the medication is given and the birth, the effects on the baby will be least harmful.

There are three categories of systemic pain medications that may be given during prelabor or during the dilation (first) stage: tranquilizers, sedatives, and narcotics (see the table on pages 332–339). Other systemic medications, called general anesthetics, are occasionally used during the dilation or birthing (second) stage. General anesthetics are discussed as a separate category on page 324.

The Partner's Role When the Laboring Person Has a Systemic Medication

Tranquilizers, sedatives, and morphine (a narcotic) are used in prelabor to reduce anxiety or cause sleep, so when one of these drugs is given, the partner's role is to keep the laboring person from being disturbed.

Other narcotics or narcotic-like drugs, however, are given during labor to help the laboring person cope with pain. They require the partner's or doula's help to work well. A narcotic may help the laboring person relax between contractions and give them a slightly longer break before the next one. The peaks, however, are about as painful with the narcotic as without. A common problem is that the laboring person dozes during the early seconds of the contraction, so the peak hits them suddenly and they

Note

We use the term *narcotic* a bit loosely here. Narcotics, technically, are drugs (such as morphine) derived from opium. Other drugs are synthetic narcotics and are not derived from opium. These narcotic-like drugs have similar properties to narcotics, but side effects and duration of action may differ. The table on page 332 lists some of these drugs. We use *narcotic* to cover true narcotics as well as the narcotic-like drugs.

can't cope. Many laboring persons who have taken a narcotic report it was "useless," even though they did get more rest after taking it.

Try to remain awake after the laboring person takes a narcotic, so you can tell from their behavior that the contraction is coming. Although they will probably be dozing, they will wince or groan before being fully aware of the contraction. As soon as it begins, get their attention: "Okay, here it is. Open your eyes. Breathe with me. That's good." This allows them to get into a rhythm before the peak. Help them over the peak by talking and moving your hand rhythmically until they drift off again. In this way, you can maximize the benefit of the narcotic.

Regional (Neuraxial) Analgesia and Anesthesia (Epidural and Spinal)

Of all the pain-relieving medications, these provide the most effective pain relief, use the smallest amount of drug, and have the fewest effects on the laboring person's mental state and on the baby's well-being. Regional, or neuraxial, medications are given in and around the spinal cord. Depending on the dosage, these drugs cause partial to complete numbness, muscle weakness, decreased control over the legs, an inability to urinate, and other effects (see page 334). As we explain in the following pages, there are numerous varieties of regional analgesia. You and the laboring person may want to talk with the doctor or midwife about the particular techniques used in your hospital.

Regional analgesia can be used for either vaginal or cesarean delivery. They usually combine a low dose of a narcotic with a low dose of an anesthetic drug. It has much less effect on the laboring person's consciousness and mental state than systemic drugs do because the narcotic in neuraxial analgesia is a much smaller dose and isn't given directly into a blood vessel. The narcotic enhances the effects of the anesthetic, allowing for lower doses of both drugs than would be effective if used separately. Regional analgesia provides the best pain relief of all the medications for labor.

Administering regional analgesia requires a high degree of skill and is, therefore, done only by specialists—anesthesiologists or specially trained nurse-anesthetists. Regional analgesia is the most costly of all obstetric pain-relieving techniques, but it is also the most popular.

Spinals and epidurals, though they are both regional forms of anesthesia, have some important differences. The spinal can be given as a single injection of a narcotic or an anesthetic or as a combination of the two. The effects last a few hours. The epidural block is usually used for more prolonged pain relief. A catheter is inserted into the epidural space in the pregnant person's low back (see illustration, page 316) and left in place. The medication is dripped into the catheter continuously, and sometimes, the laboring person can push a button to give small additional doses of the medicine whenever the pain escalates. This is called patient-controlled epidural analgesia. The equipment is designed to prevent taking too much medicine.

Both the spinal and the epidural blocks are given in the lumbar spine, in the low back. The spinal injection goes in a few millimeters deeper through the dura and into the dural space. The dura is the membrane that surrounds the spinal cord and the spinal nerves and contains the spinal fluid; the dural space is the space within the dura. The epidural injection stops just short of the dura, in the epidural space. The medicine is absorbed across the dura and has effects similar to a spinal, though usually with less effect on the laboring person's ability to move their legs.

General Characteristics of Regional Analgesia

The anesthetics used for regional analgesia are sometimes referred to as *caine* drugs; common examples are Carbocaine, bupivacaine, Marcaine, Xylocaine, Nesacaine, and ropivacaine. These drugs are quite similar in their effects on the laboring person, on the labor, and on the baby. Subtle differences in their biochemical makeup, however, affect the way they act in the body and the duration of their effects. The caregiver or the anesthesiologist usually selects the specific drug to be used. The laboring person should inform the anesthesiologist if they have a sensitivity or allergy to any drug.

The narcotics used for neuraxial analgesia include morphine, fentanyl, and sufentanil. They can be given alone in early labor or after a cesarean or in combination with the *caine* anesthetics for vaginal or cesarean birth.

Narcotics take effect more quickly than the caine drugs and interfere less with the laboring person's use of their legs. If narcotics are given alone in early labor, they are usually given as a spinal. Laboring people may be able to stand and walk a bit with help, but may not be very steady on their feet, and they could fall. For this reason, most hospitals discourage laboring people from walking with spinal narcotics. If they do walk, the partner or the nurse must stay right with them whenever they are upright.

Because the spinal narcotics administered in early labor usually are inadequate by the time a person is in active labor, an anesthetic (caine drug) may be added in the epidural space. This gives good relief when the pain becomes more intense. The two-step approach is called a *combined spinal-epidural*. It allows a birthing person to feel virtually no pain from early labor until pushing, when they may feel some perineal pain.

Narcotics administered regionally can cause side effects in the laboring person and may affect the baby, too. In many people, these drugs cause some grogginess (though less than when given systemically), itching, and nausea. Fentanyl and sufentanil, because of their biochemical properties, cross more easily to the baby than the caine drugs, and small quantities are still present in the baby's blood at 2 days of age. This may affect the baby's breathing, temperature regulation, and suckling ability. More studies of these drugs' effects are needed.

Epidural or spinal morphine (Duramorph) is often used for pain relief after a cesarean. A dose given before the birthing person leaves the operating room provides very good pain relief for about 24 hours, after which they are offered other pain medications.

In general, the desired effect of the drugs is loss of pain sensation in the affected area. Reducing the laboring person's pain during labor relaxes them and, especially in a prolonged, exhausting labor, allows them to sleep and may result in more rapid dilation of the cervix.

Possible undesirable effects depend on the area injected, the total dosage, and the choice of drugs. The effects are listed under Neuraxial Analgesia in the table "Pain Medications and Their Effects" (see pages

332–339). The table also lists precautions used to maximize the safety of each technique.

General Technique for Giving Epidural or Spinal Analgesia

There are many similarities among the techniques for administering the various types of neuraxial analgesia. The general procedure is described here. Please refer to the table "Pain Medications and Their Effects" for specific information about each type of block.

Neuraxial analgesia numbs or reduces sensation in a large portion of the birthing person's body—between the top of the uterus and the feet. The area affected can be controlled to a great extent by the amount and concentration of the drug given and by the placement of the injection. For example, the birthing person may be able to move their legs while remaining numb in the trunk. This is the procedure:

1. Before receiving the anesthetic, the birthing person is given intravenous fluids to reduce the chance that their blood pressure will drop.

2. The birthing person lies on their side or sits up and curls their body forward. An anesthesiologist scrubs the area where the injection will be given, numbs the skin with a local anesthetic, and then injects a small amount of anesthetic between the vertebrae of the low back (lumbar spine), into the epidural or dural space (see illustrations). The anesthesiologist checks to make sure the needle is placed correctly. Sometimes, more than one attempt is needed to get the needle placed perfectly.

3. For a spinal: A full dose is given in a single injection that lasts 2 to 3 hours. For an epidural: A thin tube is run through the epidural needle to allow for a continuous drip of the medicine throughout labor and birth. Within minutes, the birthing person begins to feel the effects. They are soon numb in the desired area.

4. Sometimes, pain relief is uneven or spotty and it takes some adjustment (changing the birthing person's position, injecting more doses) before the pain relief is adequate.

5. For an epidural: A catheter can be left in place and taped to the back so the medicine may drip in steadily, or, if they are using

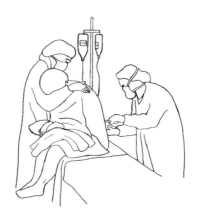

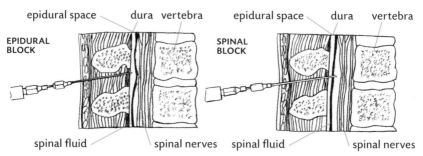

epidural space — dura vertebra   epidural space — dura   vertebra

EPIDURAL BLOCK   **SPINAL BLOCK**

spinal fluid   spinal nerves   spinal fluid   spinal nerves

Neuraxial anesthesia. Top: As the birthing person lies on one side or sits up, the anesthesiologist injects the anesthetic. Bottom: These detailed drawings illustrate the placement of the needle for an epidural block (left) and a spinal block (right).

patient-controlled epidural analgesia (see page 313), the birthing person may add some by pushing a button, if desired.

6. Once the spinal or epidural anesthetic is in place, a urinary catheter is placed in the birthing person's bladder to allow the nurse to empty the bladder because the birthing person is not able to urinate with the epidural in effect.

7. The birthing person's blood pressure is checked frequently. The blood pressure cuff remains on the arm for 30 to 45 minutes; it can be programmed to measure the blood pressure automatically every 2 or 3 minutes. Because it is not unusual for the blood pressure and fetal heart rate to drop with an epidural, frequent blood pressure checks allow for early detection and measures to quickly restore the blood pressure.

The Partner's Role When the Birthing Person Has an Epidural

An epidural usually relieves labor pain very effectively and also allows relaxation and rest; if the birthing person is exhausted, frightened, or tense, it often allows for good sleep. If labor progress is slow, the epidural makes it possible to give higher levels of Pitocin without adding pain for the birthing person. An epidural does not, however, relieve all distress. People who have epidurals are often shortchanged emotionally by their partners and the staff, who may believe that when the birthing person no longer has pain, they have no distress and no longer need support. Partners often take a break, get a meal, go to sleep, check their phone, get on the computer, or turn on the TV. Studies of birthing person's thoughts and feelings before and after epidurals indicate they still feel emotional stress and want and benefit from continuous support even when their pain is relieved.

Following are some emotional challenges for people with epidurals, and ways the partner can help:

• **The decision to ask for an epidural.** People who desire a natural childbirth may feel disappointed they cannot handle the pain. Those who have planned in advance to use an epidural may be upset if asked to wait before getting the epidural until labor has progressed more.

• **The wait.** The time from deciding they want the epidural to when they actually get it and have adequate pain relief is particularly difficult. Twenty minutes or more usually pass before the birthing person is prepared, the anesthesiologist arrives, the drug is administered, and the medication takes effect. The wait can be much longer if the anesthesiologist is busy with another patient or if the person must undergo various procedures, such as admissions paperwork or administration of intravenous fluids, before they can get the epidural. In the meantime, they must continue coping, even though they don't want to.

If you find yourself in this situation, you may feel helpless standing by while the person you love is in pain. You may feel ineffective and frustrated because they no longer find the comfort techniques and your suggestions helpful, and yet you must help persuade them to continue coping until the anesthesiologist arrives. Discuss this possible scenario together before labor and make an agreement to continue with the coping techniques in chapter 4, especially rhythmic movements, moaning, stroking, and the Take-Charge routine. These techniques can keep the birthing person from becoming panicked or overwhelmed.

Sometimes, labor progress is so fast they no longer need the extra pain relief by the time it takes effect—they may be pushing the baby out by then!

- **Getting the epidural.** Policies vary regarding the presence of partners and doulas when the epidural is being administered. Find out in advance. Administering the epidural takes 15 to 45 minutes, depending on the anesthesiologist's skill and experience, the birthing person spinal anatomy, and their ability to cooperate by lying or sitting still while curling their back—an uncomfortable position, especially during contractions. If you are there, you can help the birthing person remain still and calm and you can be encouraging.

- **Relief of pain.** Within minutes after the epidural is placed, the pain of the contractions begins to subside and will likely be gone within 15 to 30 minutes. The laboring person's mood should improve markedly; they may become chatty, optimistic, and very grateful to the anesthesiologist. If pain relief is incomplete, of course, they will be disappointed and impatient for adjustments to correct the problem. When the laboring person is comfortable, you will also be relieved and grateful, and you can rest and have a snack.

- **Feeling alone.** Once comfortable, the birthing person will no longer need intense support and close physical contact, but may feel suddenly alone and unimportant if you turn on the TV, leave to get a meal, or take a nap. Unless you have a doula or other family member to remain in the room, don't leave. Continue to show support by bringing things to make them comfortable—warm blankets, ice chips, comb, toothbrush—and asking questions and making conversation. Watch TV or play a game together. Watch the monitor from time to time and point out contractions when they occur. You may both find it hard to believe that the birthing person is really having contractions, after what they have been through.

If the birthing person goes to sleep, it will likely be light and fitful. When they wake, they may feel quite alone if you are out of the room or sound asleep. If you are exhausted, of course, you may not be able to stay awake. Before you drift off, tell them to wake you if they need anything or if the doctor comes in.

- **Almost forgetting they are in labor.** It's easy for the birthing person to be distracted from the labor when they can no longer feel it. However, the two of you may still be able to do things to prevent some possible side effects of the epidural—slowing of labor progress and malposition of the baby. Try the six positions of the Rollover (see following), changing every 20 to 30 minutes when awake. If the nurse finds problems with any of the positions, skip it and go to the next.

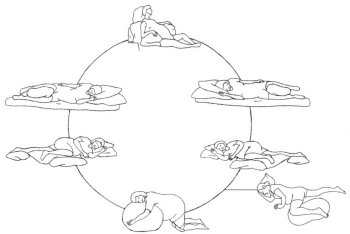

The Rollover

- **If side effects occur.** During this otherwise calm period, problems may occur that require action by the staff—for example, slowing of labor progress, a drop in the laboring person's blood pressure or the baby's heart rate, or a fever in the laboring person are all fairly common side effects of the epidural.

To speed labor, the doctor or midwife may start or increase a Pitocin (synthetic oxytocin) intravenous drip or rupture the laboring person's membranes. The nurse, watching the monitor and checking blood pressure closely, may notice the baby's heart rate slowing and have the laboring person change position and wear an oxygen mask for a while, which helps raise the baby's heart rate. If the laboring person develops a fever, the doctor or midwife may call for antibiotics because it is not possible to know whether the fever is a side effect of the epidural or due to infection. They assume it is infection causing the fever, until they know otherwise by testing the baby's blood.

- **Resting and waiting.** After the epidural takes effect, the birthing person will hardly know they are in labor until it is time to push. It feels strange to be laboring without any direct awareness of contractions, unless they press their belly. The nurse comes and goes, keeping track of blood pressure, the fetal heart rate, placing a urinary catheter and checking urine output, checking the cervix occasionally, and writing in the chart while the birthing person waits for something to happen. If not sleepy, the birthing person may feel bored or quite helpless. They may worry that labor is taking too long or the baby isn't tolerating the labor well. They need distraction, conversation, and reassurance that all is well. This is a good time to gently rehearse the bearing-down technique (breathing in, holding their breath, and gently straining) and discussing with the nurse what to expect when it is time to push.

- **Focusing on other discomforts.** Even when the birthing person's pain is under good control, other discomforts occur for some people and may be troubling, especially if they are unprepared. These include direct and indirect effects of the epidural: the heavy, numb feeling in the legs; heartburn or reflux; feeling too warm or too cold; trembling; pain in the upper back or shoulder; a small area (window) of pain that is mostly numb; dry mouth; itching; nausea; or other discomforts in position. The nurse, following hospital policy or the doctor's orders, will help relieve such discomforts. You or the doula may be allowed to provide ice chips, sips of water or juice, changes of position, warm blankets, cool cloths, and massage. Medications for itching, nausea, heartburn, or breakthrough pain will require an order from the caregiver or anesthesiologist. Some laboring people find it annoying to have to get permission before rolling over or taking a sip of water or chewing an antacid. You might help by addressing the nurse or doctor: "She always takes Tums for her heartburn, and it really helps. Do you think it's okay for her to take one?"

- **Breakthrough pain.** As labor advances, some pain may return. This can be scary for the birthing person if they have been free of pain for hours. Let the staff know so they can notify the anesthesiologist or adjust the epidural dosage to maintain good pain relief.

• **Complete dilation.** Even though the birthing person does not feel the cervix dilating, you both may feel a sense of accomplishment and optimism when the nurse tells you the cervix is completely dilated—a hurdle has been achieved! Unfortunately, however, women with epidurals typically feel unable to push effectively and find it difficult to follow directions because they can't feel what they are doing. Several options exist now: turning down the epidural to bring back sensations to guide the bearing-down efforts; directed pushing, in which the nurse coaches the birthing person in prolonged breath holding and straining—telling them when, how long, and how hard to push and when to breathe; delaying pushing until the baby is visible at the vaginal outlet or they feel the urge to push.

Turning down the epidural may appeal to a person who wanted an unmedicated birth; they may see it as an opportunity to resume an active role in the labor. But because decreases in endorphin production occur when an epidural is in effect, the pain is greater if the epidural medication is reduced than it would be if they had never had the epidural at all. Many people who have their epidural turned down find the pain of the second stage intolerable. Endorphins are the body's own painkillers and, as they diminish, the laboring person may need to turn up the epidural again. They should not feel badly about this. Of course, if they can wait a while, the endorphin levels may rise so it is tolerable to continue without the epidural.

Directed pushing is still done in some hospitals. The staff directs the pushing (see page 167), by having the person hold their breath and strain while the nurse counts to 10; they then tell them to take a quick breath and repeat until the contraction is over. The person rests until the next contraction. This does not always work well and can increase the need for forceps or vacuum extraction (see pages 266–269). A better option is to modify directed pushing: The birthing person is directed to push in the way similar to the way people push when they have no epidural (spontaneous bearing down; see page 165).

With delayed pushing, referred to as "laboring down," the birthing person rests for up to 1 hour or more, while the staff monitors the baby, until they begin to feel an urge to push or the baby's head appears at the vaginal opening. Then, they push with the contractions. The nurse may direct the pushing at this point, as described previously. Or, preferably, the nurse may modify the directed pushing, by having the birthing person hold their breath and push for only 5 to 6 seconds at a time, followed by six to eight short breaths before pushing again. Although this option may lengthen the birthing stage, it is the easiest on the birthing person and baby, and it results in fewer instrumental deliveries and episiotomies. You both should consider requesting this option in the birth plan and discussing it with the caregiver at a prenatal appointment.

- **How you can help with pushing.** When it is time to push, you or the doula can help the birthing person push well by watching the monitor for contractions, telling them when to start pushing, and cheering them on. Tell them to push when the intensity numbers go up by 20 points or so (the nurse can tell you where to look for those numbers).

  As the birthing person holds their breath and pushes, they make the numbers go up fast and high. You call out the increasing intensity readings from the contraction monitor to show how effective they are: "20, 30, 40, now press that baby down . . . 60, 73, 80, 96, 100, yes! That's the way! Now, breathe for the baby . . . and bear down again. You're at 73, 80, 91, 100, 120, 127! Yes! Wow! You're at the max! Great! Once more, same thing. . . . And now breathe your way out of the contraction. Good! Do you realize that you doubled the strength of the contraction with your pushing? That was great!"

  Responding this way shows the birthing person how well they are doing and gives them a sense of accomplishment they might not otherwise have. Have the birthing person try to hold their breath for 5 to 6 seconds, which is what women do spontaneously when they do not have an epidural. One client found this so helpful they asked the doula to continue calling out numbers even after the monitor was removed! (The monitor is usually removed a few contractions before the birth because the baby is so low that the heartbeat cannot be picked up.)

- **Rectal and vaginal pain.** As the baby's head presses on the rectum, reaches the perineum, and distends the vaginal opening, the birthing person may feel some of the same burning, stretching sensation that people without epidurals feel. This may come as an unwelcome shock after having been numb. To turn the fear to excitement, point out that the baby is almost born. If the caregiver asks the birthing person to stop pushing as the head emerges, help them pant, or "blow, blow, blow," through the contractions.

- **Vacuum or forceps delivery.** An instrumental delivery (with forceps or a vacuum extractor) is sometimes necessary with an epidural. The epidural may cause profound relaxation of the pelvic muscles, which may cause the baby to descend deep into the pelvis without rotating first. This increases the chances that the baby will not rotate to fit through the pelvic outlet. If the doctor thinks an instrumental delivery may be necessary, you can encourage the birthing person to push as hard as they can ("give it everything you have!") to help the baby be born. It may be possible to speed the delivery and avoid the vacuum extractor or forceps and cesarean. This prospect is added incentive for the birthing person to push hard. On the other hand, it may not work, and the help of instruments may be necessary to achieve a vaginal birth.

    If the doctor decides to proceed with an instrumental delivery, the birthing person may worry that the instruments will harm the baby. The doctor should describe the safety measures that protect the baby from undue force and say that, if the baby does not move with a few contractions, they will not continue with the instruments and will do a cesarean instead.

- **The birth!** The predominant emotions for the birthing person may be relief— it is over, pushing is no longer necessary—and fascination with the baby. You may have the same emotions, along with admiration and powerful love for them.

    With the sensitive support I have described here, you will contribute to a safe, satisfying birth experience that will launch you both into parenthood with a sense of competence and self-confidence.

Local Anesthesia

The local blocks are given via injection. There are three major local blocks: the paracervical, which numbs the cervix, is rarely used in North America; the pudendal numbs the vaginal canal; and the perineal block numbs the perineum. All local blocks use the caine drugs, the same anesthetics used in neuraxial analgesia.

Technique for Giving Local Anesthesia

Local blocks numb smaller portions of the body than neuraxial analgesia. Because local blocks are easier to administer, they do not require the skills of an anesthesiologist. The caregiver draws the anesthetic into a syringe and injects it into the appropriate sites within or near the vagina. For details on each type of block, see the table "Pain Medications and Their Effects," page 332.

Local blocks require larger doses of the local anesthetic (but do not use narcotics) and provide less pain relief than neuraxial analgesia. Also, with a local block, more medication enters the birthing person's circulation; the drug may thus affect the fetus and the newborn more profoundly than if administered in neuraxial analgesia. This is why the paracervical blocks have almost disappeared from use in many areas of North America, and the pudendal block now tends to be reserved for late second stage forceps deliveries. The perineal block, or local, is given either shortly before delivery for an episiotomy or immediately after delivery for stitching. If the anesthetic is administered close to delivery, the fetus may receive less of the drug and be less affected. With an epidural, usually, no local block is used.

General Analgesia and Anesthesia

This form of pain-relief medication comes either as a gas to be inhaled through a mask or a mouthpiece or as a liquid injected intravenously. It reduces pain quickly by reducing or eliminating consciousness for as little as 1 minute to several hours.

Inhalation Analgesia: Nitrous Oxide

Nitrous oxide mixed with oxygen (laughing gas or gas and air) is widely used in Canada and many other nations for labor pain. It is also becoming more available in the United States, in hospitals and out-of-hospital birth centers. Nitrous oxide has other uses, such as in dentistry, but it is used in stronger concentrations that would be unsuitable for labor.

Nitrous oxide is self-administered by the birthing person by inhaling the gas via a handheld mask or mouthpiece at the very beginning of a contraction (or a little before, if you, your doula, or the birthing person can judge when it is about to begin). Within about 15 seconds, they feel drowsy, lightheaded, or giddy. The pain isn't eliminated, but it is reduced. As one person said, "The pain was there, but I was not bothered by it." They breathe the gas throughout the contraction, and then the mask falls away as they become less conscious. They are fully conscious by the time the next contraction comes and inhale the gas again.

It is usually required that the birthing person hold their own mask or whistle, so it falls away when they become less conscious.

Nitrous oxide is considered most effective for pain in the late dilation stage, especially transition and the birthing stage. The gas is also useful in situations when quick pain relief is needed, such as manual removal of the placenta or some other painful procedure.

Nitrous oxide is also considered safe for both birthing person and baby when used intermittently over a rather short time. Many people enjoy the mental effects, although others dislike them. In any case, these effects wear off quickly. Other side effects are uncommon; they include nausea or vomiting in 1 to 10 percent of women. In the concentrations used today for childbirth and when the birthing person holds the mask themselves, the gas wears off very quickly and effects on the baby are minimal. If someone else holds it, they may hold it on for too long, and the person may stay asleep between contractions, causing undesired side effects.

The greatest drawback to nitrous oxide is also its greatest advantage: Its effects are immediate and very transient, lasting 1 minute or so. For women who want complete pain relief over many hours, nitrous oxide is not a good choice. But for those who want a quick assist for a few contractions or a brief painful procedure, nitrous oxide might be a good choice.

General Anesthetics

These systemic drugs affect the whole body. Given in the form of a gas to be inhaled or as an intravenous medicine, they rapidly enter the bloodstream and circulate to the brain, where they quickly abolish awareness of pain and cause loss of consciousness.

Though easy and quick to administer, general anesthetics carry the potential risk that the unconscious person could vomit and inhale their own vomitus, which could cause serious pneumonia. Although anesthesiologists place a tube in the birthing person's airway to prevent such a complication, neuraxial anesthesia is safer and, therefore, generally preferred. However, general anesthesia is used today in the following circumstances:

- When life-threatening complications to the birthing person (such as hemorrhage) or baby (such as a prolapsed cord) require a cesarean or other surgery to be performed within minutes

- When neuraxial analgesia cannot be performed because of specific medical conditions or anatomical anomalies in the birthing person

- When an unexpected cesarean must be performed in a hospital that does not have an anesthesiologist on duty around the clock; under such circumstances, the general anesthetic is given by the doctor doing the surgery.

- When the birthing person has expressed a strong desire to be unconscious for the birth

See the table "Pain Medications and Their Effects" (page 332) for an explanation of the effects of different concentrations of inhaled gases.

Know How the Birthing Person Feels About Using Pain Medications

It is important for you to know the birthing person's desires regarding the use of pain medications in labor and to explore how you feel about their use. While most birth partners leave the decision to the birthing person, others have strong personal feelings on the subject. Some believe deeply that natural, unmedicated birth is preferable; others believe that natural birth causes unnecessary suffering and encourage the use of medications. The most important thing is that you both share your feelings in advance and prepare together as described here. Use the "Pain Medications Preference Scale," pages 328, to thoroughly explore the way you both feel.

When you both have learned about the demands and joys of childbirth and about the medical and nonmedical methods to manage pain, it is time to create a plan regarding the use of pain medication that meets the laboring person's wishes. Both of you should examine your individual feelings about birth, pain, and the support the birthing person will need. How much help can they realistically expect from you? How do you honestly feel about taking on the role of the birth partner? Go through the list of questions headed "How Will I Feel?" (see page 22) to assess your reactions to some of the realities of labor. Consider having a doula help.

The Pain Medications Preference Scale (PMPS) offers the birthing person a systematic and realistic way to think about their preferred approach to pain relief and the kind of help they will need from you and others. Using the PMPS, the birthing person won't make a yes-no choice about the use of pain medications, but will measure the strength of their feelings. You, too, should go through the PMPS to explore your own opinion and see whether you are comfortable with the birthing person's preferences regarding pain medications.

Of course, no one knows in advance how long or painful the labor will be or whether there will be complications. A flexible approach is the only sensible one. The PMPS takes this into account by including a variety of possibilities.

After thoughtful consideration of these unknowns, the birthing person's PMPS rating will be a good predictor of whether and under what circumstances they will or will not use pain medications. The PMPS will also be a helpful guide to all who will be helping them.

Directions for Using the Pain Medications Preference Scale (PMPS)

Take plenty of time to go over the PMPS on pages 328–329. Ask the birthing person to use it to help figure out the approach to pain relief that best suits them and to discover the kind of help they will need from you, a doula, or both to make it work. In the left column, the numbers from +10 down to +3 indicate degrees of desire to use pain medication, with +10 being the highest possible (and unrealistic) desire to use them for maximum relief of pain or any other sensations. Zero indicates no opinion. The numbers from −3 to −10 indicate degrees of desire to avoid pain medication, with −10 being an impossible extreme, just as +10 is. The impossible extremes were put on the scale to ensure that everyone will be somewhere between the two extremes and to give more meaning and clarity to the points in between.

After the birthing person picks the number that reflects their preferences, you should both look in the right-hand column for the kind of support and preparation needed. Can you provide this? If either of you has doubts, the birthing person can either rethink their preferences to be more in line with the kind of support you can provide, or you can get extra help from a doula or loved one. Are they preparing adequately? Make sure they understand that avoiding pain medication requires more preparation than using it.

Pain Medications Preference Scale

Rating	What It Means for the Birthing Person	How a Partner and Doula Help
+10	• Desire to feel nothing; desire for anesthesia before labor begins	• An impossible extreme; if the birthing person indicates +10, help them accept that it is not possible to feel nothing in labor; the risks are too high. They will have some pain and you will help them cope. • Review the discussion of pain medications together. • Help them get pain medications as soon as possible.
+9	• Fear of pain; believes they cannot cope; dependence on staff for total pain relief	• Same as for +10, plus, • Suggest they discuss their fears with the caregiver. • Practice simple breathing and comfort techniques together. • Plan to remain with the person in labor.
+7	• Desire for anesthesia as soon as allowed or before labor becomes painful	• Same as for +9, plus, • Make sure staff are aware of their desire. Learn whether early anesthesia is possible in your hospital. • Inform staff of this desire when you arrive.
+5	• Desire for epidural anesthesia in active labor (at 5 to 6 cm, about 2 inches, dilation) • Willingness to cope until then, perhaps with narcotic medications	• Same as for +7, plus, • Encourage them in the 3 Rs (see pages 147–164). • Know comfort measures (see chapter 4) and how to help. • Suggest medications as they approach active labor.
+3	• Preference for using medication, but as little as possible, with some sensation; desire to use self-help comfort measures • Natural childbirth is not a goal.	• Same as for +5, plus, • Plan to be an active birth partner to help keep medication use low. • Help get medications when they are wanted. • Suggest low doses of narcotics or a light epidural (to allow some feeling).
0	• No opinion or preference • This attitude is rare among pregnant women, though not among birth partners or doulas.	• Make sure they are informed. • Discuss medications. • Respond to their requests in labor. • If no preference, let staff manage their pain.

Pain Medications Preference Scale

Rating	What It Means for the Birthing Person	How a Partner and Doula Help
−3	• Wants to avoid pain medications unless coping becomes difficult • Will not feel disappointed or guilty if they use medications	• Do not suggest medications. • Emphasize coping techniques, but do not talk them out of pain medications if requested.
−5	• Strong preference to avoid pain medications, to avoid side effects for the baby or labor • Will accept medications for a long or difficult labor	• Plan to be a very active birth partner. • If possible, hire a doula to help the two of you. • Before leaving for the hospital, call and ask for a nurse who supports natural birth. • Learn and practice all the comfort measures in chapter 4 together. Know the 3 Rs (see pages 147–164). • Choose a code word (page 330) to say if they really want pain medications. Be sure staff know the code word. • During labor, do not suggest medications. • If they ask for medications, wait for the code word or have them checked for progress; try three more contractions before deciding; use the Take-Charge routine (see page 202).
−7	• Very strong desire for natural childbirth, for a sense of personal gratification as well as to benefit the baby and the progress of labor • Will be disappointed if they need to use medication	• Same as listed for −5, but with even greater commitment • Interpret requests for pain medication as a need for more help. • If they don't use the code word, keep encouraging them.
−9	• Desire that you and the staff deny the birthing person pain medication, even if requested	• Same as listed for −7 • If worried, remind them they have a code word. • Promise to help all you can but remind the birthing person that you or staff can't deny their request.
−10	• Desire that the birthing person forego all medications, even for cesarean delivery	• Impossible choice • Same as for −9: Help them develop a realistic understanding of the risks and benefits of pain medications.

The Birthing Person's Code Word

Many partners worry that the person who has a strong desire (–5 to –9) to avoid pain medications may, especially if labor is long or complicated, change their mind. How can you know whether it's right or wrong to keep encouraging them to continue without medications? The answer is, a code word.

You and the birthing person should agree on a word they can use if they change their mind about wanting an unmedicated birth. The word should be one they're unlikely to use in conversation (for example, iguana, pumpernickel, or cosmic). As long as the birthing person does not say this word, continue helping without suggesting pain medications—even if they say they want them. If they say the code word, you know they really want to change the plan, and you must respect this.

This agreement allows the birthing person to express their discouragement ("I can't do this;" "This hurts too much;" "I want drugs"), without the partner feeling a need to rescue them with medications. One doula tells of a client whose preference score was –7, but who seemed very distressed in labor. The doula said, "I was worried. I didn't want to suggest an epidural, but I was afraid she may have forgotten about her code word. So, I finally said, 'You have a code word, you know.' She never used it, so I continued to support her. Later she told me she was glad I had asked her because it made her ask herself, 'Am I suffering?' She decided she was not suffering and kept on—crying and swearing. She was glad she could complain as much as she needed to.' Complaining—always in rhythm!—was her way of coping."

Another doula offered this story: "My client strongly desired an unmedicated birth; her sister had recently had a very traumatic cesarean, and my client wanted to do everything she could to avoid that. In early labor, they calmly slow danced during contractions and chatted quietly, sipping coconut water, between contractions. When she started to sound like she was bearing down a little with contractions, her midwife checked her cervix and said, "You're 10 centimeters! You can start pushing!" My client's first words were, "I'm so scared!" and her labor suddenly stopped despite using positions and techniques to increase contractions.

When we talked about it, my client revealed that pushing had been very long and painful for her sister. My client was afraid to push. Her fear was so strong that it stopped her contractions! We discussed her fears, she said her code word, and decided to get the epidural. Her labor picked up, and her baby was born 2 hours later!

When Are Pain Medications Used?

Medication	Dilation Stage			Birthing Stage (pushing, birth)	Third Stage (placenta)
	Prelabor to 3 cm (1 inch)	4 to 7 cm (1½ inches to 2¾ inches)	8 to 10 cm (3 to 4 inches)		
Morphine (S)	▽_____				
Sedatives (S)	▽_____				
Tranquilizers (S)	▽	▽_____			
Narcotic-like analgesics (S)	▽	▽	▽_____		
Narcotic antagonists (S)		▽	▽		▽(to baby)▽
Paracervical block (L)		▽	▽_____		
Self-administered inhalation analgesia (S)			▽	▽_____	
Epidural or spinal narcotic analgesia (N)	▽	▽	▽	▽_____	
Standard epidural anesthesia—with or without narcotics (N)		▽ -			
Segmental ("light and late") epidural anesthesia (N)		▽ -			
Combined spinal-epidural (N)	▽	▽_____			
Pudendal block (L)				▽_____	
Perineal block (L)				▽	▽_____
Spinal, for cesarean only (N)*	▽		▽	▽_____	
General anesthesia, for cesarean only (S)*	▽ - - - - - - - - - - - - -		▽	▽_____	

*These can be given whenever a cesarean is decided upon.

KEY

_____ Time when drug may safely remain in effect

- - - - - - - - Time when dosing may be continuous

▽ Time when drug may be given (some must be discontinued early to allow side effects to diminish before birth)

S systemic medication   N neuraxial anesthesia   L local anesthesia

Pain Medications and Their Effects

Drug Names and How, Where, and When Given	Desired Effects	Possible Undesired Effects	Possible Precautions and Procedures to Improve Safety
SYSTEMIC MEDICATIONS			
Morphine* • Given by injection into muscle or vein • Given in exhausting pre- or early labor	• Therapeutic rest • Temporary break from non-productive contractions • Feeling of well-being • Prefer that morphine wear off before delivery to avoid effects on baby	*Birthing Person:* drop in blood pressure, dizziness, restlessness or excessive sedation, confusion, nausea and vomiting, urinary retention, respiratory depression *Fetus:* hypoxia, drop in fetal heart rate, decreased movement *Baby:* if ill-timed, heart rate changes, respiratory depression, need for resuscitation, depression of sucking and other reflexes	Restriction to bed, continuous fetal monitoring, oxygen for the birthing person or baby, administration of naloxone (drug to reverse side effects), timing of dosage to avoid greatest risks to the baby Some hospitals send people on morphine home (with a driver) when it is clear they have no adverse reaction to it and are still in prelabor.
Sedatives/Barbiturates pentobarbital (Nembutal) secobarbital (Seconal) • Given by injection or pill • Used during the first stage before 4 cm (1½ inches) dilation to allow effects on the baby to diminish before birth	• Sleepiness, relaxation • Possible slowing of unproductive contractions • Reduction in anxiety and tension	*Birthing Person:* increased perception of pain, dizziness, confusion, restlessness, excitement, disorientation, nausea, nightmares after use, respiratory depression *Fetus:* heart rate changes. *Baby:* poor suckling, breathing problems, decreased alertness for 2 to 4 days after birth	Oxygen for the birthing person or baby; resuscitation equipment for the baby; avoidance of concurrent use of narcotics

* Indicates drugs most commonly used in the U.S.

Drug	Benefits	Possible Side Effects	Comments
Tranquilizers promethazine (Phenergan), promazine (Sparine), hydroxyzine (Vistaril), midazolam (Versed), diazepam (Valium) • Given by injection or pill • Some (not Versed or Valium) are used during the first stage before 7 cm (2¾ inches) dilation • Versed and Valium may be used for cesarean delivery for profound tranquilizing effects.	• Drowsiness, relaxation • Reduction in tension, anxiety, nausea, and vomiting • Reduction of side effects of some narcotics • Possible acceleration of labor in a tense, exhausted laboring person	*Birthing Person:* dizziness, confusion, dry mouth, blood pressure and heart rate changes; Versed causes amnesia of the birth and the first hours with the baby. *Fetus:* heart rate changes *Baby:* if ill-timed, problems with breathing, temperature, and nursing; jaundice; lack of muscle tone and alertness	Versed and Valium are considered too risky to the fetus and newborn to use during labor. They are reserved for cesarean deliveries and used in small doses.
Narcotic and Narcotic-like Analgesics* meperidine (Demerol), nalbuphine (Nubain), fentanyl (Sublimaze), butorphanol (Stadol), pentazocine (Talwin) • Given by injection or IV and also by patient-controlled IV device, especially after a cesarean • Used during first stage until 7 cm (2¾ inches) dilation, or after a cesarean	• Partial relief of pain, relaxation • Halting, slowing, or speeding of contractions, depending on amount, timing, and drug used	*Birthing Person:* nausea, dizziness, groggy feeling, hallucinations, low heart rate and blood pressure, confusion, itching, respiratory depression, temporary slowing of labor *Fetus:* heart rate changes, decreased movement *Baby:* if ill-timed, heart rate changes; depressed respiration at birth, which may require resuscitation; poor suckling; depression of other reflexes	Oxygen for the birthing person or baby; naloxone (a narcotic antagonist) for the birthing person or baby to counter depressive effects; effort to predict the time of birth to avoid giving the drug when the risks to the baby are greatest
Narcotic Antagonist naloxone (Narcan) • Given by injection into the muscle or vein • May be given to birthing person or baby after birth, if needed, to reverse side effects of a narcotic	• Reversal of some effects of narcotics on birthing person or baby, such as itching, hallucinations, respiratory depression, low blood pressure, and heart rate; diminished newborn reflexes and poor suckling	*Birthing Person:* nausea, vomiting, sweating, shivering, restlessness, increased heart rate, return of pain, high blood pressure, heart arrhythmias, pulmonary edema (rarely), tremors *Fetus:* increased activity, improved heart rate *Baby:* No apparent adverse effects observed when the drug is used to reverse respiratory depression in the newborn	Possible supplemental doses after 30 to 45 minutes or the effects of the narcotic may return

* Indicates drugs most commonly used in the U.S.

Drug Names and How, Where, and When Given	Desired Effects	Possible Undesired Effects	Possible Precautions and Procedures to Improve Safety
SYSTEMIC MEDICATIONS (cont.)			
Inhalation Analgesia nitrous oxide gas and oxygen • Self-administered by birthing person • Given late in dilation stage, in the birthing stage, and occasionally in the placental stage	• Loss of pain awareness and consciousness for about 1 minute, followed by quick recovery	*Birthing Person:* temporary grogginess and difficulty bearing down during birthing contractions *Fetus:* transient effect due to very rapid half-life *Baby:* no known effect on newborn; no known long-term effects when used in concentrations recommended for birth	*Birthing Person* tries to begin inhaling nitrous oxide a little before the onset of a contraction, to ease pain and reduce consciousness through the peak; if they wait until the contraction begins before inhaling the gas, relief comes only after the contraction has peaked.
REGIONAL (NEURAXIAL) ANALGESIA			
Standard Lumbar Epidural mepivacaine (Carbocaine), chloroprocaine (Nesacaine), bupivacaine (Marcaine), lidocaine (Xylocaine), ropivacaine (Naropin) mixed with narcotic • Injected into a catheter placed in the epidural space outside the spinal canal; given as a continuous drip • Given before 8 cm (about 3 inches) dilation or later if labor is slow or arrested	• Loss of pain sensation from abdomen to toes • Relaxation as pain is relieved • Sleep for an exhausted birthing person • Usually adequate for a cesarean	*Birthing Person:* inability to move the lower half of their body; toxic reaction (rare); after 4 hours, fever that increases with duration of the epidural; decrease in blood pressure; slowing of labor; reduced urge and ability to push; spinal headache if the drug is inadvertently injected into the dural space; prolonged birthing stage; increased chance of malpositioned baby *Fetus:* heart rate changes and lack of oxygen caused by low maternal blood pressure and fever *Baby:* subtle temporary changes in reflexes, including suckling and breathing; fussiness	*Birthing Person:* restriction to bed, frequent checks of blood pressure and blood oxygenation, withholding of food, limits on drinking, intravenous fluids, bladder catheter, oxygen mask, possible antibiotics for fever, continuous electronic fetal monitoring, Pitocin to augment contractions, forceps or vacuum extractor, episiotomy, possible increased chance of cesarean *Baby:* blood or urine cultures to detect infection, antibiotics, and 48 hours in a special-care nursery for observation if birthing person had a fever in labor (to rule out infection)

Medication	Benefits	Risks/Side Effects	What to Expect
Segmental "Light" Epidural, with or without PCEA (Patient-Controlled Epidural Analgesia)* mepivacaine (Carbocaine), chloroprocaine (Nesacaine), bupivacaine (Marcaine), lidocaine (Xylocaine), ropivacaine (Naropin), mixed with low doses of narcotics (fentanyl or sufentanil) • A lower concentration of anesthetic than for a standard epidural is injected into the epidural space outside the spinal canal. • Given as a continuous drip into a catheter and may have patient-controlled apparatus (PCEA), which allows birthing person to give small additional doses as needed; generally reduces total amount of medication used and its side effects • Given in the first stage, once labor is established	• Loss of pain sensation in the trunk, without total loss of movement and sensation in the perineum and legs • Relaxation as pain is relieved • Sleep for an exhausted birthing person • Pain reduction may reduce high anxiety from pain and may lower stress hormones, (which can slow labor), resulting in improved labor progress.	*Birthing Person* (some of these are less likely with a "light" than with a standard lumbar epidural): itching; nausea; after 4 hours, fever that increases with duration of the epidural; drop in blood pressure; slowing of labor; reduced urge and ability to push; spinal headache if the medication is inadvertently injected into the dural space; increased chance of forceps, vacuum extractor delivery *Fetus:* heart rate changes and lack of oxygen, caused by low maternal blood pressure and fever *Baby:* subtle changes in reflexes, including suckling and breathing; fussiness	*Birthing Person:* Intravenous fluids; Pitocin to augment contractions; narcotic antagonist to control side effects; Benadryl for itching; restriction to bed, frequent checks of blood pressure and blood oxygenation, withholding of food and drink, bladder catheter, oxygen mask, continuous electronic fetal monitoring, increased chance of forceps or vacuum extractor delivery and episiotomy; PCEA "lockout" mechanism controls timing of medicine (eg, once every 10 minutes) to prevent overdose *Baby:* blood or urine cultures to detect infection, antibiotics, and 48 hours in a special-care nursery for observation if birthing person had a fever in labor (to rule out infection)
Epidural Narcotics and Spinal* (Intrathecal) Narcotics meperidine (Demerol), morphine (Duramorph), fentanyl (Sublimaze), sufentanil (Sufenta) • Epidural: given by injection or continuous drip into the epidural space outside the spinal canal • Spinal: given as an injection into the dural space in the spinal canal • Used during the first stage or after a cesarean delivery	• 90 minutes to 24 hours of pain relief depending on medication used, with little change in mental state • Retention of enough muscle function in the legs that the laboring person may be able to stand and walk with help and move freely in bed	*Birthing Person:* nausea, vomiting; urine retention; itching; spinal headache (caused by leaking of spinal fluid); "breakthrough" pain at 6 to 8 cm (about 3 inches) dilation if only narcotics are used *Fetus:* heart rate changes (occurring less frequently with epidural than with IV narcotics) *Baby:* narcotics are absorbed in small amounts, but effects are unknown	*Birthing Person:* Intravenous fluids; Pitocin to augment contractions; narcotic antagonist to control side effects; Benadryl for itching; bladder catheter; blood patch (some of the birthing person's blood is injected into the dura to stop a clot to form a clot to stop leaking of spinal fluid and relieve a spinal headache), continuous fetal monitoring, increased chance of forceps or vacuum extractor delivery and episiotomy

* Indicates drugs most commonly used in the U.S.

Drug Names and How, Where, and When Given	Desired Effects	Possible Undesired Effects	Possible Precautions and Procedures to Improve Safety
NEURAXIAL ANALGESIA (cont.) **Spinal Block*** mepivacaine (Carbocaine), chloroprocaine (Nesacaine), bupivacaine (Marcaine), lidocaine (Xylocaine) • Usually given as a single injection into the dural space in the spine • Given any time before or during labor for a planned or unplanned cesarean • Rarely used for vaginal births	• 2- to 3-hour absence of sensation below chest • Easier and quicker to administer than an epidural block • More rapid onset of pain relief than with epidural • Loss of pain, other sensations, and movement from chest to toes for 2 to 3 hours after injection, with no mental effects • Relaxation and rest as pain is relieved	*Birthing Person:* toxic reaction (rare); decrease in blood pressure; spinal headache (caused by spinal fluid leaking); impaired sensation of breathing, or actual inability to breathe, requiring artificial ventilation if the level of anesthesia rises high enough to affect the chest muscles *Fetus:* heart rate changes, caused by low maternal blood pressure *Baby:* subtle changes in reflexes, including suckling; fussiness	*Birthing Person:* Frequent checks of blood pressure and blood oxygenation, electrocardiogram, intravenous fluids, bladder catheter, oxygen mask, artificial ventilation, continuous fetal monitoring until cesarean begins; blood patch (see "Epidural Narcotics and Spinal [Intrathecal] Narcotics," page 335)

* Indicates drugs most commonly used in the U.S.

Combined Spinal/Epidural (CSE)

Narcotic—fentanyl (Sublimaze) or sufentanil (Sufenta), plus anesthetic—bupivacaine (Marcaine) or ropivacaine (Naropin)

- Two separate pain-relief techniques used at one time
- The "needle-through-needle technique"—first, an epidural needle is placed in the epidural space; then, in early labor, a very thin spinal needle is run through the epidural needle into the spinal space, and narcotics are given in the spinal space. The spinal needle is removed and a catheter is run through the epidural needle into the epidural space where, later, an anesthetic can be dripped. The epidural needle is then removed. Only the catheter remains, taped to the birthing person's back.
- Given as early as 2 cm (about 1 inch) dilation with narcotics and 4 to 6 cm (2 to 2½ inches) with anesthetic

- Very fast pain relief, lasting throughout labor, with the ability to move (and perhaps walk a bit in early labor) and without mental effects
- Rest for an exhausted birthing person

Birthing Person: from the narcotic: itching, nausea and vomiting, retained urine, some weakness in the legs; from the anesthetic: fever, impaired movement in the legs, slowing of labor and the baby's descent, drop in blood pressure, impaired urge and ability to push

Fetus: from the anesthetic: heart rate changes caused by the birthing person's fever and low blood pressure

Baby: from the anesthetic: fever; narcotics are absorbed by the baby, but their effects are unknown.

Birthing Person: restriction of food and drink, intravenous fluids, check of muscle strength in legs before the birthing person tries to walk, bladder catheter; additional medications to control itching and nausea (these may make the birthing person sleepy or interfere with pain relief), Pitocin to speed labor

Baby: blood or urine cultures to detect infection, antibiotics, and 48 hours in special-care nursery for observation if birthing person had a fever in labor

Drug Names and How, Where, and When Given	Desired Effects	Possible Undesired Effects	Possible Precautions and Procedures to Improve Safety
GENERAL ANESTHESIA			
Inhalation Gas nitrous oxide; isoflurane (Forane); injected medication: thiopental (Pentothal), ketamine • To induce total unconsciousness and muscle inactivity in the birthing person, gases are administered by an anesthesiologist. (Stronger concentrations of nitrous oxide are used for total anesthesia than for self-administration during labor.) • Medications are injected into a vein to rapidly induce unconsciousness and total muscle inactivity in the birthing person. • With either method, the anesthesiologist provides oxygen and mechanically assists with respiration. • Used before labor when an elective cesarean is planned or during labor when an emergency cesarean becomes necessary	• Fastest total pain relief and loss of consciousness, for an immediate emergency cesarean	*Birthing Person:* hallucinations, postoperative excitement, amnesia, vomiting and aspiration of stomach contents, respiratory depression, drops in blood pressure and heart rate *Fetus:* unconsciousness, slowing of movements and heart rate *Baby:* depression of central nervous system and respiration, poor muscle tone, low Apgar scores, need for resuscitation	*Birthing Person:* antacid given right before surgery to neutralize stomach contents; intubation (tube placed in windpipe to protect against aspiration of stomach contents); intravenous muscle relaxants; taping of closed eyelids to protect the eyes from damage; electrocardiogram; monitoring of pulse, blood gas levels, and blood pressure; assistance with breathing; electronic fetal monitoring *Baby:* resuscitation procedures and equipment to assist breathing and alertness

LOCAL ANESTHESIA

	Benefits	Risks	Special requirements
Paracervical Block mepivacaine (Carbocaine), lidocaine (Xylocaine), chloroprocaine (Nesacaine) • Given as an injection into each side of the dilating cervix • Given after 5 cm (2 inches) and before 9 cm (about 4 inches) dilation	• Short-term localized pain relief with no change in consciousness or ability to move freely • Quick administration, can be done by the birthing person's doctor; no anesthesiologist needed	*Birthing Person:* toxic reaction (rare), sudden decrease in blood pressure *Fetus:* profound and sudden fetal heart rate abnormalities *Baby:* reduced muscle tone, decreased reflexes; fussiness	Frequent blood-pressure and blood oxygenation checks, intravenous fluids, oxygen mask, continuous electronic fetal monitoring, capability to perform rapid cesarean if the baby has an adverse reaction; rarely used in North America
Pudendal Block mepivacaine (Carbocaine), lidocaine (Xylocaine), chloroprocaine (Nesacaine) • Given as an injection into pudendal nerve endings on each side of the vaginal canal • Used during the birthing stage before application of forceps or vacuum extractor	• Numbing of the birth canal and rectum, relaxation of the pelvic floor, enabling less painful forceps or vacuum extractor delivery	*Birthing Person:* toxic reaction (rare), decrease in blood pressure, diminished pelvic floor muscle tone *Fetus:* sudden drop in heart rate *Baby:* temporary reduction in muscle tone, decreased reflexes; fussiness	Pitocin, oxygen, episiotomy, availability of forceps or vacuum extractor for delivery
Perineal Block* mepivacaine (Carbocaine), lidocaine (Xylocaine), chloroprocaine (Nesacaine) • Given as several injections into the perineum and vaginal outlet • Used during the birthing stage, before an episiotomy, or after the birth to repair an episiotomy or tear	• Numbing of perineum • Less pain during an episiotomy or stitching	*Birthing Person:* pain from injections, tearing from swelling if injections are given during the second rather than third stage *Fetus and Baby:* risks unlikely, as injections are given just before or after birth	None

* Indicates drugs most commonly used in the U.S.

CESAREAN BIRTH AND VAGINAL BIRTH AFTER CESAREAN

She dilated from 5 cm (2 inches) to complete in 2 hours, and the baby was pretty low in her birth canal, but then she pushed and pushed. We tried every position, but the contractions spaced out. She got an epidural, we tried Pitocin, but she made no progress. We waited. Then, there was nothing left but a cesarean. His head was tilted at an angle, and it was huge. She worked so damn hard—she could even see his dark hair when pushing! But he couldn't come through. She's my goddess, and we're blissed out with our baby. But we just wish . . .

—PAUL, FIRST-TIME FATHER

I wish I had read the chapter on cesareans!

—KEVIN, SECOND-TIME FATHER

Sometimes, a baby is delivered surgically, through an incision in the pregnant person's abdomen, instead of through the vagina. This procedure is a cesarean section, also called a cesarean delivery, a cesarean birth, a C-section, or, simply, a cesarean. The cesarean is the most common surgery performed in the United States. The rate in 2016 was 31.8 percent, a small decline since 2009 when the rate was 32.9 percent, the highest rate ever.

The causes for the high rate are numerous, complex, and controversial. In general, the attitude toward cesareans, while more accepting and unquestioning than ever before, is shifting. Recent research findings indicate long-term harm for the birthing person and baby from unneeded cesareans. See Recommended Resources (page 418) for further discussion of the cesarean rate in the United States.

Individual doctor's cesarean rates range from 10 to 60 percent of deliveries; hospitals also vary widely in their cesarean rates, from less than 10 percent to more than 65 percent in the United States.

The challenge of lowering the rate is enormous, but we are hopeful the rate will continue downward, now that the long- and short-term risks of this major surgery and its lack of benefits for healthy birthing parents and babies are becoming well known. At the same time, however, we must recognize the judicious use of the cesarean operation has, over the years, saved or improved the lives of millions of birthing persons and babies and continues to do so.

You and the pregnant person need to be able to recognize when a cesarean will improve the chances of a healthy parent and baby and when a cesarean can do more harm than good. Clear communication and covering the Key Questions for Informed Decision-Making (see page 237) with a caregiver whom you both trust, a birth setting that has a relatively low cesarean rate, and a doula are probably your most important assurances that there will not be an unnecessary or ill-advised cesarean. Numerous research studies report that birth settings in which high priorities are placed on a low cesarean rate and the presence of a doula have lower rates of cesareans and better parent and infant outcomes.

Know the Nonmedical Reasons for Cesarean Birth and Factors to Consider

Cesareans are often done even when there is no medical reason. Among the numerous reasons are:

1. Belief that the nonmedically indicated cesarean is as safe, or safer, for the baby than vaginal birth and risks to the birthing person, though greater, are minimal. Ignorance of the risks may lead to regret over the choice.

   • Risks to the birthing persons from nonmedically indicated cesareans include surgical risks (that occur with any surgery), such as infection, hemorrhage, or bladder or bowel injury; complications in recovery; problems with incision healing; and development of abdominal adhesions, excessive internal scar tissue that binds to other structures, possibly causing chronic pain and problems with future childbearing (including more stillbirths and abnormal placental implantation). Though most people have good outcomes from cesarean deliveries, these risks should be considered, especially when there is no medical need for the surgery.

- Risks to infants (when compared to babies born vaginally) include increased chances of serious respiratory problems; more autoimmune diseases in childhood; or more asthma, allergies, and type 1 (childhood) diabetes.

2. Deep fear of labor and vaginal birth in the birthing person (tocophobia). Every birthing person deserves education, sensitive counseling, and birth planning that addresses their fears and provides practical strategies for avoiding or minimizing those fears; these often give them the confidence to plan a vaginal birth. If, however, there is no such counseling available or they cannot come to terms with the fear, they should have the right to make the informed choice for a cesarean.

3. Fear of incontinence (involuntary loss of urine or feces) or pelvic floor damage caused by vaginal birth. These problems are rare after vaginal birth, especially with birth practices such as those discussed on pages 38–39, 40–42 and 164–165. However, they do sometimes occur in difficult vaginal births or in people with friable vaginal tissue, which is more easily injured or bleeds more easily than normal. After a few months, there is no difference in incontinence rates between those who had vaginal births and those who had cesareans. General health and fitness and body type play a greater role than mode of birth. It is true, however, that the pelvic floor is not stretched during a cesarean.

4. Convenience. The appeal for busy people and doctors of being able to plan the date and time for a cesarean is great—especially if they think the risks are acceptable. While it is undeniably more convenient for doctors, women should weigh the potential risks to themselves and their babies against this benefit, as the prolonged recovery time may negate the convenience of planning the date.

5. Inadequate hospital facilities. Many hospitals do not offer the choice of a trial of labor after a previous cesarean (TOLAC) because they do not have the capability to perform an emergency cesarean at all times of the day. ACOG's (the American Council of Obstetricians and Gynecologists) 2017 Practice Bulletin No. 184 says, "ACOG recommends that TOLAC be attempted in facilities that can provide cesarean delivery for situations that are immediate threats to the life of the [pregnant person] or fetus." These hospitals would seem to be subpar, not only for women wishing a VBAC, but for all laboring women because the need for a cesarean can arise at any time, with any person, whether there staff are available or not. It seems that the pregnant person might be forced to go to another hospital that can provide TOLAC or, more likely, to plan a cesarean for a time when the hospital can provide adequate care.

Know the Medical Reasons for Cesarean Birth

You and the birthing person should understand the reasons for the cesarean before it is done and agree it is the right thing to do. If you find out in advance that the birthing person or the baby has a medical problem requiring a cesarean delivery or making it highly likely, you both can learn all about the surgery and adjust emotionally beforehand. If the need for the cesarean arises in labor, you both will have to do much of the adjusting afterward. Either way, the birthing person should have the opportunity to talk about the experience with you, your doula, the doctor, and the nurses.

See chapters 6 and 7 for information about problems that sometimes arise in labor and how they are detected and treated; a cesarean becomes the solution if other treatments are unsuccessful.

Following are the most likely medical reasons for a cesarean. Although cesareans are not always necessary in these circumstances, they are always considered and very often done.

1. Preexisting conditions that lead to planning a cesarean in advance. Most cesareans are unplanned and the need becomes clear once labor is underway. There are, however, some situations

better handled by planning a cesarean for a few days before the due date. For example, some chronic illnesses or conditions: heart disease; some cases of diabetes; asthma; physical disability; some cases of twins or triplets; fetal growth restriction; placenta previa; breech presentation; deep fear of vaginal birth; previous cesarean delivery; and others. While some of these are controversial, they are among the labors considered to be at higher risk and more unpredictable than when these conditions do not exist. Parents should ask the key questions (see page 237).

If a decision is made to have a planned cesarean, read this chapter because planned and unplanned cesareans have much in common. The one bit of advice we want to add is, when setting the date and time for a planned cesarean, try to schedule it early or as the first case of the day, for two reasons: It is less likely to be a delayed (from earlier surgeries taking longer than expected) and the birthing person will likely be instructed to eat nothing after midnight; if they do not have to wait until late in the day, they'll be much more comfortable.

2. Emergencies that arise in labor, including:

 • Prolapsed cord (see page 290)

 • Serious hemorrhage (excessive bleeding) in the birthing person (see page 283); in these situations, there is no time for questions. Rapid action is essential.

3. Arrested labor. This is the most common reason for a first cesarean. Failure to progress in labor may be caused by the following:

 • Abnormal position or presentation of the baby

 • Uterine inertia (inadequate contractions)

 • A poor fit between the baby's head and the birthing person's pelvis (see page 287)

 • A combination of more than one of the above indications

According to many experts, far too many cesareans are performed because of arrested labor, or "failure to progress" (see "Complications with Labor Progress," page 285). Many of these cesareans are actually done because of failure to *wait* rather than failure to progress. In fact, the American College of Obstetricians and Gynecologists has recently published several documents offering evidence-based guidelines for reducing primary (first) and repeat cesareans (see Recommended Resources, page 418).

4. Problems with the fetus, including:

- Fetal intolerance of labor. Many experts believe this is another reason for which cesareans are too often performed (see "Diagnosing Fetal Distress," page 293).

- Breech presentation (see "A Breech Baby," page 226)

- Prematurity, postmaturity (when the baby is overdue), or other conditions that might make vaginal birth too stressful for the baby. Through fetal movement counting, by which the birthing person keeps track of how much the baby moves (see page 42), nonstress testing (see page 242), and ultrasound (see page 241), the caregiver tries to predict whether the baby can tolerate labor.

5. Problems with the birthing person, including:

- Serious illness (such as heart disease, diabetes, or preeclampsia) or injury. Sometimes, in these cases, a cesarean is planned in advance. Otherwise, a "trial of labor" is planned. The birthing person is watched carefully and, if all goes well, they give birth vaginally. If the problem worsens, they have a cesarean.

- A genital herpes sore (see page 280)

6. A previous cesarean delivery. This is a major reason for the high cesarean rate in the United States and Canada. Today, approximately 86 percent of people who have had a cesarean will have another, even though most are good candidates for a VBAC. With the right doctor and hospital, a VBAC is possible. Furthermore, there is good reason to believe that VBACs will increase now that ACOG and other professional organizations strongly support VBACs under safe conditions. If the birthing person wants to try for one, you both should read "A Previous Disappointing or Traumatic Birth Experience," page 231, and "Vaginal Birth After Cesarean (VBAC) & Trial of Labor After Cesarean" (TOLAC); see pages 356 to 362.

Once the decision to perform a cesarean is made, concentrate on helping the birthing person and greeti ng the baby as lovingly and gently as possible.

Know What to Expect During Cesarean Birth

You may be surprised by how quickly the staff move once the decision is made to do a cesarean and by the number of people involved: Besides you, possibly a doula, and the birthing person, there is the doctor who will do the surgery; an assisting doctor or midwife; a "scrub nurse," who gives instruments to the doctor; a "floating nurse," who prepares the room and looks after the surgical team; an anesthesiologist; a pediatric nurse or two to look after the baby; and possibly a pediatrician or neonatologist, if problems with the baby are anticipated. They all work together as an efficient, businesslike team.

You may feel frightened and worried for the birthing person or baby. You may feel relieved to know the end is in sight, especially after a long, difficult labor. You may be impressed and reassured by the teamwork and competence of the staff. You may feel left out or even shocked by their apparently casual attitude. They may talk and even joke among themselves, paying little attention to you and the birthing person, as if you are not there. You may feel overwhelmed by the sounds, smells, and sights of the operating room. You may be confused about your role. Should you ask questions and try to make sure the birthing person's wishes are being followed, or should you stay out of the way and let them proceed in their customary manner? Just a few minutes before, your role was essential to the birthing person's ability to handle the contractions; now you feel much less important. Be assured: you are still most important, but in a different way. The following descriptions of the surgery and your role will help you help the laboring person.

Preparations for Surgery

Preparations for cesarean delivery include the following steps:

• The birthing person signs a consent form.

• A nurse starts intravenous fluids in the birthing person's arm, which is placed on a board that extends out to the side of the operating table. The nurse checks the birthing person's blood pressure frequently.

- The birthing person may be offered a sedative, which can be refused if they want to remain aware during the surgery and immediately after birth. At any time, if they change their mind, they can tell the doctor and get the sedative.

- An anesthesiologist, nurse-anesthetist, or, rarely, the obstetrician gives the anesthetic (spinal, epidural, or general; see chapter 8). The choice of anesthesia depends on the birthing person's situation, training and qualifications of the staff, and the facilities. General anesthesia, being fastest, is chosen if the cesarean must be done immediately—which is very rare. Regional anesthesia is safer if time allows.

- The birthing person will probably receive oxygen, administered with a face mask or nasal prongs (tubes that blow oxygen into the nose).

- A pulse oximeter, a small device that tracks the oxygen content in the birthing person's blood, will be clipped to a finger or toe.

- Electrocardiogram (EKG or ECG) leads are placed on the chest. These keep track of the birthing person's heart function throughout the surgery.

- The birthing person's body is draped so only the abdomen can be seen. The end of the drape is raised to form a screen between their head and abdomen. Even if conscious, the birthing person cannot see the surgery. Some hospitals have a clear window in the drape so the birthing person can see the baby being removed from their abdomen.

- Most hospitals now welcome the birth partner (and sometimes a doula or other person) in the operating room for a cesarean. You sit on a stool at the head. The anesthesiologist remains at the head also.

- Some birth partners want to watch and even photograph the surgery. Discuss this option with the birthing person and the caregiver, if it interests you and the birthing person. It is quite likely for staff to refuse to let you photograph the surgery, but you can photograph the baby's first contact with their gestational parent and other tender moments. To see or photograph the baby's birth, you will have to stand up and look over the drape or hold your camera high.

- The birthing person's abdomen is scrubbed and shaved. Some pubic hair is usually removed.

- A catheter is placed in the bladder to keep it empty and out of the way of the scalpel.

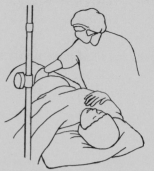

The birthing person's abdomen is scrubbed in preparation for the surgery.

Surgery Begins

This is how a cesarean delivery starts:

- Once the anesthetic takes effect, the doctor makes the incisions with a scalpel.

- The skin incision is usually low and horizontal, or transverse (this is called a "bikini incision" meaning it is so low that later, even when wearing a bikini, the scar will not be visible). Rarely, the incision is vertical and in the mid-abdomen (called a classical incision).

- The muscles of the abdomen are not cut; there is a connective tissue line (the "linea alba") down the middle of the abdominal muscles. These often separate spontaneously and painlessly during late pregnancy, as the muscles stretch around the growing uterus. During the cesarean, the surgeon spreads the muscles further, without cutting them. The incision in the uterus is made through the gap between those muscles.

- The uterine incision is usually horizontal, or transverse, in the lower segment of the uterus, but it can be made higher if speed is essential or if the higher opening is needed to get the baby out (for example, in the case of twins, a premature baby, or an unusual presentation).

- The amniotic fluid is suctioned from the uterus with a plastic tube. You will hear the sucking sound.

- To prevent excessive bleeding, the cut blood vessels are cauterized. You may hear the high-pitched tone of the cautery device or notice a slight odor as it burns the ends of the blood vessels to close them. The birthing person cannot feel this.

- If at any time during the procedure the birthing person indicates they feel pain (as opposed to pressure or tugging), make sure the doctor knows it and stops working until more anesthetic can be given. This does not happen often, but sometimes the anesthesia is spotty and the birthing person is not numb where they need to be.

The Baby Is Born!

The baby is usually delivered within 15 minutes after surgery has begun. This is how:

- The doctor either places one hand in the uterus to grasp the baby's head or buttocks or may instead attach a vacuum extractor to the baby's head if it is accessible (vacuum extraction allows for a smaller incision in the birthing person's abdomen). The assisting doctor pushes on the birthing person's abdomen to move the baby down to the incision. The first doctor removes the baby. The birthing person may feel pressure and tugging, but should not feel pain. Help them use relaxation and slow rhythmic breathing (see page 161). Make sure the doctor and anesthesiologist know if they complain of pain, so more anesthetic can be given.

- The doctor or nurse suctions the baby's airways and clamps and cuts the cord. You may want to ask the doctor to lower the drape so the birthing person can see the baby, or the baby may be briefly held up for you both to admire. Then, the baby is usually taken to an infant care area in the corner of the delivery room or in an adjacent room, for evaluation and any necessary treatment. By this time, the baby is probably crying lustily. You may wish to go take a look at the baby, especially if your doula can remain with the birthing person.

- The oxygen apparatus is removed from the birthing person's face.

In some hospitals, some caregivers now delay clamping and cutting the umbilical cord for a short time or "milk" the cord to allow some placental blood to return to the baby (see page 142).

Some hospitals have adopted practices (sometimes referred to as the natural or gentle cesarean), that keep the baby and birthing parent together skin to skin, starting right after the cesarean or shortly after a brief observation in the infant care unit located in or close to the operating room. They value the practice of placing the unwrapped baby on the birthing person's bare chest and then covering the baby (see page 299).

If so, the birthing person might be trembling and feel weak, so help them hold the baby on the chest, and you both can sing your baby's song

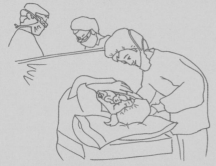

While the incision is being repaired, you may hold the baby so the birthing person can see and talk to the baby.

(see page 44) or talk to the baby. These practices that encourage parent-baby contact from birth have the advantages of keeping the baby warm and enhancing bonding, feeding, and breast-seeking behaviors, Furthermore, skin-to-skin contact early after birth, enhances the birthing person's and baby's own production of oxytocin (the "love hormone").

The Placenta Is Removed

While you are greeting the baby, the doctor reaches into the uterus, separates the placenta from the wall of the uterus, and removes it.

Some doctors then lift the uterus out of the abdomen to check it thoroughly before beginning to close the incision. The birthing person may feel this as uncomfortable pressure and may feel nauseated and vomit, turning their head to the side and using the basin that you, the doula, or the anesthesiologist holds for them. Because the benefit of removing the uterus is questionable and because it causes the birthing person much discomfort (even with anesthesia), many physicians have safely discontinued the practice. Others believe it is the only way they can repair it well. You might discuss this with the doctor ahead of time, and the birthing person might state in the birth plan that they prefer not to have the uterus lifted out for inspection.

The Repair Begins

The repair phase takes 30 to 45 minutes. These procedures are involved:

- The uterus and other internal layers are sutured with absorbable suture thread. You might ask ahead of time whether the caregiver does a single-layer or double-layer repair of the uterine incision. Some doctors use the single-layer repair because it is quicker, but studies have found that single layer suturing leaves the uterine scar weaker and more likely to separate in a future pregnancy or labor. Consider asking for a double-layer repair in the birth plan.

- The skin is closed with stitches or, less frequently, stainless steel clips. You may hear the clicking of the stapler as the clips are placed.

- A bandage is applied over the incision.

- The birthing person may develop a pain in their shoulder. This is "referred pain"—pain felt a distance from where the cause lies. Shoulder pain is usually caused by air entering the internal abdomen or pelvic area. The anesthesiologist may be able to help by raising the head of the operating table slightly, which sometimes moves the air bubble. There is little else that can be done—rubbing the shoulder is unlikely to help much—but knowing the pain is not a sign that something is wrong and that it will soon fade, may reduce the birthing person's anxiety.

- The birthing person may be very shaky, trembling all over, or nauseated—normal reactions after major surgery—so they might be given a relaxing, sleep-inducing medication via the intravenous line, without either of you knowing it. If it is important to the birthing person to be awake after the birth to experience the first hours with the baby, ask ahead of time and again just after the birth, that these medications not be given without first checking with the birthing person. The nausea and trembling usually subside within 30 minutes. If the nausea and trembling are extreme, the birthing person can always change their mind and ask for medication. It takes effect within 2 minutes.

  There is one medication, Versed, that the birthing person should be warned about. Along with being an effective sedative, it is also a potent amnesiac. It wipes out all memory of the birth and related events for hours afterward. The birthing person will not remember having the baby, nor will they remember their first impressions or the first feeding. The absence of memory of the momentous event might haunt them and cause much regret later.

  Zofran is an effective antinausea medication that does not make a person groggy or take away their memory. Ask about it or other medications that do not cause drowsiness.

- The birthing person is cleaned and taken to the recovery area.

The Recovery Period

This is what you can expect during the recovery period:

• The birthing person remains in the recovery room or in the labor room for a few hours with a nurse close by, until it is clear the recovery is going well and the anesthetic is wearing off as expected.

• The nurse frequently checks the birthing person's pulse, temperature, blood pressure, uterine tone, and state of anesthesia.

• The baby may remain with their parents or go to the nursery for observation or treatment, depending on the baby's condition and hospital custom. You might go with the baby; it is very helpful if the birthing person has the company of a friend, relative, or doula if you leave.

• A pain medication regimen will be established to keep the birthing person comfortable; see pages 333 and 335 for explanations of narcotics used after a cesarean.

• If they haven't already done so in the operating room, the birthing person can breast-feed the baby now. The nurses or doula can help position the baby and get started. It is a good idea to begin breast-feeding before the anesthesia wears off, as it will be a little easier to get started when not in pain.

• If the birthing person is asleep or groggy from the medication for nausea and trembling, it will be difficult to breast-feed. This is why some people refuse medication for nausea and trembling, preferring to put up with it for 30 minutes to 1 hour—they do not want to miss the first few hours with the baby.

• If the birthing person is unable to nurse or hold the baby, you do it. Hold the baby close (skin to skin, if possible) and talk or sing to them.

• The nurse checks the baby's breathing, skin color, temperature, and heart rate frequently.

• Once the anesthesia wears off and the birthing person's condition is stable, they will go to the postpartum room, where they will stay until they go home. See chapter 10 for information about the first few days after birth.

Your Role During and After a Cesarean Birth

For one who plans a vaginal birth, a cesarean is unexpected and may be disappointing, even if they know the surgery has made it possible to have a healthy baby. Some get over these feelings quickly; others do not. A birthing person often needs time afterward to adjust emotionally, to talk about and even grieve over the experience, especially if they had a strong desire to give birth vaginally. It is sometimes surprising to loved ones, nurses, and caregivers how deeply disappointed some people are and how much patience and understanding they may need from loved ones, the doula, and staff to come to terms with their baby's cesarean birth.

They are less likely to grieve for a long time if they have been able to participate thoroughly in the labor and in the decision to have a cesarean. Prolonged anger, depression, or guilt may result if the birthing person was caught by surprise and could do nothing or if they did not understand the need for it. How you respond to the birthing person's worries and feelings, both during and after the cesarean, can make a big difference in how well they adjust. Here are guidelines:

- Your perceptions of what happened will be very important to the birthing person as they put the pieces together. Try to stay with them during surgery, hold their hand, and talk to them. They may want you to take pictures, especially after the baby is born; check with staff before doing so. Many people, especially if unaware during and after the surgery, treasure such photographs later; the photos help fill in the parts they missed. It is quite likely that staff will not okay photos during the actual surgery, citing legal concerns. However, early pictures of the baby and the first feedings will be treasured.

- The birthing person will probably feel some discomfort during surgery. If it is painful, not just pressure or tugging, ask for more anesthetic to be given. You should help them focus on relaxing and breathing in a slow rhythm to handle the anxiety and sensations of pressure and tugging.

- After the birth, you will probably be able to get close to the baby and to get a good look, see, touch, stroke, talk to, and sing to the baby. The thought of talking or singing to the baby in the operating room may seem strange, but, if you are the baby's parent or the birthing person's spouse, the baby knows your voice and will respond when hearing it. You may be able to soothe the baby as no one else can besides the birthing person.

Think of this birth from the baby's point of view—an abrupt tug out of the warm and familiar womb to a bright, cold, noisy place. They are handled competently but perfunctorily and hear only strangers' voices. Then, you come close and say, "Hi, Baby! I'm so glad to see you. Everything is all right, and I'm here to take care of you." Or, you sing a song, perhaps the one you sang aloud often during the pregnancy (see page 44). You stroke the baby's arm and put your finger into the palm of their hand. The baby stares into your eyes and clings to your finger. At last, a familiar voice and loving touch for the baby! You will always cherish this moment.

• As we said earlier, it may be possible for the baby to go straight to the birthing person. If the baby goes first, though, to the infant warmer for examination, you might go there, too; bring the baby to the birthing person as soon as possible, so they can see, touch, and kiss the baby.

One of the most beautiful welcomes we ever heard about for a cesarean-born baby was this: When the parents learned early in pregnancy they were having a boy, they started singing, "Here Comes the Sun!" to him every day. When their baby emerged and was held up so the father could see him, the father was so overcome with joy he began singing loudly, in a choked-up voice, "Here Comes the Son!" The mother joined in weakly, despite her nausea and trembling. The baby stopped crying and looked right at his dad. Everyone in the operating room was very moved, and the doula was in tears. What a lucky child! See page 44 and Recommended Resources for more on this delightful custom.

• Help the birthing person breast-feed or chest-feed in the recovery room. They may need your help holding the baby to the breast.

If the baby must go to the nursery for special care, you may want to go along to see for yourself what is being done and fill in these gaps for the birthing person later. Or, you can stay with the birthing person, to give comfort and ease your own worries about their well-being. This is a difficult choice. If a family member or doula can stay with one, then you can be with the other and have some peace of mind.

- Physical recovery from a cesarean can take weeks or months. Pain, weakness, and fatigue are great at first, and the birthing person may require narcotics or other pain medication (injections, pills, or IV) for days or longer. It may take weeks or months for the last step—from functioning fairly well to returning to their pre-pregnant condition. Encourage them to rest and focus on feeding the baby while you take over the housework or get help from others. Many new parents enlist the help of friends and family to provide meals, run errands, and do household chores.

- It may take the birthing person longer to recover emotionally than it takes to recover physically. Be patient. Give them time and fill in any gaps in their memory or understanding of what happened and why.

  People vary in how long it takes them to integrate and accept the cesarean birth experience. For some, a cesarean is a positive experience; for others it is not. If the birthing person is disappointed, accept their feelings as valid and normal. Too often the birthing person's loved ones try to distract them from thinking about the birth by pointing out "all that matters" is the baby is healthy—but that is not all that matters. How one gives birth also matters, and their loved ones' patience, acceptance, and concern for these feelings will help the birthing person work through them.

- If the birth experience was particularly negative or traumatic for the birthing person, they may benefit from professional counseling or therapy. Call the caregiver or childbirth educator or doula for referrals; see "Unhappiness After Childbirth," page 393 and Recommended Resources (page 418).

- See chapter 7 for more suggestions about the birth partner's role when problems arise during labor.

Despite feeling possible disappointment with the birth experience and the slower recovery, which is usual after a cesarean, it is unlikely that the birthing person will extend that disappointment to the baby. A cesarean birth is, after all, a birth, and all the emotions that come with birth and meeting one's baby also come with cesarean birth. The birthing person's ability to love, feed, enjoy, and care for the baby are not altered by the fact that the baby was born by cesarean. Enjoy this child together.

Vaginal Birth After Cesarean (VBAC) and Trial of Labor After Cesarean (TOLAC)

A pregnant person who has had a previous cesarean birth may be able to have a vaginal birth (VBAC) the next time. The term *TOLAC* (trial of labor after cesarean) includes those who attempt a vaginal birth after a previous cesarean; some of these develop problems in labor and must change course and have a cesarean. In the past, if a person had one or more cesareans, it was policy to deliver all subsequent babies by cesarean. That made sense because surgery techniques at the time were very invasive and left a large scar high in the uterus, which was at significant risk for reopening (rupturing) in a subsequent labor. Over the years, however, cesarean surgery has improved. Now, the American College of Obstetricians and Gynecologists (ACOG) states it is not only possible, but safer, for many to have a vaginal birth for the second child because the risks of a repeat cesarean for a healthy person are greater than those of a vaginal birth. Their 2017 Practice Bulletin supports VBAC and TOLAC. It provides safety guidelines for obstetricians and describes best practices to incorporate VBAC and TOLAC and improve outcomes.

Not all people are candidates for a TOLAC. ACOG recommends careful evaluation of each pregnant person who had a cesarean for their suitability for a TOLAC. The following criteria are considered:

• Pregnant person's current health status

• Reasons for the first cesarean

• Whether those reasons (for example, some chronic illnesses; anatomical abnormalities in the pelvis, uterus, spine, etc.) still exist

• The person's recovery after the cesarean

• A hospital and staff that support VBAC and who can perform a cesarean day or night

• A hospital within a reasonable distance from the parents' home

If these criteria are not positive, ACOG recommends a repeat cesarean. If these factors are positive, the odds of a successful VBAC are high, and the benefits of a TOLAC outweigh the risks. Despite these safeguards, it is not possible to guarantee that everyone who meets these criteria will have a VBAC. The decision to have a TOLAC should be made after complete discussion between the caregiver and birthing parents.

There are many significant benefits to having a VBAC, including:

- It allows the birthing person to avoid the many short- and long-term risks of major abdominal surgery.

- Following a vaginal birth, recovery is easier and faster than after a cesarean; this is a blessing especially when there will be both a toddler and a newborn to look after.

- If the cesarean was a great disappointment for the birthing person, they may find a VBAC emotionally healing.

In the Unites States, between 60 and 80 percent of those who have a TOLAC are able to have a VBAC. Despite the safety and long-term advantages of VBAC, very few people in the U.S. are offered the opportunity or choose a TOLAC and, as a result, only about 12 percent of all pregnant people who have had a cesarean birth will have a VBAC.

By contrast, in many European countries, there is a higher percentage of attempts (TOLACs), and the VBAC rates in six European countries range from 29 to 55 percent.

The reasons for the low VBAC rate in the United States, compared to other industrialized countries, are manifold but, actually, it is likely the rate will increase, partly because the American College of Obstetricians and Gynecologists has published Practice Bulletins over the years and each has supported VBAC and TOLAC more positively than the ones that came before (the most recent was published in 2017, just prior to this book's publication). See Recommended Resources (page 418) for more on VBAC.

With this support from the professional society representing obstetricians, more of them feel comfortable doing VBACs. In other words, if the birthing person wants a VBAC, they can probably find a supportive caregiver, at least in most urban areas. With modern surgical techniques and a supportive birth environment and caregiver, between 60 and 80 percent of women who attempt a VBAC will have one.

Improving One's Chances for a Vaginal Birth

Though professional attitudes are becoming more accepting of VBACs, obstetricians and hospitals still vary in their enthusiasm, and their attitudes are reflected in their rates of repeat cesareans and VBACs. An unsupportive doctor will have a high rate of repeat cesareans and is likely to warn the pregnant person against getting their hopes up or emphasize potential complications instead of offering encouragement. Such a negative attitude may undermine the person's confidence and lead them, in the words of one person who wanted a VBAC, "down the garden path to another cesarean."

It is wise for the pregnant person to learn which hospitals maintain relatively low cesarean rates and to interview some doctors and midwives who work there. They should also check their health plan to find out which caregivers are covered by insurance. They might also ask a childbirth educator (preferably one who is self-employed or one who is employed by the hospital the pregnant person is considering) for advice on which caregivers to interview.

Attend these interviews with the pregnant person, to give moral support and to help ask questions such as: Do you support VBACs? What percentage of your clients who have had cesareans plan to have VBACs? What percentage succeeds? What are the most likely reasons for a VBAC attempt to end in a cesarean? Can you recommend ways I can improve my chances for a VBAC? Do your associates share your opinions about VBACs?

After comparing the attitudes of the various caregivers, they can choose one who seems most supportive.

It helps if the birthing person is surrounded by people who respect their desire for a VBAC and assume they can and will do it. Family and friends, the professional caregiver, the nursing staff, and you, most of all, should have confidence in the birthing person. A doula can supply emotional support and concrete practical advice. A doula with experience supporting VBACs will inspire confidence in both of you.

Knowledge of ways to deal with some of the challenges inherent in VBAC labors will arm both of you with self-confidence and helpful coping strategies. Childbirth classes are valuable preparation, especially if you can attend ones specifically for VBAC preparation. There are also valuable books, websites, and internet news groups that focus on VBAC (see Recommended Resources, page 418).

Lastly, if the birthing person suffered emotional or physical trauma in the previous birth, counseling with a perinatal social worker, a trauma therapist, a seasoned doula or childbirth educator, or a sensitive midwife or doctor may help them develop strategies to prevent troubling thoughts and feelings from undermining their self-confidence (see page 231).

Fears About VBAC

Although most VBAC labors proceed normally, they carry a small extra risk because the uterus bears a scar from the cesarean. The greatest fear about a VBAC is the risk of scar separation, sometimes referred to as uterine rupture. The risk of scar separation is about 0.5 percent, or 1 in 200 VBAC labors, and is somewhat higher in people who have had more than one cesarean. With careful monitoring of the fetal heart rate and observation of the birthing person, however, a scar separation can usually be detected in time for a cesarean to be performed and the separation mended. Though worrisome when they occur, most scar separations end well, with a healthy birthing person and baby because of immediate and appropriate action. On very rare occasions, the scar separates enough to cause a fetal crisis (or death) and/or serious bleeding in the birthing person. Careful screening of the birthing person ahead of time helps the caregiver identify people at greater risk for such complications. A uterine scar sometimes thins during labor without separating, but, in this case, the uterus heals itself as it returns to its nonpregnant state.

Emotional Concerns Surrounding VBAC

Once one becomes pregnant after having had a cesarean, one may feel less confident about giving birth than the first time. They may feel they were naive before and are now realistic enough to recognize they might have another cesarean this time. Preparation for a vaginal birth should include exploring emotions involving the cesarean and the upcoming birth and also seeking resources that provide the best chance of a safe and satisfying experience.

Once the birthing person has prepared as well as possible to optimize the chances for a VBAC, they will know they will give birth vaginally unless a cesarean is truly appropriate. You can help the birthing person prepare for a VBAC in the following ways:

- Explore any strong emotions associated with the first cesarean: Was it necessary? Was it traumatic? Did the birthing person feel well cared for? Are there concerns about the baby being injured or harmed during the previous birth or about the upcoming one?

- Explore any fears about the next labor: a fear of pain or exhaustion or a fear that something could go wrong for the baby or pregnant person (the scar could separate, they could have another cesarean, or a lack of support from the caregiver, nurses, or even from you).

- Explore their feelings about the caregiver and the hospital where the first child was born: Does the birthing person want to go back there? Were they a part of the problem? Can the birthing person find a caregiver whom they trust?

- Explore how much the birthing person wants a VBAC: Are they willing to prepare by learning self-help measures for comfort and aiding labor progress? Are they willing to use medications and other interventions judiciously? Will they be surrounded by truly supportive friends and relatives?

For a person who has had a long, exhausting labor that ended in a cesarean, the thought of attempting a VBAC may raise all kinds of fear. They may say, "I can't put myself through that again," or "I'd rather just plan a cesarean." After a traumatic or disappointing first labor, they may be very reluctant to try again, even though they also dread the thought of having to recover from major surgery while taking care of an infant and an older child.

In such a situation, you might suggest that the birthing person think about conditions under which they would be willing to labor—for example, if they don't have to go through the same things as before (such as pushing "forever" to exhaustion before the cesarean was done or waiting through many hours with a painful stalled labor). If they conclude they would prefer to try for a VBAC as long as they do not have to go through an ordeal like the first birth, then they might discuss the idea of setting limits with the caregiver and prepare a birth plan for a VBAC that reflects these limits.

Knowing this labor will not be allowed to happen as the first one did, they can put their mind at rest and focus on a positive birth experience over which they have some control. If the labor does exceed the limits the birthing person and caregiver have set, they have the option of proceeding with a cesarean.

After a traumatic birth, setting limits for an upcoming labor frees the person to go ahead with a positive attitude, without fear that the same trauma will be repeated. Even if the birthing person needs another cesarean, their position of control, not helplessness, will save them from emotional trauma. Here is an example:

One person, who very much wanted a natural childbirth, had prepared fully—excellent diet, weekly massages, pregnancy fitness classes, excellent childbirth education, practiced relaxation and comfort measures with her partner, prepared a birth plan, hired a doula—everything that was in her power. Yet, the labor stalled for many hours at 7 centimeters (2¾ inches). They tried everything, certain they could find a way to speed the labor along. It didn't happen. The birthing person became exhausted and discouraged and had an epidural and Pitocin. Even those did not move the labor along. Eventually, after many hours, she "gave up" and had a cesarean. Afterwards, she felt shame she had not been strong enough to continue and saw herself as a failure. She felt "ripped off" that no one had said this could happen and suffered depression after the birth.

Three years later they became pregnant again and, at first, thought they'd have a planned cesarean to avoid repeating all they had gone through, without success.

However, they met with a wise educator who, knowing how important a natural birth had been to this person, asked her to think about setting limits on the next labor. If labor exceeded those limits she would have a cesarean, a chance to bow out if labor exceeded her limits of coping. That would give them an opportunity to go for their desired goal, but with a sense of control over how much difficulty she'd accept. This freed them to participate in the labor, knowing it would not happen as the first labor did.

As it turned out, the labor slowed for a while as it had the first time, but she knew it would not be the same. She decided when the time limit was up, to go for a repeat cesarean. She felt much better about being the decision maker this time—sad it had not worked out, but not traumatized like the first time. It turns out she had a painful bicycle accident in childhood that altered the flexibility of her pelvis.

As the birth partner, you may have mixed feelings about the pregnant person's trying for a vaginal birth, especially if the first labor was distressing for you. It will help to prepare yourself to fully support the pregnant person's efforts by reading this chapter, getting answers to your questions from the caregiver, attending a VBAC support group or class, and sharing your concerns with a doula.

The Special Challenge of a VBAC

Beyond the usual emotional challenges that come with most labors (see chapter 3), a person having a VBAC may have to deal not only with disappointment, but with other challenges such as posttraumatic stress; see page 231 for a description of these challenges and how to deal with them.

If, during labor, you become worried or are reminded of some of the unhappy events of the previous labor that ended in cesarean, it is best to talk to someone else about this. Do not increase the pregnant person's anxiety with your own. If you have a doula, you might talk with them; if not, you might talk to the nurse, out of earshot of the laboring person. If the doula or nurse knows you are troubled, they can reassure you in nonverbal ways.

We are in an era in which the cesarean rate is very high and not because cesareans are safer than vaginal births, except in selected circumstances. If you and the birthing person want the best chance of a vaginal birth without giving up the option of a cesarean when it is truly indicated, you may have to actively seek out the right caregiver and setting and prepare well for the experience. Then, your odds for a vaginal birth or at least for a satisfying birth are very good.

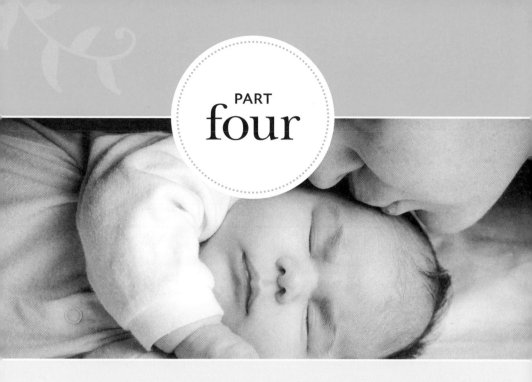

AFTER THE BIRTH

ONCE THE BABY AND PLACENTA ARE BORN, the pace slows. The staff seem preoccupied with finishing medical tasks and cleaning up. You, the birthing person, and the baby are engrossed with the appearance, the touch, and the smell of one another. The doula takes photos, helps with breast-feeding, brings beverages and snacks, and makes the new family comfortable.

The baby's every gurgle, every grimace, every squirming stretch brings fascinated exclamations from both of you. Some babies are quiet, calm, and alert, captivated by your faces and voices. Others fuss and cry at first as they adjust to their new surroundings.

If you are the co-parent, this is the beginning of a honeymoon for all of you. What happens is much like a honeymoon for lovers: withdrawal from the everyday events of the world, intense preoccupation and fascination with one another, profound feelings of love, lack of sleep, and deep contentment.

chapter 10

THE FIRST DAYS
POSTPARTUM

Through the labor, I was struck by the thought I would be meeting my child later that day. I had done a lot of thinking about the birth ahead of time and about being a parent, but I was surprised at how instantly we moved from one to the other. I realized afterward it was as if I had expected someone to hit the pause button, let us relax, check in with each other, get some sleep, and then start parenting. This was obviously not the case.

—MATT, FIRST-TIME FATHER

During the first few days after the birth, there is much going on physically, medically, and emotionally with both the birthing parent and the baby. This chapter explains what to expect—what the caregiver does, some important choices, and your role in all this. Your primary duty, of course, is to stay with your family and give them as much emotional support and practical help as possible.

The First Few Hours

Immediately after the birth, the baby's well-being is quickly assessed. The nurse or midwife checks the baby's Apgar score, temperature, pulse and respiration, state of alertness, and general behavior (see page 135). Assuming all is well, the baby is dried and placed naked on the birthing parent's chest. Both are covered with warm blankets. This skin-to-skin contact is really the best way to keep the baby warm—better than wrapping or placing the baby under warming lights. It is also the perfect setting for beginning life outside the womb. The birthing parent's smell, voice, warmth, touch, and heartbeat provide familiarity and a gradualness to the baby's adjustment. The baby is also giving important gifts to the parents. When the baby is alert and staring into the parents' eyes— they can't take their eyes off each other— they're falling in love! The baby's wiggling squirming limbs massage the soft warm abdomen of the birthing parent, stimulating the uterus to contract and aiding the birthing parent's first steps in recovery.

The baby's nuzzling at the breasts also helps the uterus contract and initiates the process that ends with the baby grasping the birthing parent's nipple and suckling vigorously. As parents, you will likely be focused completely on the baby—except when reality reenters in the form of the caregiver or nurse's necessary intrusions. Their agenda is different from yours: Their main concern is the physical well-being of the birthing person and baby. So, while the two of you are engrossed in the baby, they are dealing with the following immediate clinical concerns.

Care of the Birthing Parent's Perineum

After a vaginal birth, the caregiver carefully inspects the vagina and perineum to determine whether stitches are necessary. This examination is often somewhat painful if there has been no anesthesia. An episiotomy (see page 263) or a sizeable tear will require stitches. If needed, and the birthing parent is not already anesthetized (see page 339), the caregiver places a local anesthetic in the perineum. The stitches will be gradually absorbed as the incision heals; they do not have to be removed. An ice pack applied to the perineum now brings great relief.

Care After a Cesarean Birth

Following a cesarean birth (described in chapter 9), the birthing parent leaves the operating room and spends a few hours in a recovery room or labor room while the anesthetic wears off. They may be very sleepy, depending on the drugs given. There will be a nurse close by all the time. You can remain with the birthing person and, unless the baby has a problem that requires care in the nursery, the baby will be with you, too. If the baby is in the nursery, you may be with the baby.

The Vital Signs of Birthing Parent and Baby

The caregiver frequently checks the vital signs (pulse, respiration, temperature, and blood pressure) of the birthing parent and baby and performs other routine assessments. If either the birthing parent or baby had medical problems during the pregnancy or labor, the nurse or caregiver watches even more closely. They will also check the birthing parent's lochia (see page 283).

The Birthing Parent's Uterus

The nurse checks the uterus frequently to make sure it is contracting firmly. If it is soft and relaxed, it will bleed too much. It usually contracts well on its own, but, if not, there are three ways to cause it to contract:

1. **Nipple stimulation:** When the baby suckles at the breast, the hormone oxytocin is released, which makes the uterus contract. If the baby is not ready for a feeding, you or the birthing parent can stroke or roll their nipples, which has a similar effect.

2. **Fundal massage:** The nurse or midwife does this, but the birthing parent can learn to do it, too. This massage involves firmly kneading the low abdomen until the uterus contracts (they can feel it becoming firm as they massage it) to the size and consistency of a large grapefruit. This is painful for the birthing parent, which is one reason they may want to do it; they can do it less vigorously and get the same results.

3. **Injection or intravenous administration of Pitocin or another uterine stimulant:** This is often done routinely as the baby is being born, but may also be done later, if necessary. This is the most reliable way to contract the uterus; it may be used along with the methods described previously, although it is not needed in most cases.

Cord Blood Removal and Storage

Umbilical cord blood contains stem cells that can be used to treat the same conditions that bone marrow is used for—various cancers and other serious diseases such as blood, immune disorders, and metabolic disorders. Cord blood can be donated to public blood banks by birthing parents, where it is stored for research and for treatment of people with these conditions. Cord blood has saved many lives due to the generosity of such parents. If this interests you, check with your care provider or check our Recommended Resources (page 418) for more information on cord blood donation and how to arrange it. This should be arranged by the week 34 of pregnancy.

You may also arrange to have your baby's cord blood stored privately for possible later use by the child or other family members. There are many issues to explore with regard to storing or donating your baby's blood, such as costs, actual likelihood of needing to use the stem cells, reliability and ethical standards of the private for-profit companies, and public availability of stem cells from blood banks.

Another issue is the timing of cord cutting and removing cord and placental blood: Usually, the cord is cut immediately to extract the blood; now, though, that delayed cord cutting is known to benefit the baby, other methods to extract cord blood after the delayed cutting have been devised. Ask that the blood extraction techniques allow your baby to get their share of placental blood (see chapter 1, page 48, and Recommended Resources, page 418).

Placental Encapsulation

A growing trend among pregnant and postpartum families is to have the placenta prepared and encapsulated for consumption after the baby is born. There are numerous ways to prepare the placenta, but most include steaming, dehydrating, pulverizing the desiccated placenta into powder, and placing the powder into capsules for consumption. The thought is that consuming the placenta, rich in iron and hormones, imparts many health benefits such as minimizing postpartum depression, providing additional energy, and increasing milk supply. It is important to know there is scant scientific evidence to support these claims, though there are numerous positive personal stories from parents who have tried it. There are currently studies underway to investigate the composition of desiccated placenta powder, as well as at least one carefully controlled scientific trial comparing possible benefits and risks of consuming capsules containing placenta with placebo-filled capsules during the postpartum period.

If having the placenta encapsulated appeals to you and the birthing parent, you can either search online for ways of preparing it yourselves, or you can hire a placenta encapsulation specialist to do this for you. The cost varies from about $150 to $500 depending on experience and where you live. When selecting someone to prepare the placenta, ask about their experience and training, safety protocols, where the placenta will be prepared (in your home or their preparation space), the preparation method used, and how their equipment is cleaned (see Recommended Resources, page 418).

There are some circumstances under which it is not considered safe to encapsulate the placenta. If the placenta cannot be properly refrigerated or kept cool following the birth or if it has been refrigerated longer than 4 days, it should not be encapsulated. If you were diagnosed with chorioamnionitis (infection of the bag of waters) or if your placenta needed to be sent to the hospital pathology department for testing, it is not considered safe to encapsulate. Finally, if you have a blood-borne pathogen such as hepatitis or HIV/AIDS, the hospital will generally not release the placenta for preparation. Some placenta specialists have additional contraindications such as Group B streptococcus or meconium staining of the amniotic fluid. Discuss these scenarios with your specialist. It bears repeating: there is no scientific evidence to support the claims of placenta encapsulation. However, at the time of writing, studies are underway.

Common Procedures in Newborn Care

In the first few minutes or hours after birth, the baby is examined and a number of procedures are done. Many of these are routine; others are optional. Some are required by law to detect or prevent certain serious conditions. Because the birthing parent may be exhausted or preoccupied with the procedures they are still undergoing, it will be up to you to keep track of what is happening to the baby, remind staff of the birthing parent's preferences regarding newborn care, and help the birthing parent make decisions, if necessary.

Suctioning the Baby's Nose and Mouth

The baby's airway may contain mucus, amniotic fluid with or without meconium, or blood. There are two ways to deal with this fluid: the caregiver observes the baby and suctions only if the baby is not breathing or is not vigorous. It may also be done routinely—the caregiver inserts the tip of a rubber bulb syringe several times into the baby's nostrils and mouth and suctions the secretions out.

Sometimes, if the amniotic fluid was stained with meconium, deeper suctioning is done via a long tube passed through a nostril and down the baby's trachea (windpipe).

Purposes of suctioning: Suctioning is done to clear the airway of secretions, especially if the baby is unable to cough or sneeze to remove them, or to assist a baby who is not breathing.

Until recently, it was recommended that deeper suctioning be done if the baby had passed a meconium bowel movement while in the uterus. The concern was that the meconium, mixed with amniotic fluid, might be inhaled by the baby. The caregiver would try to suction it out before the baby's first breath, to keep the baby from breathing the meconium into the lungs, and repeat the suctioning as soon as possible after the birth. A recent, large scientific trial of early deep suctioning when the baby's head is out, compared with no suctioning, found this does not improve outcomes. There was no difference in the number of babies who inhaled meconium. This finding comes as a relief to caregivers because sometimes the baby comes out too quickly to accomplish the first suctioning.

Disadvantages of suctioning: The baby may experience brief discomfort and stress and may gag, flinch, or struggle or possible abrasions of the mucous membranes in the baby's nose and throat may occur if the tip scrapes them. Usually, suctioning is unnecessary because healthy babies are fully capable of coughing or sneezing the fluids out. The American Academy of Pediatrics recommends reserving any type of suctioning only for babies who have obvious obstruction or who require positive pressure ventilation (mechanically assisted respiration).

Alternatives to consider: Parents can ask the caregiver to withhold suctioning of the mouth, nose, and throat unless the baby is unable to rid their airway of secretions. If suctioning is necessary, the caregiver can use the syringe gently.

Cutting the Umbilical Cord

Once the baby is out, the cord is clamped in two places and cut with scissors. You might wish to cut the cord. The nurse will give you the scissors and show you exactly where to cut.

Pros and cons of early versus late clamping and cutting the umbilical cord: Until recently, the custom was to clamp and cut the cord immediately after birth—for efficiency and to enable removal of the baby from the birthing parent to a newborn unit where the baby could be assessed and given the initial procedures (described in these pages). It was believed that early cord clamping prevented newborn jaundice. This practice came into question when research studies comparing early and late cord clamping found that the likelihood of jaundice does not increase with late cord clamping.

Studies have also found that the baby benefits from delaying cord clamping in many ways:

1. Because the size of the placenta diminishes as the blood drains from it into the baby, delivery of the placenta occurs sooner.

2. The baby continues to receive oxygen from the blood in the cord until the cord stops pulsating—especially helpful for babies who are slow to start breathing.

3. The increased volume of blood circulating to the baby's lungs hastens optimal respiration.

4. The baby's iron stores increase by as much as 45 percent, and anemia is less likely to occur in the baby for as long as 6 months.

5. Premature babies are less likely to require blood transfusions (see Recommended Resources, page 418).

All this occurs because the blood in the placenta is the baby's blood and amounts to approximately 150 milliliters (5 fluid ounces; about one-third of the baby's total blood volume). Until the cord is clamped or stops pulsating, this blood is transferred from the placenta to the baby. The best way to make sure the baby has its full allotment of blood is to place the baby on the birthing person's belly and wait for the cord to stop pulsating.

An exception to delaying cord cutting is when the baby is very ill and needs immediate medical attention (because of prematurity, breathing in large amounts of meconium, or a low Apgar score; see page 244). Then, the baby is removed to a resuscitation bed.

Note: Now that professionals recognize the importance of letting the baby receive its full allotment of oxygenated blood, the custom of early cord cutting with compromised infants is being replaced in North America. Hospitals are beginning to invest in bedside resuscitation units (from Europe) that allow the baby to remain near the birthing parent with the cord intact. With this practice, the baby still gets oxygenated blood via the cord, while resuscitation procedures are being carried out. (Interestingly, home birth midwives have always done newborn resuscitation with the baby connected by the cord to the birthing person, using portable equipment to aid the baby's breathing. While not as sophisticated as the new bedside resuscitation beds, they saved many babies by not cutting the baby off from its only source of oxygenated blood—the placenta.)

Eye Medication

An antibiotic (usually erythromycin ointment) is placed in the baby's eyes within the first hour after birth.

Purposes of eye medication: The antibiotic prevents serious eye infection or even blindness due to the bacteria that cause gonorrhea or chlamydia—two common sexually transmitted diseases. These bacteria are sometimes present in the vagina and can be transmitted to the baby during birth.

Eye medication is medically indicated if the birthing parent tests positive for chlamydia or gonorrhea or if either parent may have been exposed to the diseases (via sexual contact with someone who has the disease). Because the lab tests are not 100 percent reliable and the organisms can appear if sexual contact occurred after the lab tests were done, the eye medication is required by all states and provinces.

Disadvantages of eye medication: The medicine blurs the baby's vision for a short time, until the warmth of the baby's eyes melts the ointment.

Alternatives to consider: Getting the doctor or nurse to accept your refusal of the treatment may be difficult because the most worrisome organisms, chlamydia and gonococcus, although tested for during early pregnancy, sometimes are present at birth. Because these do not always cause symptoms in adults, they sometimes go untreated. Unfortunately, the newborn can be seriously infected by these organisms. But if you and your partner have both been tested for them and found negative and you both have been monogamous, the odds of having these organisms are extremely low. Still, your nurse or caregiver may feel very uncomfortable if you refuse the eye treatment, as many states and provinces may hold the caregiver, not the parents, responsible if the treatment is not given and the baby develops one of these infections.

A very popular alternative is to ask the nurse or midwife to postpone putting the ointment in the baby's eyes until an hour or two after birth, so the baby will be able to see your faces clearly in the meantime.

Vitamin K

Required in most U.S. states and Canadian provinces, vitamin K is given as an injection shortly after birth. This vitamin is essential in blood clotting. Newborns are relatively slow in clotting their blood for the first week or so, although once they start consuming and digesting colostrum and milk, they begin making their own vitamin K. Until then, they are at a very small risk for excessive bleeding (called vitamin K deficiency bleeding, or VKDB). Giving vitamin K to tide them over reduces the risk of bleeding problems.

Until recently, vitamin K was sometimes given by mouth, but it was found that oral vitamin K does not prevent later onset of VKDB, so the American Academy of Pediatrics now recommends only injectable vitamin K, although they call for more research on the oral form. The injection is given once, in the thigh, within an hour after birth.

Purposes of giving vitamin K: The injection is quick, easy, and inexpensive and is very effective in preventing VKDB. Giving vitamin K is especially important when a baby is at greater risk of bleeding, for example, after a difficult or instrumental birth, prematurity, or plans for circumcision before the baby is 1 week old.

Disadvantages of giving vitamin K: The injection is briefly painful. The safety of the low dose given to newborns is well established.

Alternatives to consider: Refusing vitamin K altogether is a somewhat risky option because it is not possible to predict which babies will or will not develop this rare condition—vitamin K deficiency bleeding (VKDB). The Canadian Paediatric Society does suggest giving oral vitamin K if parents refuse the injectable form, perhaps thinking it may be better than nothing.

Blood Tests

Virtually every newborn has at least two blood tests in the first two days. Blood samples are obtained in two ways:

1. A few drops of the baby's blood are drawn from the heel or a vein to check for:

   - Bilirubin levels, a yellowish blood pigment that, at high levels, causes jaundice (see page 301)

   - Blood sugar (glucose) levels

   - Infection, if the birthing parent had a fever in labor or if the baby has one now

   - Numerous genetic or congenital disorders (see "Newborn Screening Tests," page 378)

2. Blood from the baby's umbilical cord may also be collected at birth for:

   - Blood typing

   - Rh determination

   - Storage or donation to a blood bank (see page 366 and Recommended Resources, page 418)

Purposes of blood tests: The general purpose of testing the newborn's blood is to record the baby's blood type and detect rare but potentially serious problems early enough to treat them and prevent dangerous effects on the baby. Tests for congenital disorders are mandated by state laws. Early identification of many congenital disorders often means early treatment with very good outcomes. Without treatment, some disorders become increasingly severe and disabling for the child.

Disadvantages of blood tests: The heel stick is painful to the baby, and some of the tests (such as those for bilirubin and blood glucose) may have to be repeated many times.

Also, results of some blood tests are sometimes confusing and can lead to overtreatment. Caregivers sometimes disagree on when bilirubin and blood glucose levels require treatment. Ask the key questions (see page 237) to learn enough to make an informed decision about any recommended tests.

Alternatives to consider: You and the birthing parent can ask the caregiver about less painful ways to gain the information provided by blood tests. For example, observe the baby's skin and the whites of the eyes and have a blood test for jaundice done only if they appear yellow. Or, if your baby is at low risk of hypoglycemia (born full term and the birthing person is not diabetic), ask whether the nurse can look for early symptoms of hypoglycemia (such as jitteriness and low body temperature) before doing the blood test and have the birthing person nurse the baby as soon as possible.

If the caregiver prefers the blood test to these other approaches, they should explain the reasons. There are some ways the blood draws can be made less stressful for the baby: for example, warming the baby's heel brings more blood to the heel before the blood draw; holding the baby upright so gravity causes blood to go to the heel; breast-feed during the procedure. All these techniques can reduce the stress for the baby (and the parents!). Weigh the benefits of the recommended test and treatment against the risks of the test and the problem it is designed to detect. There are no alternative ways to get the important information provided by the state-mandated blood tests.

Warming Unit

A warming unit is a special bed with a heater above it. A baby placed in a warming unit has a small thermostat taped to the abdomen; the thermostat automatically turns up the heat if the baby becomes chilled. Small or premature babies become chilled more easily than average-size or full-term babies.

Purpose of the warming unit: The unit is used to prevent a temperature drop and the potentially harmful aftereffects of hypothermia (sluggishness, abnormal blood sugar levels, lung problems, and others) or to warm a baby who has become chilled.

Disadvantages of the warming unit: The baby is separated from the parents. Also, warming units are not risk-free; they may cause the baby to lose fluids through evaporation of moisture from the skin and lungs (breathing out moist air). This is a greater potential problem for premature babies, but fluid loss and signs of dehydration must be monitored carefully. Breast-feeding often, feeding water or formula, or giving IV fluids to the baby and adjusting the heat in the warming unit are the most common solutions, but being held skin to skin with the birthing person is the best solution (see page 299).

Alternatives to consider: Prevent chills in the baby by drying with towels right after the birth and protecting the baby from cool air. The baby should be kept warm by staying skin to skin with the birthing parent (see "Kangaroo Care," page 299 and Recommended Resources, page 418), putting on a hat, and covering the birthing person and baby with a warm blanket. The baby's temperature should be checked frequently with a quick-action thermometer. If it is not possible to do these things because the baby needs medical attention, the warming unit becomes a necessity. If the birthing person is not ready to hold the baby, you might hold the baby skin to skin with a blanket around the two of you.

Cleanup

The birthing parent's bed linens are changed; the caregiver or the nurse helps them wash up and put on a clean gown. The gown should open in the front for convenience when feeding the baby. The birthing parent wears a sanitary pad to catch the bloody vaginal discharge (lochia, which will be present for several days or weeks; see page 383). The baby is wiped dry and diapered.

First Feeding

The following applies to those who plan to breast-feed or chest-feed, discussed at length in the next chapter. During all this cleanup activity, the birthing parent should lie back in a propped position, with pillows beneath both arms, and hold the baby on their chest so they can nurse as soon as they are ready. This is called the laid-back breast-feeding position (developed by Suzanne Colson; see Recommended Resources, page 418). If not rushed, the newborn is fully able to self-attach, that is, find their way to the breast. In their own time, they'll nuzzle, mouth the breast, salivate, and bob their head until they open their mouth wide and place it right on the nipple. Then, they begin to suckle. The nurse, doula, or midwife can help the baby "latch on" (form the connection between mouth and breast tissue) to the breast by leaving the birthing parent and baby together for up to an hour while resisting the urge to take the breast in one hand and direct the baby's mouth onto it with the other hand. Modeling patience and reassurance and not rushing the process is the best way to help the breast-feeding pair get started.

If staff are in a hurry to get the baby nursing or if the birthing parent becomes upset, ask the nurse or doula for help to gently encourage the baby to take the nipple. See chapter 11 for more on breast-feeding/chest-feeding.

Care of the Birthing Parent for the Next Couple of Hours

When the immediate postpartum care is over, the three of you may be left in privacy for a while. Dim the lights to encourage the baby to open their eyes; enjoy these quiet moments together. The baby may want to continue feeding at this time or may be ready to take a nap. You and the birthing parent both will soon be ready for a meal.

If the birthing parent had a cesarean delivery, they may be allowed small amounts of solid food when they want it or may have to wait several hours before being offered anything more than clear liquids. Caregivers' orders vary. The birthing parent may continue receiving intravenous fluids for up to a day after the cesarean.

The First Few Days for the Baby

Once both birthing parent and baby are settled, the three of you can relax together, cooing, cuddling, exploring, and nursing—or simply sleeping. There is usually no reason to be separated after birth, although for a long time it was (and still is in some places) a hospital custom to do so. If the birthing parent or baby is not well, the baby may have to go to the nursery or may stay in the room but the birthing parent may be unable to hold the baby.

You are the perfect person to hold the baby if the birthing parent cannot (and even if they can) or to remain with the baby in the nursery, as long as both you and the birthing parent wish for you to do so. If you cuddle with the baby sometime during the first day or so after birth, you will have even stronger feelings for your child. There is something magical about holding your baby close—especially skin to skin—gazing at each other and talking or singing to your beautiful child. We overheard one father saying to his baby as he held him close, "And when you're six, we'll take you horseback riding in Montana!" The baby seemed to approve. They were planning their lives together.

Physical Exam and Assessment

A doctor or a midwife will give the baby a thorough physical exam, checking the entire body and all systems. It is interesting to watch the exam, which can teach you a great deal about the baby. Over the next few days, you, the birthing parent, or staff will make these observations of the baby: the number and quality of bowel movements; frequency of urination; frequency and length of time in feeding; respiration rate; temperature; pulse; and so forth. The staff will teach you how to do so because they will be your responsibility for the first few days at home with the baby.

Bowel Movements

The baby will have a bowel movement within a few hours after birth. This and the next several bowel movements are composed of meconium, and they are different from bowel movements that will come later. Meconium is thick, black, sticky, and hard to clean. If you think of it, soon after birth, rub some vegetable oil or massage oil all over the baby's buttocks and genitals. This will make cleaning off the meconium easier, and you will thank us.

Over the next few days, as the birthing person's milk shifts from colostrum (see page 378) to mature milk, the baby's bowel movements will change from black to brown to green to yellow and will become very runny and almost odorless or slightly sweet-smelling. After the first few days, the baby may have a bowel movement after almost every feeding and should have at least four per day. This is a good sign they are getting enough to eat.

Bathing the Baby

The baby will have a bath within the first couple of days. As we have gained knowledge of the baby's microbiome, it has become clear that the substances on the baby's skin at birth—vernix, amniotic fluid, including the vaginal secretions the baby picked up coming through the birth canal—contain microbes that provide protection for the baby against some potentially harmful bacteria, such as Group B streptococcus, *E. coli*, and others. The vernix also protects and moisturizes the baby's skin. Many people now wait 24 hours or more before giving the first bath.

Unless you or the birthing parent is accustomed to bathing newborns, the nurse or midwife will probably give the bath, teaching you both at the same time. The usual advice is to start at the top and work

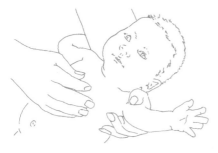

The safe way to hold a baby during a bath

down, always holding the baby securely with your arm around the baby and your hand holding the baby's upper arm.

Caring for the Cord

Before being cut, the umbilical cord is either tied tightly with umbilical cord tape or clamped with a plastic clip. The cord stump needs to be kept clean and dry. Arrange the baby's diaper so it does not touch the cord. Clean the cord with tap or bottled water. The nurse or midwife will show you how. The cord clamp is removed by the nurse or midwife, usually on the second day, leaving a black, dry stump that remains for a week or two and then drops off. The cord usually has a faintly foul smell, but call the baby's doctor if pus or red blood oozes from it.

Feeding the Baby

For the first six months, breast-fed babies need no food but colostrum (the first "milk" to come from the breasts) and breast milk. They do not need formula or water, and they do not need glucose water unless they have low blood sugar that is not corrected by breast-feeding. It is a good idea to begin breast-feeding as soon after birth as the baby is interested, usually within 20 to 60 minutes (see page 375).

Babies who will be formula-fed should begin receiving formula when they seem ready to suck and when their condition is stable.

For more information about your role in feeding the baby, see chapter 11.

Newborn Screening Tests

Every state and province has a newborn screening program. Through the heel-stick test, these programs can detect numerous rare endocrinological, metabolic, and hematologic disorders, most of which, if detected early, can be treated to prevent mental, developmental, and other serious disabilities or early death. As of this writing, the March of Dimes recommends screening for at least 34 specific congenital health problems, and 30 states do that, while other states screen for fewer disorders.

One heel stick can usually provide enough blood for the tiny samples needed for all these tests.

Some of the disorders the March of Dimes recommends screening for are PKU (phenylketonuria), congenital hypothyroidism, congenital adrenal hyperplasia (CAH), biotinidase deficiency, maple syrup urine disease, galactosemia, homocystinuria, sickle cell disease, and medium-chain acyl-CoA dehydrogenase deficiency (MCAD). See Recommended Resources (page 418) for more information and for a site that reports screening tests by state.

Hearing Screening Test

Approximately 2 to 4 babies per 1,000 are born deaf or hard of hearing. Within the first few days, your baby will probably be given a hearing test to identify any hearing problem much earlier than you and the birthing person would notice them (the average age at which hearing problems are identified without the screening test is 14 months, by which time the child already has fallen behind in speech development). Identifying hearing problems early allows for early therapy.

Most hospitals do the hearing test routinely, but if you give birth outside the hospital, you may have to arrange a test yourself. Ask your midwife how and where to do this and check whether your insurance will cover the cost.

The test is done while the baby is asleep. The baby wears headphones, and several electrodes are placed around their head. They record brain-wave activity and middle-ear activity in response to sounds transmitted into the baby's ears and via the bones of their head.

If the test indicates a problem or the results are unclear, there is more testing. If repeat tests indicate the baby has impaired hearing, you will be referred to a hearing specialist and speech therapist. Early detection and treatment of hearing loss has greatly improved the hearing and communication skills of affected children.

Circumcision

In this section, we address the custom of circumcision of male infants. Although female circumcision is a common practice in many countries, it is rare among Western countries. For those who wish to study female circumcision, we suggest an internet search on the topic.

The decision whether to circumcise a male baby is a highly personal one. Most major medical groups, including the American Academy of Pediatrics (AAP) and the Canadian Paediatric Society, advise that parents learn about the pros and cons, explore their own values, and decide as they see fit. The following section outlines the health benefits listed in the AAP statement. The statement calls for health insurance companies to cover circumcision. (See Recommended Resources, page 418 for a link to the 2012 statement and other information on circumcision.)

If the baby will be circumcised, the procedure is done in the hospital on the first or second day after birth or, in the Jewish tradition, in the home or synagogue on the eighth day. When circumcision is done in the hospital, and sometimes as part of the Jewish bris ceremony, the penis is usually numbed with local anesthetic. The foreskin is separated from the underlying glans (the end of the penis) and removed from the glans with a scalpel.

The incidence of circumcision in the United States is now estimated at about 55 percent, with regional variation—lowest in the western United States and highest in the Midwest. Rates are lower in states where the procedure is not covered by Medicaid insurance. In Canada, the rate is considerably lower, about 20 percent.

Purposes and benefits of circumcision:

• The surgery changes the appearance of the penis according to the parents' preferences.

• The surgery is done to observe Jewish or other religious customs.

• The surgery reduces the child's later chances of acquiring some sexually transmitted diseases (STDs) from an infected person. Studies in developing nations in Africa indicate that circumcised heterosexual men have a lower incidence of many kinds of STDs, including HIV/AIDS. There is controversy over the applicability of these studies to the culture of North America.

• The surgery reduces the risk of cancer of the penis in later life. Although this cancer is very rare, affecting only 1 to 2 males in 100,000, it is almost nonexistent in circumcised males. Long-term poor hygiene and old age are the other factors associated with penile cancer. The American Cancer Society does not recommend newborn circumcision to prevent cancer of the penis.

Urinary tract infections in the first year of life are rare, but more frequent in uncircumcised babies. It may be that instruction in proper care and hygiene for the uncircumcised penis would lower that risk.

Other health-related reasons for circumcision have been less well studied, and their validity hasn't been established. For more information about these, see Recommended Resources, page 418.

Disadvantages of circumcision: Circumcision carries the same risks as all surgery—infection, hemorrhage, adhesions, pain, and injury due to human error.

• The procedure is very painful unless anesthesia is used. A local anesthetic is usually injected in several places at the base of the penis to reduce the pain. Although the injections are painful, they prevent pain during the circumcision itself. Sometimes, instead of being injected, anesthetic cream is applied to the penis, but a wait of 20 minutes is needed for the cream to take effect, so it is not widely used in hospitals.

• Infection or hemorrhage occurs in about 1 in every 200 circumcisions. These conditions can usually be well controlled with medications and extra time in the hospital.

• There is a small possibility, especially with an inexperienced, unsupervised doctor, that the surgery will be done poorly—too much or too little foreskin may be removed.

• The circumcised penis usually takes 7 to 10 days to heal. Parents are taught how to care for the penis during this time by avoiding wet diapers and other irritations, applying a lubricating ointment to the penis, and observing the penis for signs of poor healing.

• If the newborn child is ill or if their penis is abnormal in structure, circumcision may be harmful.

Alternatives to consider. The baby's parents can:

• Leave the baby uncircumcised. If you do, learn proper care of the uncircumcised penis (see Recommended Resources, page 418). Do not forcefully retract your baby's foreskin to clean it or for any other reason. When most male babies are born, their foreskin adheres to the glans. Over a period of months or years, it gradually loosens and becomes easily retractable. Many of the problems attributed to being uncircumcised are really caused by parents and others who do not know to leave the foreskin alone. As your child grows, teach them proper hygiene; washing the penis is about as complicated as washing the ears.

- Decide to have the baby circumcised, with appropriate anesthesia and an experienced doctor or *mohel* (a Jewish person with training in circumcision). If possible, remain with the baby to comfort them. Learn proper care for the newly circumcised penis to promote healing.

- Leave the decision for the child to make himself when they reach adulthood.

Whether you choose to circumcise your baby or not, you will later want to teach them responsible sexual practices to protect themselves and their partners from sexually transmitted infections.

Baby Care

The nurse or midwife and friends and family who are experienced parents can teach you many baby care skills not covered in this book, such as safety measures, changing diapers, bathing, and soothing a fussy baby. Books, videos, and classes are also available; see Recommended Resources, page 418.

The First Few Days for the Birthing Parent

For the birthing parent, the early postpartum period is marked by fatigue, emotional highs and lows, preoccupation with the baby, curiosity, some pain, and an array of physical changes that affect most parts of the body.

They may be tired and excited at the same time, finding it difficult to sleep, but unable to do very much without feeling worn out. A shower or a short walk is enough to send them straight back to bed.

They may be surprised by the variety of physical changes they experience; these physical changes will require more attention than they ever expected.

The Uterus

The nurse or midwife and the birthing parent should check the uterus frequently in the first few days to make sure it remains contracted (see page 366). Remind them to continue checking until it feels contracted at every check over 2 or 3 days.

Afterpains

These are uterine contractions that come and go. Especially if this is the second child or more, the birthing parent's afterpains may be quite intense when suckling the baby. Afterpains are a good sign that the uterus is returning to its pre-pregnant size. Remind them to use relaxation and breathing techniques. If the pains are severe, they can request pain medications. Afterpains go away in a few days.

Vaginal Discharge

The birthing parent will have a bloody vaginal discharge, called lochia, which is similar to a menstrual period. It starts as a heavy red flow containing some clots and gradually diminishes; it lasts from two to six weeks.

In the first few days after the birth, the birthing parent may notice they pass very little blood while lying down, but when they stand up after a few hours in bed, they may suddenly lose a lot of blood. This can be alarming, but it is probably because blood may pool in the vagina until gravity causes it to flow out. If heavy bleeding continues longer than a few minutes, however, or if the birthing parent feels faint, call the caregiver or the hospital's maternity floor.

After the lochia has clearly subsided but then suddenly increases or if the birthing parent passes large, golf ball–size clots, call the caregiver because they may be bleeding from a blood vessel in the former site of the placenta. Sometimes, heavy physical exertion causes one to bleed heavily after the lochia has decreased. Rest usually puts an end to the heavy bleeding, but you should call the birthing parent's caregiver if you are concerned.

The Perineum

After a vaginal birth, the perineum will be sore, especially if stitches were needed. Even with no stitches, there may be swelling and bruising. The birthing person can try the following comfort measures:

- Apply an ice pack, especially during the first 24 hours. Damp washcloths, folded and placed in a plastic bag in the freezer for 1 hour or so, make great ice packs. Make up several at a time, so you'll always have one available.

- Sit in a bath of warm water for 20 minutes, two or three times a day. They should not wash in this water; it should be kept clean.

- After using the toilet, carefully pat the perineum dry (starting at the front and moving toward the anus) or squirt it with warm water from a bottle. This is less irritating than wiping with toilet paper.

- Apply witch hazel–soaked pads to the perineum and to hemorrhoids for soothing. For other hemorrhoid treatments, consult the caregiver.

- Do the 10-second pelvic-floor contraction exercise (Kegel exercise) ten times per day to promote healing, reduce swelling, and restore strength. They should always do these while sitting, which helps keep the buttocks from spreading and putting painful stress on the stitches. The birthing parent tightens the muscles around the vagina and urethra as when trying to hold back urine (see page 38). They should do ten per day, probably not all at once. Also, they should follow the directions on page 38 to restore pelvic floor muscle tone. The good news is, improvement can be detected rapidly when exercising these muscles.

Emptying Bowels and Bladder

You may be surprised how preoccupied the birthing parent becomes with bowel movements and urination! These functions are more difficult than usual because the perineum is sore, abdominal muscles are temporarily weak (making straining to move the bowels difficult), and the interruption in food and fluid intake during labor may have caused constipation.

If unable to urinate, try all the tricks—run a faucet, have them urinate in the bath (and get out when done) or shower, and encourage them to press in on their low abdomen just above the pubic bone, putting pressure on the bladder—but not if they had a cesarean!—which may encourage emptying. These almost always work; in the unlikely event that the birthing person does not urinate within a half day or so, call the caregiver. They may need to have a catheter placed in the bladder to empty it. This is unpleasant, but it is better than letting the bladder become distended.

On a positive note, one very welcome change is that the bladder, no longer crowded by the baby, has much greater capacity than during pregnancy, so the birthing parent will need to urinate less frequently.

To help the birthing parent avoid or reduce difficulties with the first bowel movements after giving birth, remind them to eat and drink high-fiber foods: prune juice, other juices, raw fruits and vegetables, bran breads or cereals, and so forth. Bulk-producing stool softeners or laxatives are also helpful. In addition, it might reduce discomfort if they support their sore perineum by pressing toilet paper against it as they have a bowel movement. These measures also help if a person has painful hemorrhoids.

It may take a week or two for the birthing parent to resume their usual bowel patterns. If they're feel uncomfortable or constipated despite the measures described, they should contact the caregiver.

Pain Following Cesarean Delivery

Post-cesarean pain results from the incision, from the stitches or clamps closing it, and from gas that commonly builds up in the abdomen after this surgery. Activities such as turning over, getting out of bed, walking, and nursing the baby are usually very painful for a few days, even though some activity of that kind hastens recovery. Help as much as you can to make these activities easier for the birthing parent by reminding them of how to roll from back to side, giving a helping hand as they get out of bed, offering a supportive arm as they walk, and providing a pillow for their lap as they nurse the baby. The birthing parent will begin feeling better gradually each day.

To reduce pain when rolling from back to side, the birthing person who has had a cesarean should raise the hips and rotate the hips and legs to the side before turning the shoulders.

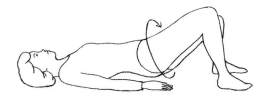

Clamps are removed from the incision site on the second or third day after the delivery. The procedure is not very painful, and the pain from the incision will then decrease. If the birthing parent had stitches, they may dissolve over time or be removed within the first week, depending on the material used for suturing. The birthing parent may feel itching and soreness at the incision site and should not use any soothing cream except what the doctor suggests.

Keep an eye on the scar as it heals. If it becomes inflamed or produces pus or a fever develops, call the caregiver.

To help reduce abdominal pain, encourage the birthing parent to do the following:

- When rolling from back to side, they first bend the knees so their feet are flat on the bed. Then, lift their hips (so only their head, shoulders, and feet are on the bed), twist them to one side, and roll their shoulders to the side (see illustration on page 385). This is much easier and far less painful than rolling over the usual way.

  To sit up from the side-lying position, they should push themselves up with their hands. These techniques avoid strain on the incision.

- The birthing parent should avoid gas-producing foods such as lentils and beans, foods in the cabbage family, and cold or carbonated beverages.

- To avoid feeling faint when getting of bed the first few times, the birthing parent should first circle their ankles, raise their arms above their head several times, and then sit up and raise their arms several more times. As they stand, you should stand close by so they can hold on to you.

- When holding the baby on their lap, they should place a pillow over the incision to protect it.

- The birthing parent should ask the nurse or lactation consultant to show ways to hold the baby to avoid pressure on the incision.

Homecoming

Check the birthing parent's insurance plan ahead of time to learn what to expect and what options they have after the birth. The usual hospital stay after a normal vaginal birth is 24 to 48 hours; after a cesarean, it is 48 to 72 hours. If the birth takes place in a birth center, the birthing parent will likely go home 3 to 6 hours afterward. After a home birth, the midwife usually stays for 3 to 4 hours.

The caregiver should make sure you both have clear instructions about observations to make of the birthing parent and baby, special care needs of each, and numbers to call in case you have any concerns. Also, make sure you know the name and phone number of the baby's doctor.

Ideally, a follow-up appointment should be scheduled within the first week (preferably 3 or 4 days) after the birth to check on breast-feeding and on the birthing parent's and baby's health and well-being. Unfortunately, with all the cutbacks in services that hospitals and insurance companies are making to save money, a follow-up appointment may not be offered. In this case, it is especially important to make sure you know whom to call if you or the birthing parent has any problems before the first scheduled postpartum checkup.

If the baby was born at home, the midwife will make two or more home visits within the first several days and have office appointments over the next weeks.

Before the birth parent comes home from the hospital or birth center, take a moment to think about what they are coming home to. Is the house a mess? Is the sink full of dishes? Is the bed unmade? Is the baby's place (basket, bassinet, cradle or crib, and changing area) ready? There is nothing more disheartening for the birthing parent than returning home to chaos. You want them to feel glad to be home, so provide a pleasant homecoming.

Consider going home alone for a few hours to prepare the home. Better yet, get friends and family to help. These are things they might do:

• Make the bed with fresh linens.

• Tidy up the house and wash any dirty dishes.

• Make sure good food is available.

- Have a stack of fresh diapers ready (call a diaper service or buy some).

- Have a few welcoming touches around the house—fresh flowers, a "Welcome Home" poster.

    Also, prepare for the ride home:

- Install the infant car seat (see page 34) if this hasn't been done already.

- Tidy up the inside of the car.

- Have enough gas so you don't need to stop on the way home.

- Make sure the birthing parent and the baby have clothes to wear home and that the baby has a blanket or two.

    When you arrive home, you both may feel like celebrating—and with good reason! You're introducing the baby to their new world. The birthing parent may feel they have has been away a long time (even though it has probably been only a few days!) and may be relieved to be in familiar surroundings. Fatigue is likely to set in very soon. Perhaps the best thing for the birthing parent to do is get right into bed, snuggle with their loved ones, and bask in the warm feelings. Consider asking visitors not to come until at least the next day.

After a Home Birth

If the baby has been born at home, there may be a cleanup operation ahead—dishes, laundry, trash, a bath to empty, a bed to make with fresh linens. The midwives, doula, and others attending the birth should leave things reasonably clean, but after they leave to give you and your family some quiet time together, there may still be a lot to do. Friends and family can be recruited to help over the next few days. Plan in advance so you're not overwhelmed with cleanup and putting the home back to normal.

- Ask the midwife and the assistant about cleanup ahead of time: How much do they do? What needs to be done? What happens to the placenta? Sometimes, the caregiver disposes of it. Some families bury it and plant a tree as a memento. You might store it in the freezer (mark it well!), until you have time to do this. Some are interested in placental encapsulation (see page 367 and Recommended Resources, page 418 for further discussion); ask your midwife about this practice. If you used a birthing tub, how is it emptied, cleaned, and removed, and who does it?

- Have large trash bags available during labor—for recyclables, for trash, and for laundry. As items are used, they can go right into the appropriate bags.

- If extra people are available, assign ongoing and after-birth cleanup tasks: picking up and washing dishes, putting food away, doing laundry, taking out trash, and straightening up the house. They can do these things while you and your family rest undisturbed.

Getting Help and Advice

The two of you will have your hands full, maintaining the household, feeding yourselves, and getting to know and care for the new baby, especially as all these tasks must be carried out in the midst of disrupted sleep schedules and the birthing parent's postpartum adjustments. The brightest spot in all this is your baby. The baby certainly makes it all worthwhile, but is there anything that could also make it a bit easier? The answer is yes—help!

Accept any and all offers of help from family and friends. Errand running, meal preparation, phone calls, housework—all can be done by someone else. The best kind of help, however, is availability whenever you need it—day or night. Getting such help may not be possible unless you are fortunate enough to have a relative or close friend who can fit comfortably into the chaos. If you are very lucky, grandparents or other helpful relatives or friends will come every day to help as needed. Or maybe, the baby's grandmother or aunt can come to stay for a week or two. She can keep the household running smoothly, feed you both, and answer questions about baby care. You will want to make sure this person can foster the postpartum parent's self-confidence in meeting the baby's needs. This is no time for parental strife to rear its ugly head. See page 57 for more ideas on accepting help from family and friends.

One way to ensure harmony is to invite the person most preferred by the birthing person and to plan the visit for when they prefer it—perhaps immediately after the birth or perhaps one or two weeks later. It also makes sense to specify what you think you need from this person: "We are going to need help running the household and cooking because Jane gets really upset when the place gets messy." Or, "We've never been around babies. We need someone who can show us what to do, what's normal, how to take care of our baby."

Postpartum doulas are a great solution to the problem of new family adjustment. These trained helpers can be hired for blocks of several hours every day or every other day for a period of a week or many weeks. Some offer overnight support. It's like having your favorite aunt (who had lots of kids!) helping with whatever you need; see page 59 for more on postpartum doulas and check Recommended Resources (page 418) to locate one.

For more discussion of ways to smooth the adjustment to becoming parents, see chapter 1.

Postpartum Emotions

During the early postpartum period, the birthing parent's emotions are changeable and unpredictable. One moment, they may be rapturous and full of energy; the next, tired, frustrated, and in tears. The sudden changes in hormone production and body functions—as they go from supporting the growth of a fetus during pregnancy to expelling the baby to producing milk while returning to a nonpregnant state—take an emotional toll. Add to this the inevitable fatigue from loss of sleep during labor and for weeks after the birth, as well as the stress of a profound role change, and it is not surprising there are emotional ups and downs.

If you are the birthing parent's life partner as well as birth partner, you have your own share of emotional adjustments—the role change to parenthood, your own fatigue, and a complete disruption in lifestyle. Even if you are a relative or a friend helping out temporarily, you are probably tired from the birth experience and from the strain of caring for the birthing parent and the new baby.

As two tired people with a great many needs, you will be sustained through this stressful time by your underlying feelings for each other and by the joy and commitment you share in having your new baby. It helps to know this situation *will* get better. Following are suggestions for getting through the emotional ups and downs of the first few days after the baby is born.

Baby Blues

You may be caught off guard if the birthing parent seems sad or cries a lot or has mood swings from depressed to very happy or irritable, without an apparent reason. You may feel helpless or guilty, believing you are to blame or that it is up to you to make things right. You may worry about the birthing parent; you may feel angry or wonder whether this situation is permanent.

When a new postpartum parent experiences these kinds of emotional ups and downs in the first week or two after the birth, we first think of the "baby blues," a common state in the early postpartum period, with all its physical, emotional and hormonal changes, new responsibilities, lack of sleep, and a mysterious totally dependent little person to feed and care for. What can you do to help? Here are some suggestions:

- First of all, ask what you can do to help. The birthing parent may or may not have an answer. They may not know why they are crying. It may simply be a need to cry without you and other people feeling you must help them get over it. Accept their need to cry with patience, tenderness, and empathy. They might appreciate a warm hug while the tears flow.

- Do not blame yourself if you did nothing to cause the crying.

- Know that almost every birthing parent sheds tears and goes on an emotional roller coaster for a few days after childbirth. Emotions are close to the surface at this time, likely because of the abrupt changes in hormone production that take place with birth.

- Realize this will likely not last more than a few days. Be patient.

- Encourage naps and rest (see "Recipe for Getting Enough Sleep," page 395). Lack of sleep can interfere with anyone's mood and confidence.

- Ask friends and relatives, especially those who have given birth, to visit, if the birthing parent seems to feel isolated or lonely.

- Call the caregiver, childbirth educator, or lactation consultant if you are worried.

- Enlist the assistance of a postpartum doula or someone else who understands and can help the birthing parent and give you perspective.

• Look into new parent groups or postpartum classes. They are becoming very popular as settings where people get support from others and can share and discuss feelings and practical tips.

Sometimes, blue feelings continue without letup for more than a week. If this is happening or if you feel under undue pressure, the birthing parent may have postpartum depression, anxiety, or another mood disorder. Discuss your concerns with them and call the resource people already mentioned.

Ask the birthing parent to go over "Unhappiness After Childbirth: A Self-Assessment" (see page 393) with you, as a way to clarify feelings. This self-assessment is an adaptation of a very widely used questionnaire to help a health care professional diagnose a postpartum mood disorder. We include it here to help the birthing parent think about their current feelings and help them recognize that they are not "themselves" and that they deserve some support in overcoming the unhappiness they are feeling. A referral from their caregiver to a social worker, psychologist, or psychiatrist for counseling or therapy may be appropriate and very helpful. A complete physical exam, with blood tests to check levels of various hormones, including thyroid tests, might reveal a physical condition contributing to depression. Or, a support group alone might help the person recover from the depression. Consider these options if the birthing parent is unhappy most of the time. See Recommended Resources (page 418) for online support.

What About Your Feelings?

Becoming a parent has its thrills and joys, but if you are the baby's parent and/or the birthing parent's life partner, you are also making huge emotional adjustments and lifestyle changes in a state of fatigue and constant demands. Many partners find this rather chaotic and unpredictable time exciting and satisfying, but others feel depressed or stressed at times. Even though your needs seem to rank low in the hierarchy, you deserve time for yourself—to sleep, see your friends, and get a break. Why don't you and the postpartum parent plan for you to take a few hours' break when someone else is there? Make a date with yourself and do something you like to do. You'll be refreshed and glad to reconnect with your family!

Unhappiness After Childbirth: A Self-Assessment

Circle the answer that comes closest to how you have felt in the past 7 days, not just how you feel today.

1. I have been able to laugh and see the funny side of things . . .
   a. as much as I always could
   b. not quite as much as I used to
   c. definitely not as much as I used to
   d. not at all

2. I have looked forward with enjoyment to things . . .
   a. as much as I always could
   b. not quite as much as I used to
   c. definitely not as much as I used to
   d. not at all

3. I have blamed myself unnecessarily when things went wrong . . .
   a. not at all   b. very little   c. some of the time   d. most of the time

4. I have been anxious or worried for no good reason . . .
   a. not at all   b. very little   c. some of the time   d. most of the time

5. I have felt scared or panicked for no good reason . . .
   a. not at all   b. very little   c. some of the time   d. most of the time

6. I have been feeling overwhelmed . . .
   a. not at all; I've been coping very well.
   b. very little; I've been coping pretty well.
   c. some of the time; I haven't been coping as well as usual.
   d. quite a lot; I haven't been able to cope at all.

7. I have been so unhappy that I've had difficulty sleeping, even when the baby is asleep and the house is quiet . . .
   a. not at all   b. very little   c. some of the time   d. most of the time

8. I have felt sad or miserable . . .
   a. not at all   b. very little   c. some of the time   d. most of the time

9. I have been so unhappy I've been crying . . .
   a. not at all   b. very little   c. some of the time   d. most of the time

10. The thought of harming myself or my baby has occurred to me . . .
    a. not at all   b. very little   c. some of the time   d. most of the time

After reviewing this form, if you have feel something isn't right or if you have any questions about your emotional well-being, please contact your caregiver, childbirth educator, doula, or a mental health therapist. Or contact Postpartum Support International (www.postpartum.net or 1-800-944-4773).

Adapted from Cox, J. L., Holden, J. M., and Sagovsky, R. 1987. Detection of Postnatal Depression: Development of the 10-Item Edinburgh Postnatal Depression Scale. *British Journal of Psychiatry* 150:782–86.

Sometimes, the partner's feelings are more than just needing some time to relax and refresh. Approximately 10 percent of fathers have been found to experience postpartum depression. Other co-parents may have similar challenges. You might benefit from going over the Unhappiness After Childbirth Questionnaire (page 393) and seeking help if you feel you're suffering more than you realized.

Practical Matters at Home

Much of the turmoil of the postpartum period can be avoided if you're prepared for it in advance and if you can simplify your lives for a while. The following suggestions will help all of you get through these first days until the household becomes more settled.

Fatigue and Sleep Deprivation

The birthing parent is tired. You are probably tired, too. If after being the birth partner you are now the "at home" support person, you are probably running out of energy. Sleep deprivation is a serious problem among new parents that is often ignored. In the lactating parent, it may cause inadequate milk supply; severe mood swings (including postpartum mood disorders); and the inability to deal with the baby's crying, other minor annoyances, and even simple decisions (what to have for dinner, for instance). Fatigue makes *everything* worse, and adequate rest makes *everything* better—the lactating parent's appetite, feelings toward the baby and toward you, their mood, their milk supply, their patience, and so on.

And yet, people simply resign themselves to the belief that all new parents, especially birthing parents, cannot possibly get enough sleep. This is not true. It is possible, but to do so you and the birthing parent must give sleep a very high priority (right after making sure the baby is fed and cared for) and restructure your lives to ensure you both get enough. It does not work for the birthing parent to simply "sleep when the baby sleeps," as most are advised to do.

Until things settle into a comfortable routine, give a high priority to getting enough sleep. Unplug the phone and keep a DO NOT DISTURB sign on the front door until one of you is ready to get up. For the first several weeks after the birth, try very hard not to schedule any appointments before noon—any earlier is too early!

The "Recipe for Getting Enough Sleep" (see following) is very effective for ensuring sufficient sleep for both parents. It is based on the requirement that neither of you gets out of bed in the morning until you have had the amount of sleep you need to function well. This is most helpful if the baby is the only child in your family.

Recipe for Getting Enough Sleep

This advice applies to both parents until the breadwinner(s) returns to employment. Then, that person will have to get more sleep at night and less during the day. Start this technique the first night you are home.

Ask yourselves how many hours of sleep you each need every 24 hours to function well. Six hours? Eight hours? Nine? That is the amount of sleep you owe yourselves every day. The recipe spells out how to get that amount of sleep.

As you cannot get this amount of sleep in one stretch, due to interruptions for feedings and baby care, you will require more hours in bed to get your allotted amount of sleep. It is likely that if you spend 8 hours in bed as a new parent, you may sleep only 4 or 5 hours of that time.

Keep a mental note of approximately how much time you have slept at each stretch and stay in bed in your nightclothes until you have slept the required number of hours. Plan to stay in bed or keep going back to bed until you have slept your allotted number of hours. It might take 12 hours or more! This means that, except for meals and trips to the bathroom, you do not get up in the early morning.

Then, brush your teeth, take a shower, get dressed, and greet the day! You might even want to stay in bed all day for the first few days after birth. The good news is, over time, the nursing parent and baby become more efficient at nursing and sleep for longer intervals, so it takes less time to get the necessary amount of sleep.

Many parents find it easier to follow this advice if the baby sleeps with them or nearby.

At first glance, it may seem impossible to follow this recipe. It does require putting a very high priority on sleep. Keep in mind that fatigue or sleep deprivation contributes to reduction in milk supply, mood swings, anxiety, strained relationships, and less joy in parenting.

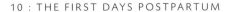

Adapting the Recipe with Two or More Children in the Family

Of course, if there are other children, it may be impossible to avoid morning activities. Then, the two of you will have to adapt (such as urging the birthing parent to go to bed 11 or 12 hours before they need to get up in the morning). Also, it is very helpful to have relatives, friends, or a postpartum doula look after the older child in the mornings to allow more sleep for both of you.

You can also combine the recipe with "platoon sleeping" (see following), in which one parent goes to bed earlier and gets up earlier in the morning than the other parent. For example, if you have an older child, one of you may have to look after them while the other goes to sleep with the baby.

Platoon Sleeping

This arrangement may be the best way to increase sleep for both of you. It works this way: Right after the baby is fed in the early evening, one parent is in charge of the baby (awake or asleep) and any older children while the other parent sleeps in the evening; then, the parent who sleeps in the evening gets up early in the morning, so the other can sleep in the morning.

When it is your turn to stay up, rock and talk and bounce and walk and soothe the baby as long as they are awake. If the baby is asleep, you can doze, watch TV, or get something done. Try to give the early-to-bed parent 2 to 3 hours of sleep, but when the baby really wants to eat, take the baby to the lactating or feeding parent. Then, you both sleep, or try to, with intermittent feedings and diaper changes. You carry on in this way until the early-to-bed parent has had the amount of sleep required. They then get up with the baby, allowing you a few extra hours of sleep.

With platoon sleeping—theoretically, at least—you each get a stretch of unbroken sleep, plus several hours of intermittent sleep.

Fussy, Crying Baby

Entire books have been written about fussy babies, and comprehensive baby care books contain sections on the topic (see Recommended Resources, page 418). In the first few days, you can usually soothe a fussy baby in these ways:

- Feed or burp the baby.

- Change the diaper.

- Let the baby suck on your (clean) little finger: Place your finger in their mouth with your fingernail touching baby's tongue and the soft pad of your finger touching the roof of the baby's mouth. The baby might take your finger more eagerly at first if you wet it. (Offer your finger only if baby has been fed within the past hour. At any other time, the crying may be because they are hungry!)

- Swaddle the baby snugly in a blanket.

- Pick them up, rock or walk them. "Wear" the baby by carrying them close to your body in a baby carrier or sling.

- Hold the baby against your shoulder while bouncing on a birth ball (see illustration, page 182). This works wonders.

- Reclining on your back, hold the baby with their belly against your chest and sing.

- Create "white noise"—the sounds of a dishwasher or a washing machine, "shushing" (that is, saying "shhhh, shhhh," for a few minutes very close to their ear), play peaceful recorded music, or croon lullabies in the baby's ear.

To learn a successful step-by-step approach to soothing a crying baby, see Recommended Resources, page 418.

Don't leave a tiny baby crying. The first few days after birth are a time of major adjustment for the baby, as they are for the birthing parent and for you. A newborn needs the comfort and security of feeling your warm bodies and hearing your voices close by. Do not worry about spoiling the baby: You cannot spoil someone by meeting their basic needs.

Scheduling the Baby's Sleeping and Feeding

Don't even try to get the baby on a schedule in the first few weeks. Instead, discover the baby's own schedule and pattern your life around that. Focus on meeting the baby's needs; figure out how they tell you they are hungry, curious, interested, bored, uncomfortable, or overstimulated. Let the baby call the shots. It is much easier for the household to adjust to the baby at first than to make the baby adjust to the household. Make it your goal to meet the baby's needs, as they express them—you will all be happier if you do. Read *Your Amazing Newborn* and *Your Baby Is Speaking to You* (see Recommended Resources, page 418) to help you understand the baby.

Meals

Time for meal preparation hardly exists during the busy first days at home, yet good food, quickly available, is a must. Try the following:

- **Prepare meals in advance**. Before the birth, prepare a few dishes—such as soups, casseroles, and stews—that will either keep for several days or can be frozen.

- **Purchase quick, nutritious, tasty foods**. Foods that need little or no preparation—that you can grab and eat—are good choices for the first few weeks. Such foods include yogurt, fruit, granola and nuts, cottage cheese, hard cheeses, raw vegetables, cold cuts, and whole-grain breads and crackers. Plan to have these on hand before the birth so you won't have to go shopping right away. This is the time, too, to search the deli counter and frozen food section at the grocery store for nourishing, delicious prepared food.

- **Prepare foods that last for a while**. For example, you can roast a turkey and pick from it for a week or wash, cut, and chill raw vegetables to keep in the refrigerator for munching.

- **Accept food from friends and relatives**. If people ask how they can help, tell them you'd love a main dish. Sometimes, a group of friends establishes a "meal train" in which each signs up to provide one or more meals over the course of a week or two. Visit Mealtrain.com to prepare an online sign-up schedule. One hint: Ask your friends to bring food only every other day. People usually bring more than one meal's worth, so you can find your refrigerator overflowing after a few days of daily contributions. Besides, if you ask for meals only every other day, your friends may keep the meal train going for a longer period, or they may be willing to offer services other than food, such as walking the dog, running errands, doing laundry, etc.

- **Remember the birth parent's dietary needs**. The postpartum diet should be as good as the pregnancy diet. If breast-feeding, they will need 200 to 300 calories more than normal each day. They will also need at least 2 quarts (1.9 L) of liquids each day.

Household Chores

The first few days at home are busy and full of adjustments. Do yourselves a big favor: If you have no help, plan to do the minimum in the way of household chores—just enough to maintain sanity. It may be easier if you have "supercleaned" before the baby was born; if you haven't, just close your eyes and let things accumulate for a while. Simplify your lives so you are free to care for and enjoy the baby and to get enough rest.

If you do have help, do not be shy about asking for what you really want done. One advantage of a postpartum doula is they are there to do what you need done, not to enjoy the new baby (though they will!) and your company, and you don't need to worry about offending them. They won't even mind wearing the baby in a sling while doing some chores or preparing a meal, allowing the two of you a chance for a nap!

In conclusion, the first days and weeks postpartum are a time of adjustment: for the birthing parent as their body returns to a nonpregnant state and begins making milk and feeding the baby; for you both, as you get to know your baby, develop baby care skills, adjust to the changes in sleep, learn your parenting roles, take on a new lifestyle, and explore your relationship with each other; and for your baby, who must learn about their new world, their parents, and the sights and sounds outside the womb. You will never be the same—nor will you want to be.

CHAPTER 11

GETTING STARTED WITH FEEDING YOUR BABY

Before Elliot's arrival, we could never understand why anyone wouldn't breast-feed their baby. One session with a bad latch, and Heather's nipple hurt terribly. Dread and fear of feeding led to brief moments of resentment. We stayed with it, though, and feel wonderful about the quality and quantity of his intake. It is a great relief to us to know he is getting the best thing for him.

—MATT, FIRST-TIME FATHER

From the first moment my wife held my son, they both seemed to know instinctively what to do. He wriggled up to her breast and began to drink. Her breast milk was his sole nourishment for the first few months of his life. Two and a half years later, nursing is still his source of comfort when he is upset, and the only thing he looks for when he is tired. The power of their bond and my wife's perseverance continue to amaze me every day.

—ALLIE, FIRST-TIME MOTHER

Throughout this section we use the terms *breast-feeding* and *chest-feeding*—often combined as *breast-feeding/chest-feeding*, to describe the act of feeding one's baby from one's breast or chest. We also use other lactation-related terms, including "nursing." This is a move toward inclusivity for all who care for and nourish their babies with their bodies regardless of gender identity or anatomy.

For a family with a breast-feeding/chest-feeding baby it may seem unclear what the partner's role is because it is not as simple as taking over the feeding when the lactating parent is tired. It is more a matter of supporting feeding holistically and helping simplify life so it can happen. It really helps if you have some knowledge and conviction about the advantages of breast-feeding.

Reasons for Breast-Feeding/ Chest-Feeding

Families choose to breast-feed/chest-feed for many reasons, including:

• It costs much less to feed human milk than formula.

• Time-consuming chores of formula preparation and bottle washing are avoided.

For the breast-feeding/chest-feeding parent, reasons include:

• Lactation hastens the return of the uterus to its normal state by causing it to contract with feedings during the early postpartum period.

• Hormones associated with successful lactation can help with relaxation and feelings of contentment.

• Lower rates of type 2 diabetes, certain types of breast cancer, and ovarian cancer for the lactating parent

• After the initial learning period, most parents find nursing a pleasant way to connect with and nurture their baby.

• It's quick and convenient—simply lifting a shirt and offering the breast/chest; there's no frantic bottle preparation while your baby cries impatiently.

For the baby, reasons include:

• Human milk is perfectly suited to the baby's nutritional requirements.

• Human milk changes in composition as the baby grows and nutritional requirements change.

• The milk is always at the right temperature and instantly available.

Breast-feeding/chest-feeding and human milk feeding are important parts of establishing a baby's microbiome. At least one study has found that 30 percent of the beneficial bacteria in a baby's intestinal tract comes directly from their parent's milk, and an additional 10 percent comes from skin on their parent's breast/chest.

- Human milk contains substances (human milk oligosaccharides) that feed the bacteria and provide important protection against illness (immunoglobulins and antibodies).

- Fewer problems with allergies, lower respiratory infections, ear infections, eczema, indigestion, diarrhea, vomiting, and overfeeding, necrotizing enterocolitis, SIDS, childhood leukemia, childhood obesity, and type 2 diabetes occur with human milk than with formula.

- Other long-term health benefits, such as jaw development, reduced likelihood of asthma, and better ability to handle dietary fats

For these reasons, most families today decide to breast-feed/chest-feed their baby.

While there may be challenges to overcome in the first days or weeks, for most families, it becomes easy, quick, and convenient. It's not uncommon for new parents to worry whether the baby is getting enough milk and whether their baby nurses too often or not enough. They may not trust the process. To get off to a good start with breast-feeding—before the baby is born—identify helpful resources, such as:

- A good book or website can be an amazing resource in the middle of the night (see Recommended Resources, page 418).

- A lactation consultant, for ongoing support. Your baby's doctor or childbirth educator can likely refer you to a lactation consultant who can provide support at any stage of your feeding journey. You can also search online for lactation or breast-feeding services, counselors, or lactation consultants in your area.

- Peer-to-peer support groups, La Leche League International chapters, and other perinatal or parenting support groups meet regularly in most communities. La Leche League International and Breastfeeding USA can be found online (see Recommended Resources, page 418).

- Your baby's doctor will help you know whether your baby is thriving and can suggest helpful resources, if needed.

- The Special Supplemental Nutrition Program for Women, Infants, and Children (WIC) provides lactation support, health care referrals, supplemental foods, and nutrition education for low-income families during pregnancy and for up to five years after birth.

- Friends who have nursed their babies can advise on helpful products and resources and can empathize and assist with problems.

- Internet sites provide products and information, and news groups offer advice and support (see Recommended Resources, page 418).

- Videos are available online or for purchase that teach and illustrate basic principles (see Recommended Resources, page 418).

Make a list of names, phone numbers, and addresses of all these helpful resources. Post it on the refrigerator for reference.

If possible, your family should take a breast-feeding or lactation class to learn the basics before the birth. Most organizations and hospitals offering childbirth classes also offer related classes.

Even if you do not know very much about breast-feeding or lactation, being a supportive partner is very valuable. Your partner needs your belief in breast-feeding/chest-feeding and your help to make it easier. You can do this by providing an extra pair of hands to help position the baby for feeding; keeping your partner fed and their thirst quenched; helping your partner stay as rested as possible; changing diapers; bathing, soothing, rocking, or bouncing the baby; taking the baby for short walks or rides outside; and being patient and loving through the early adjustments.

Above all, your partner needs you to recognize that nursing is giving your baby the best possible food for the best possible start. Show your partner how much you appreciate their role as the lactating parent by helping as much as you can and offering encouragement if any challenges arise. If needed, find professional guidance to support your family.

Getting Off to a Good Start

A good start with breast-feeding depends on:

- Frequent, responsive feeding of the baby whenever they give cues they want to nurse, beginning soon after birth, as soon as the baby will suck. Babies need to nurse at least eight times per 24 hours and usually more.

- Recognition of baby's feeding cues: bringing hand to mouth, turning their head side to side, opening their mouth and turning their head toward anything that brushes their cheek (rooting), making sucking sounds and motions with their mouth and tongue, fussing, or sucking avidly on a finger placed in their mouth. A baby usually indicates the desire to nurse long before crying from hunger.

- A good "latch" between the baby's mouth and the breast

- A comfortable position for the lactating parent, with pillows for support, so they can release tension and remain relaxed for the entire feeding

- Availability of advice from a lactation consultant or other knowledgeable person

- *Your* help and positive support

- Freedom from excessive difficulty

We mention the last item because, on rare occasions, a family who wants very much to breast-feed has one problem after another, even when working closely with a lactation consultant. If, based on the level of challenges faced, the decision is made to stop breast-feeding, some people feel disappointment, depression, uncertainty, and shame over the decision. But each family must balance the advantages and disadvantages of their situation. Getting the best support and advice available is the first step. If feeding problems are still insurmountable, explore alternatives such as pumping milk and feeding with a bottle or formula-feeding.

Having support in those steps can make a great difference in the experience and ability to move forward confidently. Your understanding and support of these decisions will help immensely. Most important, try to deal with overzealous advocates of breast-feeding who may not understand your family has made the right decision for its circumstances.

How to Offer Support Related to Infant Feeding

Research shows that breast-feeding/chest-feeding parents feel more capable and confident about breast-feeding if their partners are supportive with encouragement and active assistance.

Sincere encouragement comes from the heart; spend some time thinking about why you appreciate your partner's role in nursing your baby. Then, talk about it. Consideration and communication go a long way!

Active involvement in *supporting* feeding doesn't have to be just directly feeding your baby. Here are some other ways to offer support:

- Caring for your baby's needs—including diaper changes, burping, and holding, babywearing, or settling baby down between feedings

- Caring for your partner's needs—bringing water, food, and restocking any needed supplies within arm's reach

- Positioning—during feedings, checking on your baby and partner's position can keep them both comfortable; place pillows nearby, offer a footstool or ottoman, and give gentle reminders about the baby's positioning and the breastfeeding/chestfeeding parent's comfort including posture, ergonomics, and any sources of tension.

- Keeping a cozy environment—tidying up, keeping your space a comfortable temperature, taking care of other household responsibilities your partner typically does

Early Concerns

At first, nursing a baby does not come easily to most parents. It can take 2 to 4 weeks to reach the point where all the nursing parent needs to do is put the baby near the breast to get them to latch on and suck. In the meantime, possible early challenges such as temporary nipple soreness, lack of sleep, and concern about the milk supply may have to be overcome. Both you and your partner need information and guidelines on what is normal and how to solve these problems. The resources you have lined up will help with these concerns.

Milk Supply

How can you know whether your baby is getting enough milk? If the baby needs to nurse frequently, does it mean there is not enough milk to satisfy the baby's hunger? It can sometimes feel difficult to trust such an imprecise process. Knowing these facts may help:

- For the first 2 to 4 days after birth, there is a small quantity of colostrum. With frequent nursing sessions, it is typically enough to satisfy the baby's nutritional requirements during this period.

- Between approximate days 2 and 7 after birth, the colostrum is replaced by transitional milk. The frequency and total amount of time spent suckling help determine when the milk "comes in" and how much milk is produced.

- Young babies typically nurse often—eight to twelve or more times each 24 hours. This may surprise new parents. Expect that breast-feeding will take a number of hours every day and plan accordingly. Generally, the more the baby suckles, the more milk that will be made.

- Babies do not nurse at regular intervals; they "bunch up" several feedings in a row (called cluster feeding) and then may go without feeding for a relatively long stretch. It is normal for a baby to nurse four times in 6 hours and sleep for 3 to 4 hours before the next feeding.

- Ample milk supply can be indicated by these signs: how the breasts feel (heavier and more "full" before a feeding than afterward); whether milk can be expressed or drips from the breasts; whether the baby is wetting their diapers and having bowel movements (after the milk comes in, six to eight wet diapers and four or more bowel movements a day are good signs for the first 4 weeks); and whether the baby noticeably swallows after every few sucks. Weight gain is a clear sign the baby is getting enough milk—although the baby may not begin to gain until a few days old.

If the baby appears not to be getting enough milk, try the 24-Hour "Cure" (see page 412) or consult your baby's doctor or a lactation consultant.

Fatigue and Lack of Sleep

Because young babies nurse frequently and sometimes fuss during the night, long stretches of sleep are not possible for the breast-feeding parent or for you if you're trying to help. Sleep tends to come in the form of 2- to 3-hour naps between feedings. This normal change in sleep patterns is not a major problem if new parents can catch up during the day with a nap or two. If not, fatigue sets in and interferes with all aspects of parenting and daily living. Follow the instructions for "Recipe for Getting Enough Sleep" on page 395.

The breast-feeding parent may get more sleep and the baby may fuss less if they nurse in bed at night and nap or sleep with or near the baby. This way, they can doze while feeding the baby and do not have to get up as much. A good discussion of this subject appears in *Sleeping with Your Baby*, by James McKenna (see Recommended Resources, page 418). If, however, your partner is uncomfortable bed-sharing, this solution will not work.

Public health officials are very opposed to bed-sharing with a baby, but under certain conditions, according to Dr. James McKenna, an anthropologist who has thoroughly studied co-sleeping, it can be safe and beneficial under strict safety conditions. He suggests the following to ensure safe sleeping with your baby:

- Neither parent smokes and the pregnant parent did not smoke during pregnancy.

- The parents are not obese.

- The room is not overheated.

- Neither parent is under the influence of recreational or medical drugs or alcohol.

- No pets, other children, or stuffed animals are in the bed.

- Baby sleeps on their back, on a firm mattress, and without multiple pillows, a feather mattress, waterbed, sagging sofa, heavy bedding, or a sheepskin.

If these conditions cannot be met, the baby should not sleep in the parents' bed, but in a safe separate baby bed or crib nearby.

Breast/Chest and Nipple Concerns

Following are some causes of breast pain in the first few days of breast-/chest-feeding:

- **Engorgement:** The transition from colostrum typically begins after 2 to 4 days as breast milk "comes in" over a period of 8 to 12 hours. This, combined with extra fluids in the breast tissue, can lead to the breasts becoming extremely full and painful, or engorged, making it difficult for the baby to latch on.

  Frequent breast-feeding, even before this transition, helps prevent severe engorgement, but the baby's appetite and ability at the breast may not match the milk supply at first. If the breasts are too firm to allow the baby to get a good latch, steps can be taken to soften the nipples before feeding: expressing a small amount of milk by hand or with a pump, applying warm compresses, or letting the shower run over the breasts to start the flow of milk. The goal is to express just enough milk to soften the nipples so the baby can take them into their mouth.

  After feeding, the breast-feeding parent may want to apply a cool pack to the breasts/chest to reduce any engorgement. A pain reliever such as ibuprofen may also help (it is a good idea to check this with a health care provider).

  After a few days, the engorgement should subside and a balance will eventually be reached between the amount of milk needed by the baby and the amount produced.

  Engorgement occurs even in people who do not breast-feed, but a lack of suckling or milk expression and a supportive, but not too tight, bra will stop milk production.

Nipple pain may be caused by the following:

- **Prolonged, vigorous suckling with a poor latch:** Some babies suck harder and longer than others. Early nipple soreness may be greater with such babies, but it should pass after the milk comes in or within a week or so if the latch is good. Soreness is considered within normal limits if it occurs in the first minute of the feeding but subsides for the rest of the feeding. If soreness persists throughout a feeding, it may be caused by a poor latch (see latch quality, following).

Limiting suckling time may not reduce soreness, but will likely reduce the amount of milk the baby gets. If the baby sucks steadily at one breast for 15 minutes, switch sides.

It is important not to fall into the trap of giving a bottle to "rest" the breasts, unless the soreness is extreme. In cases of extreme soreness or cracked, bleeding nipples, without delay seek help from a professional lactation consultant, one of the recommended books on breast-feeding (see Recommended Resources, page 418), or someone experienced with breast-feeding.

- **Latch quality:** A good latch is key to comfortable and efficient nursing. Improper suckling is the number one cause of nipple soreness. If the baby nibbles or "clicks" (breaks the suction with each suck), it is more likely to cause nipple pain and lead to less time with the baby on the breast. This may reduce the amount of milk produced. A nurse or midwife, lactation consultant, childbirth educator, or a good book on breast-feeding (see Recommended Resources, page 418) can help with the quality of latching.

A good latch means the baby opens their mouth wide and takes a large amount of the areola (the dark circle around the nipple) into their mouth. If the baby is held comfortably to the chest while the breast-feeding parent sits back with their arms resting on pillows, they can both relax and let baby seek and latch on. While at first this takes time while the baby learns to do it efficiently, the baby becomes an expert and there is usually little pain. This is the laid-back breast-feeding position, described by Dr. Suzanne Colson (see page 375 and Recommended Resources, page 418).

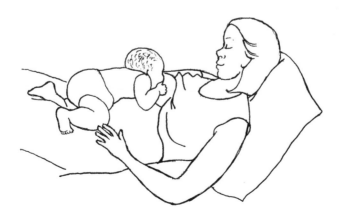

To find a comfortable nursing position, the baby should lie on their side ("tummy to tummy") rather than on the back. Other good positions are side lying or lying side by side on a bed and the "football" or "clutch" hold, in which the breast-feeding parent sits up and holds the baby beside and facing the breast. The baby's head can be supported by the breast-feeding parent. In all positions, ordinary pillows or the now popular horseshoe-shaped nursing pillows may be useful for comfortably propping the baby and supporting the breast-feeding parent's arms. In all positions, too, the baby's face is held very close to the breast to keep it close with every suck. Any good breast-feeding book contains instructions and illustrations of breast-feeding positions and aids.

Sometimes, despite one's best efforts, a baby has a challenging time latching deeply, which causes pain and frustration for all involved. One possible cause is wry neck (torticollis), in which the baby's head is tilted to one side and they have trouble turning their head freely. The position of the baby and neck in the uterus may cause torticollis. Another possible cause is tongue-tie (ankyloglossia), a condition in which there is an unusually short, thick, or tight frenulum (the membrane that extends from the bottom of the baby's tongue to the floor of the mouth). This restricts the tongue's mobility. It may be important to work with a lactation and/or health care professional to rule out or address these concerns.

- **Thrush:** This is a yeast infection that can be present in both the baby's mouth and the areola and cause pain. A thrush infection is most likely to occur if the lactating parent or baby has recently taken antibiotics or is prone to yeast infections. If you suspect thrush, check the baby's mouth for patches of white film on the gums, tongue, and the roof of the mouth and the parent's areola for irritated or whitish patches. Deep pain in the breast tissue can be caused by other factors. Call a lactation consultant and the baby's doctor if you suspect thrush or have other concerns, as there are treatments available.

Treating sore nipples. Here are some strategies for treating sore nipples:

- Rub a little colostrum or milk into the nipples and the base of the areola.

- Rub a topical emollient, such as a nipple balm or unscented purified lanolin (or another ointment recommended by a knowledgeable caregiver), into the nipples and the base of the areola.

- Begin each nursing on the less sore side.

- Try different nursing positions to determine if one is more comfortable than any other.

- If the soreness is extreme and the nipples are cracked or bleeding, it could be because of the quality of the baby's latch. Immediately seek professional lactation support. Reducing or stopping breast-feeding without pumping milk can lead to engorgement and reduced milk production. If your lactation consultant or other health care professional advises a change in breast-feeding, they should also advise pumping and bottle-feeding during this time.

- Try nipple shields—thin silicone nipple covers with holes that allow the milk to flow out. They may protect the nipples from further damage during nursing sessions. It is best to consult a lactation consultant if considering these shields (see Recommended Resources, page 418).

- Check with your health care provider about pain medications, if needed.

If these measures fail, consult a lactation consultant, childbirth educator, the baby's physician, or a good book on breast-feeding (see Recommended Resources, page 418).

The 24-Hour "Cure"

During the first few weeks after birth, the breast-feeding parent and baby are mastering the art of nursing. The 24-hour "cure" can solve some problems that arise, such as:

- Doubts about whether there is enough milk being made

- Fatigue, lack of sleep, or anxiety

- Lack of appetite, poor nourishment, or low fluid intake

- Slow weight gain in the baby

- "Nipple confusion"—that is, the baby seems to prefer a bottle nipple or nipple shield to the breast/chest.

The "cure" promotes frequent, efficient suckling and an abundant milk supply by nurturing both the lactating parent and baby. The parent gets complete rest, plenty of good food and drink, and freedom from all responsibility other than feeding and cuddling the baby. The baby gets prolonged skin-to-skin contact with the breast-feeding parent, constant access to the breast/chest, and nurturance.

Before starting, make sure the baby is gaining weight—slowly, at least—by comparing weights recorded over a few days. If not gaining weight, consult the baby's doctor or a lactation consultant before beginning the cure. Make sure, too, there are no sore, blistered, or cracked nipples, which should be addressed before the cure begins (see treating sore nipples, page 411).

Here is how to do the 24 Hour "Cure:"

- Set aside a full 24 hours when the breast-feeding parent and baby can have support during the cure. Use your day off or get a friend, relative, or postpartum doula to take your place for part of the 24 hours. Around-the-clock help is essential.

- The baby and breast-feeding/chest-feeding parent go to bed. They both wear as little clothing as practical under the bedcovers so the baby gets lots of warm skin-to-skin contact, which stimulates the suckling reflex and interest in feeding. Be sure to follow the safety guidelines for sleeping with the baby on page 407.

- The breast-feeding parent may read, watch TV, chat with you or other support people (but no visitors, please), and, most important, doze. The extra sleep will make a big difference, although it will come in short snatches. Even if it takes a long time to fall asleep, the nursing parent should stay in bed. Some sleep-deprived people take a long time to relax and give in to sleep. The goal should be that the nursing parent gets out of bed *only to go to the bathroom*—not to eat, answer the phone, do housework, or anything else.

- Supply plenty of liquids—place water or juice within reach with a goal of having the lactating parent drinking about 2 to 3 quarts (1.9 to 2.8 L) during the 24 hours.

- Offer tasty, nutritious meals. If your family has been relying on take-out fast foods or cold ready-to-eat foods, a hot, home-cooked meal or two will be appreciated. If cooking is not your forte, there are many healthful alternatives you can consider.

- The baby should stay in bed with the nursing parent, except when a diaper change is necessary or when the baby is fussy (but not willing to nurse) and needs to be briefly walked or rocked. Then, you should take care of the baby.

- Whenever the baby awakens or seems at all interested in suckling, they should breast-feed/chest-feed. Do not give the baby a bottle of either formula or breast milk, unless the baby's doctor or a lactation consultant advises doing so because the baby is underweight.

The combination of rest and nourishment for the lactating parent and skin-to-skin contact and unlimited suckling for the baby almost always results in a marked increase in milk production, improved sucking by the baby, a well-rested parent, and a much happier family.

If your family is unable to closely follow the 24-Hour "Cure" or if it fails to solve the problem, consult the baby's doctor, a lactation consultant, or peer-to-peer support such as La Leche League International.

Special Circumstances for Infant Feeding

As mentioned at the start of this chapter, there are many ways to care for and nourish a baby at their parent's body. Chest-feeding is a term often used within the transgender community by parents who choose to feed or nurse at the chest.

Some families choose to use at-breast supplementation, sometimes referred to as an SNS, which stands for "supplemental nursing system." This involves using a small tube connected to a bottle that holds pumped milk from the lactating parent, donor milk, or formula. The tube is then placed in the baby's mouth and, when they suck, they receive the liquid. This method can also be used in cases where the parent does not have milk-making tissue (due to anatomy or surgery), when a baby needs additional nutrition, or in the case of inducing lactation.

Inducing lactation may be considered by adoptive parents or LGBTQ co-parents. The process of encouraging the body to make milk in absence of a pregnancy may be undertaken with the support of herbs, medications, pumping, and/or nursing the baby. Finding a supportive lactation professional to offer guidance as early in the process as possible may be beneficial. Regardless of the timing and method chosen, many parents who do not birth their babies share that nursing can be a source of connection regardless of the volume of milk they may make and transfer.

"Co-nursing" is a term sometimes used by LGBTQ parents who choose to share the role of nursing a baby. It is important to make sure that adequate stimulation and removal of milk is happening to meet the needs of the baby and the milk-making goals of each parent.

If a baby needs supplementation, the family needs support and information to be successful. A knowledgeable lactation professional may be an asset to your family if you're considering inducing lactation, co-nursing, or any situation for which you feel you need additional support.

When to Give the Baby a Bottle

Most parents want their babies to be able to get milk from a bottle eventually, especially if the nursing parent will be away from home regularly. You may have heard stories about babies who won't take a bottle and about how distraught the parents become when they need the baby to do so. For a smooth introduction to bottle-feeding, timing can be crucial. Bottle-feeding too early may interfere with the baby's learning to breast-feed. But if the bottle is introduced too late, the baby may refuse it.

It is wise not to rush bottle-feeding with a breast-fed baby, for two reasons. First, while the baby is getting used to the feel and flow of milk from the human nipple, it may be confusing to go back and forth with a different method. Different sucking techniques—different mouth and jaw motions—are required for human and bottle nipples. The baby may not be able to transition smoothly from one to the other. (Of course, there are circumstances when a very young infant must be bottle-fed. A lactation consultant can be very helpful in teaching a baby who has been bottle-fed to suck at the breast, when able to do so.)

Second, when a baby skips breast-feeding sessions and takes milk from a bottle, they spend less time suckling at the breast. This may slow milk production, especially at the time when lactation is still becoming established because it is the suckling that stimulates milk production, and may result in less milk over time. Pumping during these gaps between nursing helps maintain the milk supply.

If you plan to bottle-feed the baby at some time, it is best to wait until the baby is able to latch on and suckle at the breast/chest easily, without coaxing, and until the milk supply is clearly plentiful. Most babies are good latchers and sucklers by 3 to 4 weeks of age (although some may need several more weeks). If the bottle is introduced at this time, the baby will probably adjust easily. You can then continue to offer the bottle regularly— three to five times a week—so the baby won't forget how to bottle-feed and ensure the baby continues to feed willingly from the bottle and the breast. Feed the baby expressed milk or, if needed, formula.

It usually works better if someone other than the nursing parent gives the bottle to the baby. If the nursing parent tries to give the bottle or is present while someone else does so, the baby may refuse the bottle and insist on nursing at the breast. Many people advise introducing a bottle when the baby is very hungry. This doesn't always work, however. A very hungry baby may be so upset that they have difficulty adjusting to the different sucking required with a bottle. They just want their nursing parent. Instead, offer the bottle when the baby is not hungry but awake and content. Stroke the baby's lips with the bottle nipple and let them "play" with it and mouth it. Out of curiosity, they may suck on it a bit. Do this several times. Then, they may be ready to take the bottle when they are hungry.

If the baby is reluctant to take the bottle after becoming accustomed to nursing, allow a couple of weeks for the baby to learn to use the bottle before the breast-feeding parent is absent for a significant length of time. Don't wait until 2 days before the nursing parent goes back to work!

With persistence, the baby will eventually take the bottle. But if it ever happens that the breast-feeding/chest-feeding parent is unavailable to nurse and the baby will not take the bottle, try squirting milk into a corner of the baby's mouth with an eyedropper or even using a tiny cup, such as a shot glass, to feed.

Once Breast-Feeding/ Chest-Feeding Is Established

By 3 to 6 weeks of age, most babies and their parents find breast-feeding to be a pleasant, quick, convenient method of feeding. By this time, you and your co-parent probably function as an efficient team as you divide the work and pleasure of integrating the baby into your lives. Although there are more hurdles to come, any lactation challenges you faced should be behind you, and the closeness and joy you all share are most satisfying.

PARTING WORDS

The family is launched. The baby is born and getting used to the world; your co-parent is no longer pregnant and is adjusting to being on constant call. Your job as birth partner is over, and your new role has begun. The excitement is over, and you may feel strangely let down.

Now what? It will take a while to absorb and integrate all that has happened. This birth has transformed you into a parent, or grandparent, or more-special-than-ever friend. You will never be the same, and you will always treasure this experience.

We wish you well.

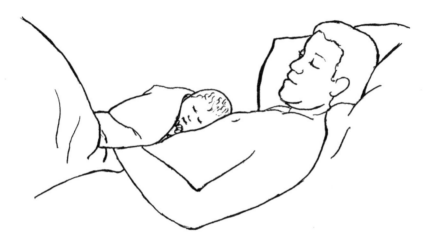

Recommended Resources

The following topics are listed alphabetically and include books, video recordings, and websites that provide helpful information to supplement this book.

To contact Penny Simkin:
www.pennysimkin.com
info@pennysimkin.com

Penny Simkin's Social Media:
YouTube Channel: www.youtube.com/psfrompenny
Facebook: www.facebook.com/PennySimkinChildbirth
Instagram: @penny.simkin

To contact Katie Rohs:
www.birthtastic.com
katie@birthtastic.com

Aids for Relaxation

Schardt, Dana. 2000. *Pregnancy Relaxation: A Guide to Peaceful Beginnings.* CD.

Simkin, Penny. 2008. *Comfort Measures for Childbirth.* DVD. www.pennysimkin.com.

Simkin, Penny. *Relaxation, Rhythm, Ritual: The 3 Rs of Childbirth.* Downloadable video. www.pennysimkin.com/shop.

Aromatherapy

Aromatherapy for Childbirth: www.aromatherapyforchildbirth.org.

Clark, Demetria. 2015. *Aromatherapy and Herbal Remedies for Pregnancy, Birth, and Breastfeeding.*

Baby Care, Supplies, and Infant Sleep

American Academy of Pediatrics website for parents: www.kidshealth.org.

BabyCenter: Clothing, supplies, equipment for baby www.babycenter.com/baby-products-and-gear.

Klaus, Marshall H., and Phyllis H. Klaus. 2000. *The Amazing Talents of the Newborn.* DVD. www.pennysimkin.com.

Klaus, Marshall H., and Phyllis H. Klaus. 2000. *Your Amazing Newborn.*

Leach, Penelope. 2010. *Your Baby & Child: From Birth to Age Five.*

McKenna, James J. 2007. *Sleeping with Your Baby: A Parent's Guide to Cosleeping.*

Nugent, Kevin. 2011. *Your Baby Is Speaking to You: A Visual Guide to the Amazing Behaviors of Your Newborn and Growing Baby.*

Pantley, Elizabeth. 2003. *Gentle Baby Care: No-Cry, No-Fuss, No-Worry— Essential Tips for Raising Your Baby.*

Sears, William, Martha Sears, Robert Sears, and James Sears. 2013. *The Baby Book: Everything You Need to Know About Your Baby from Birth to Age Two*, revised ed.

Bed Rest Support

Sidelines: www.sidelines.org.

Breast-Feeding/Chest-Feeding

Birth International. *Biological Nurturing—Laid-Back Breastfeeding.* DVD. www.birthinternational.com/product/biological-nurturing-dvd.

Breastfeeding USA: www.breastfeedingusa.org.

Find a lactation consultant:
www.uslca.org/resources/find-a-lactation-consultant-map#!directory/map.

Getting Started with Breastfeeding from Stanford Medicine has lots of outstanding videos about early breastfeeding:
med.stanford.edu/newborns/professional-education/breastfeeding.html.

Huggins, Kathleen. 2017. *The Nursing Mother's Companion*, 7th ed.

KellyMom: www.kellymom.com.

La Leche League International: www.llli.org.

Mohrbacher, Nancy, and Kathleen Kendall-Tackett. 2010. *Breastfeeding Made Simple: Seven Natural Laws for Nursing Mothers*, 2nd ed.

Newman, Jack. *Dr. Jack Newman's Visual Guide to Breastfeeding*. DVD. www.breastfeedinginc.ca.

Newman, Jack, and Teresa Pitman. 2006. *The Ultimate Breastfeeding Book of Answers*, revised ed.

Special Supplemental Nutrition Program for Women, Infants, and Children (WIC): www.fns.usda.gov/wic/about-wic.

Breech and Baby's Positions In-Utero

Breech Version: How a Doula or Partner May Help.
www.pennysimkin.com/download

Evidence Based Birth: www.evidencebasedbirth.com.

Simkin, Penny, and Ruth Ancheta. 2011. *The Labor Progress Handbook: Early Interventions to Prevent and Treat Dystocia*, 3rd ed.

Spinning Babies: www.spinningbabies.com.

What Your Baby's Position in the Womb Means: www.healthline.com/health/pregnancy/baby-positions-in-womb.

Cesarean Delivery

Childbirth Connection. 2016. *What Every Woman Needs to Know About Cesarean Birth*. National Partnership for Women & Families.
www.nationalpartnership.org/research-library/maternal-health/what-every-pregnant-woman-needs-to-know-about-cesarean-section.pdf.

Childbirth Connection. 2016. *Why is the C-Section Rate so High?*
National Partnership for Women & Families.
www.nationalpartnership.org/research-library/maternal-health/
why-is-the-c-section-rate-so-high.pdf.

Haelle, Tara. 2018. "Your Biggest C-Section Risk May Be Your Hospital."
Consumer Reports. www.consumerreports.org/c-section/
biggest-c-section-risk-may-be-your-hospital.

Circumcision

American Academy of Pediatrics. 2012. Policy statement.
"Circumcision Policy Statement." Task Force on Circumcision.
pediatrics.aappublications.org/content/pediatrics/130/3/585.full.pdf.

Canadian Paediatric Society. 2015. "Newborn Male Circumcision."
Position Statement. www.cps.ca/en/documents/position/circumcision.

Kass, Elias. 2018. "Circumcision." https://drdadsays.com/2018/02/09/
circumcision.

Comfort Advice and Aids for Childbirth

Pregnancy and Labor Ice Pack: www.pennysimkin.com/shop/
pregnancy-and-labor-ice-pack.

Simkin, Penny. 2007. "Comfort in Labor." Available at no cost from
www.childbirthconnection.org/pdfs/comfort-in-labor-simkin.pdf.

Simkin, Penny. 2008. *Comfort Measures for Childbirth.* DVD.
www.pennysimkin.com.

Cord-Blood Storage

American Academy of Pediatrics. 2007. Policy Statement. "Cord Blood
Banking for Potential Future Transplantation."
pediatrics.aappublications.org/content/pediatrics/119/1/165.full.pdf.

KidsHealth. 2015. The Nemours Foundation. "Cord-Blood Banking."
kidshealth.org/en/parents/cord-blood.html

Cutting the Umbilical Cord

Bakalar, Nicholas. 2011. New Cochrane Review. "Childbirth: Benefits Seen in Clamping the Cord Later." The *New York Times*. www.nytimes.com/2011/11/29/health/research/delay-in-clamping-umbilical-cord-has-benefits-months-later.html.

Science & Sensibility. 2017. *New Cochrane Review*. "Delayed Cord Clamping Likely Beneficial for Healthy Term Newborns." www.scienceandsensibility.org/blog/new-cochrane-review-delayed-cord-clamping-likely-beneficial-for-healthy-term-newborns.

Simkin, Penny. 2012. *Penny Simkin on Delayed Cord Clamping*. www.youtube.com/watch?v=W3RywNup2CM.

Fussy, Crying Babies

Brazelton, T. Berry, and Joshua D. Sparrow. 2003. *Calming Your Fussy Baby: The Brazelton Way*.

Karp, Harvey. 2003. *The Happiest Baby on the Block*. (Also available on DVD.)

Nugent, Kevin. 2011. *Your Baby Is Speaking to You: A Visual Guide to the Amazing Behaviors of Your Newborn and Growing Baby*.

Pantley, Elizabeth. 2002. *The No-Cry Sleep Solution: Gentle Ways to Help Your Baby Sleep Through the Night*.

Sears, William, and Martha Sears. 1996. *The Fussy Baby Book: Parenting Your High-Need Child from Birth to Age Five*.

Plooij, Frans X. 2017. *The Wonder Weeks: How to Stimulate Your Baby's Mental Development and Help Him Turn His 10 Predictable, Great, Fussy Phases into Magical Leaps Forward*. Also has an outstanding app for baby milestones: www.thewonderweeks.com.

Gender Neutral Information

Canadian Midwives Trans Inclusivity Statement: www.canadianmidwives.org/2015/09/25/trans-inclusivity-statement.

MANA Statement on Gender Inclusive Language: www.mana.org/healthcare-policy/position-statement-on-gender-inclusive-language.

The *New York Times* Gender Neutral Glossary: www.nytimes.com/2015/02/08/education/a-gender-neutral-glossary.html.

Gestational Diabetes

Diabetic Mommy: www.diabeticmommy.com.

Geil, Patti Bazel, Patricia Geil, and Laura Hieronymus. 2003. *101 Tips for a Healthy Pregnancy with Diabetes.*

Grief and Traumatic Birth

Church, Lisa, and Ann H. Prescott. 2004. *Hope Is Like the Sun: Finding Hope and Healing After Miscarriage, Stillbirth, or Infant Death.*

Douglas, Ann, John R. Sussman, and Deborah Davis. 2000. *Trying Again: A Guide to Pregnancy After Miscarriage, Stillbirth, and Infant Loss.*

Faces of Loss: A place for mothers to share their story of miscarriage, stillbirth, and infant loss. www.facesofloss.com.

HopeXchange Publishing: www.hopexchange.com (on miscarriage, stillbirth, and infant death).

Kitzinger, Sheila. 2006. *Birth Crisis.*

Madsen, Lynn. 1994. *Rebounding from Childbirth: Toward Emotional Recovery.*

Now I Lay Me Down To Sleep: free remembrance photography services for stillbirth: www.nowilaymedowntosleep.org.

P.A.T.T.C.h (Prevention and Treatment of Traumatic Childbirth). *The Traumatic Birth Prevention and Resource Guide,* a collection of reflections written by many of the PATTCh Board members, explains the components of traumatic birth, increases awareness, and promotes prevention. www.pattch.org/resource-guide.

Schweibert, Pat, and Paul Kirk. 2012. *When Hello Means Goodbye,* 3rd revision.

Simkin, Penny, and Phyllis Klaus. 2004. *When Survivors Give Birth: Understanding and Healing the Effects of Early Sexual Abuse on Childbearing Women.*

Hypnosis for Birth

Mongan, Marie. 2015. *HypnoBirthing: The Mongan Method: A Natural Approach to a Safe, Easier, More Comfortable Birthing*, 4th ed.

O'Neill, Michelle Leclaire. 2000. *Hypnobirthing: The Original Method: Mindful Pregnancy and Easy Labor Using the Leclaire Childbirth Method*.

Tuschhoff, Kerry. "Hypnobabies Home Study Course." www.hypnobabies.com.

Labor Support Tools and TENS Unit Purchase

Apollo Massage Roller: www.amazon.com.

TENS unit rentals/sales in Europe (also ships to U.S.): www.babycaretens.com.

TENS unit rentals in the U.S. and Canada: www.midwiferysupplies.ca/products/elle-tens-machine. (Many doulas have TENS units available for loan or low-cost rental.)

TENS unit sales in the U.S.: www.sharonmuza.com.

Locating a Birth or Postpartum Doula

DONA International: www.dona.org.

DoulaMatch.net: www.doulamatch.net.

Klaus, Marshall H., John H. Kennell, and Phyllis H. Klaus. 2012. *The Doula Book: How a Trained Labor Companion Can Help You Have a Shorter, Easier, and Healthier Birth*.

Meal Trains and Chore Sign-Ups

CareCalendar: www.carecalendar.org.

Lotsa Helping Hands: www.lotsahelpinghands.com.

Take Them a Meal: www.takethemameal.com.

Newborn Screening Tests

March of Dimes. "Newborn Screening Tests for Your Baby." www.marchofdimes.org/newborn-screening-tests-for-your-baby.aspx.

Screening tests by state: www.babysfirsttest.org/newborn-screening/states.

Pelvic Floor Self-Assessment Pamphlet

Dr. April Bolding: www.aprilbolding.com.

Placenta Encapsulation

Dekker, Rebecca. 2017. "The Evidence on Placenta Encapsulation." www.evidencebasedbirth.com/evidence-on-placenta-encapsulation.

Find placenta specialists and other questions to ask: www.findplacentaencapsulation.com.

Postpartum Depression Online Support

Postpartum Support International (PSI) online support: www.postpartum.net/learn-more/help-for-moms.

Solace for Mothers: www.solaceformothers.org.

Postpartum Doulas

Kelleher, Jacqueline. 2002. *Nurturing the Family: The Guide for Postpartum Doulas.*

Pascali Bonaro, Debra. 2014. *Nurturing Beginnings: Guide to Postpartum Care for Doulas and Community Outreach Workers.*

Webber, Salle. 2012. *The Gentle Art of Newborn Family Care: A Guide for Postpartum Doulas and Caregivers.*

Postpartum Emotions and Depression

Postpartum Support International (PSI). Dedicated to helping women suffering from perinatal mood and anxiety disorders, including postpartum depression. www.postpartum.net.

Pregnancy Apps for Tracking Fetal Movements and Contractions

Full Term: www.fulltermapp.com.

Ovia Pregnancy (and others): www.ovuline.com.

Sprout Pregnancy: www.sprout-apps.com.

Prematurity and Kangaroo Care

Bergman, Nils M.D., Ph.D, and Jill Bergman. www.kangaroomothercare.com.

Bradford, Nikki, Jonathan Hellman, Sharyn Gibbins, and Sandra Lousada. 2003. *Your Premature Baby: The First Five Years*.

March of Dimes: www.marchofdimes.org.

Sears, William, Robert Sears, James Sears, and Martha Sears. 2004. *The Premature Baby Book: Everything You Need to Know About Your Premature Baby from Birth to Age One*.

Preparing Older Children for the Birth of a Sibling

Overend, Jenni, and Julie Vivas. 1999. *Welcome with Love*.

Simkin, Penny, Janet Whalley, Ann Keppler, Janelle Durham, and April Bolding. 2016. *Pregnancy, Childbirth, and the Newborn: The Complete Guide*, 5th ed. (chapter 16).

Simkin, Penny (producer and writer), and Walter Zamojski (videographer and film editor). 2013. *There's a Baby: A Children's Film About a New Baby*. DVD for children (shows a birth). www.pennysimkin.com.

Proper Care of the Uncircumcised Penis

Most comprehensive infant-care books contain a section on this topic.

WebMD. 2017. "How to Care for Your Baby Boy's Penis." www.webmd.com/parenting/baby/tc/your-newborn-boys-genitals-care-of-penis.

Singing to Baby Before and After Birth

Chamberlain, David. 2013. *Windows to the Womb: Revealing the Conscious Baby from Conception to Birth.*

Fink, Cathy, and Marcy Marxer. 2011. *Sing to Your Baby.* (CD/playbook).

Simkin, Penny. 2013. Singing to the Baby. www.youtube.com/watch?v=gsdEK6OxucA.

Vaginal Birth After Cesarean (VBAC)

Churchill, Helen. 2010. *Vaginal Birth After Caesarean.*

International Cesarean Awareness Network: www.ican-online.org.

American College of Obstetricians and Gynecologists. 2017. Practice Bulletin No. 184: Vaginal Birth After Cesarean Delivery. *Obstetrics & Gynecology* 130 (5): 1167–1169. https://journals.lww.com/greenjournal/Fulltext2017/11000/Practice_Bulletin_No_184_Vaginal_Birth_After.51.aspx.

VBAC Facts: www.vbacfacts.com. www.vbac.com.

Vitamin K

American Academy of Pediatrics. Policy Statement. "Controversies Concerning Vitamin K and the Newborn." http://pediatrics.aappublications.org/content/112/1/191.full.

Canadian Paediatric Society. Position Statement. "Routine administration of vitamin K to newborns." www.cps.ca/en/documents/position/administration-vitamin-K-newborns.

Waterbirth Information, Tub Rental, and Sales

AquaDoula: www.aquadoula.com.

Waterbirth International: www.waterbirth.org.

Waterbirth Solutions: www.waterbirthsolutions.com.

Your Water Birth: www.yourwaterbirth.com.

Index

Amniotic fluid. *See also* Bag of waters

Abdominal lifting, 220

Active labor phase
  arrest of, 286–289, 344
  baths and, 178
  birth partner and, 101, 106–108
  caregivers and, 101, 104–105
  contractions, 102
  doulas and, 102, 108–109
  duration of, 103
  feelings, 100–101, 103–104
  loss of control and, 100–101
  pain management, 102, 108–109
  slow progress, 221–224
  summary of, 139
  "3 to 6 phase," 100
  visualization and, 160

Acupressure
  for comfort, 193–194
  for induction, 214

Acupuncture
  breech presentation and, 228
  for induction, 214–215

Afterbirth. *See* Placental stage.

Amnioinfusion, 256

Amniotic fluid. *See also* Bag of waters.
  amount, 71, 241, 242, 244
  color, 71, 244
  leaking, 63
  meconium and, 293, 369
  observations of, 243–244
  odor, 71, 244
  testing, 71, 254, 273

Anesthesia
  general anesthesia, 324–326, 338
  local anesthesia, 323–324, 339
  nitrous oxide, 324–325

Anesthesiologists, 313, 314, 347

Antibiotic treatments, 240–241

Apgar score, 129, 244–245

Aromatherapy, 196–197

Arrested labor, 286–289, 344

Artificial Rupture of the Membranes
  (AROM), 254–255

Attention focusing
  checklist, 198
  methods, 158

Augmentation of labor. *See* Induction.

Baby. *See also* Complications (baby);
    Fetal positions; Fetus; Postpartum
    care (baby).
  Apgar score, 129, 244–245
  bathing, 377–378
  bed-sharing, 407
  bilirubin, 301–302, 373
  birth injuries, 300
  blood sugar, 301
  bowel movements, 377
  breathing problems, 299
  caregiver for, 54–56
  circumcision, 379–382
  cleanup, 375
  clothes, 52–53
  crowning and birth phase, 127–128
  death, 49–50, 302–303
  drug side-effects, 300–301
  electronic fetal monitoring
    (EFM), 249–252
  eye medications, 371–372
  first days, 376–382
  first feeding, 375
  first hours, 364–365
  formula-feeding, 54, 378, 414
  fussiness, 397
  GBS infections, 240
  gestational diabetes mellitus (GDM)
    and, 278–279
  health supplies, 53
  hearing screening test, 379
  hydrotherapy and, 179
  homecoming supplies, 34
  home space for, 56
  infections, 299–300
  internal fetal monitoring, 249–250
  jaundice, 301–302
  kangaroo care, 299
  low birth weight, 302
  nonstress test, 242
  nose and mouth suctioning, 368–369

observing, 244–245
physical exam and assessment, 376–377
portable fetal monitoring (telemetry),
   250, 252
postpartum blood tests, 372–374
postpartum period, 368–375
recover and bonding stage, 135
safety classes, 51
screening tests, 378–379
sleep schedule, 398
temperature of, 299
umbilical cord cutting, 369–371
umbilical cord stump, 378
vitamin K, 372
warming unit, 374–375
weight, 302
Back pain. *See also* Comfort measures; Pain.
baby position and, 222
checklist, 198
counterpressure, 194
criss-cross massage, 188
Double Hip Squeeze, 195
hands-and-knees position, 172
pelvic rock position, 38
prolonged labor and, 67
rolling pressure, 196
sitting leaning forward position, 172
slow dancing, 170
slow labor progress and, 221
squatting position, 174
standing and leaning forward
   position, 169
standing lunge position, 170, 222
Transcutaneous Electrical Nerve Stimulation (TENS), 185, 186
Bag of waters
amnioinfusion, 256
Artificial Rupture of the Membranes
   (AROM), 254–255
feelings, 292
hydrotherapy and, 179
infection and, 71–72
labor and, 64
observations of, 71, 243–244
pre-labor rupture of, 71–72
prolapsed cord and, 290
very rapid labor and, 208
Baths
active labor and, 178
bath vs. shower, 177
infection and, 179
newborn baby, 377–378
pain management with, 177
ruptured membranes and, 179

slow-to-start labor and, 219
timing of, 178
water births and, 180
water temperatures, 178–179, 219
Bearing-down. *See* Pushing.
Bed restriction, 224–226
Bed-sharing, 407
Bilirubin, 301–302, 373
Biotinidase deficiency, 379
Birth balls, 180–183
Birth centers
early labor and, 95–96
supplies for, 33, 35
tour of, 24
Birthing beds, 168
Birthing stage
caregivers and, 116–117
crowning and birth phase, 127–131
descent phase, 121–127
duration of, 117
overview of, 116
resting phase, 117–120
slow progress, 221–224
summary of, 140
Birthing tubs, 35
Birth partner
active labor and, 101, 106–108
arrest of active labor and, 288–289
breast feeding and, 354, 405
breech version and, 230
cesarean births and, 347, 353–355
communication with, 32
complications with mother and, 271
complications with newborn and, 297
crowning and birth phase, 130
descent phase, 125–126
early labor and, 94–95, 97–99
epidurals and, 317–323
excessive bleeding during labor, 283
feelings during active labor, 106
feelings during crowning and birth
   phase, 130
feelings during descent phase, 124–125
feelings during early labor, 96–97
feelings during onset of active labor, 101
feelings during placental stage, 133
feelings during postpartum period,
   392, 394
feelings during recovery and bonding
   stage, 136–137
feelings during resting phase, 119
feelings during transition phase, 112
fetal distress and, 294–295

gestational diabetes mellitus (GDM)
and, 280
herpes lesions and, 281
high blood pressure and, 277
lacerations and, 296–297
narcotics and, 311–312
natural birth and, 21
pain medication and, 311–312
postpartum period, 392, 394
prelabor and, 88–89
premature labor and, 274–275
pushing and, 322
qualifications of, 31–32
recovery and bonding phase, 137
resting phase, 120
rituals and, 149–151
role of, 21–22
self-care, 106, 197, 200
slow labor progress and, 224
supplies, 33–34
systemic medications and, 311–312
traits of, 31–32, 61
transition phase, 113–114
Vaginal Birth After Cesarean (VBAC)
and, 362
Birth plan
caregivers and, 234
cesarean births, 49
death and, 49–50
illness and, 49
labor options, 47
medical care decisions, 47
overview of, 45–46
pain medication directives, 146, 205,
326–327
personal choices, 50–51
personal information, 46
positions and, 47
postpartum care, 48
premature births and, 49
staff message, 46
stillbirth and, 49–50
support team, 47
Bladder control, 316, 384–385
Blood
excessive bleeding after birth, 283–285
excessive bleeding during labor,
281–283
excessive postpartum bleeding, 295
lacerations, 296–297
placenta, 133, 282, 295
tests, 372–374
umbilical cord, storing, 48, 366–367
vaginal discharge and, 383

Bottle-feeding, 298, 414–416
Bowel movements
first days (mother), 384, 385
first hours (baby), 377
incontinence, 38, 342
meconium and, 369
Bowel stimulation, for induction, 215–216
Braxton Hicks contractions, 73
"Breaking the ice pop" foot massage,
191–192
"Breaking the ice pop" hand massage, 190
Breastfeeding
birth partner and, 354, 405
bottle feeding and, 415
colostrum, 378
concerns, 408–411
co-nursing, 414
engorgement, 408
establishment of, 416
first feeding, 375
laid-back position, 375
latch quality, 409–410
milk supply, 406
reasons for, 401–403
resources for, 402–403
schedule, 398
sleep and, 407
sore nipples, 411
starting, 403–404
supplies for, 53
terminology, 400
thrush, 410
24-hour "cure," 412–413
vigorous suckling, 408–409
Breathing
hyperventilation, 163–164
light breathing, 207
problems, 299
rhythmic breathing and moaning,
161–164, 204–205
slow breathing, 204
Breech presentation. *See also* Fetal
positions.
acupuncture, 228
breech-tilt position, 227–228
cervix and, 226
prolapsed cord and, 290
rate of, 226
sound and, 228
version, 229–231

Caregivers
active labor and, 101, 104–105

for baby, 54–56
birthing stage, 116–117
birth plan and, 234
crowning and birth phase, 129
descent phase, 123–124
dilation stage and, 91–92
incompatibility with, 233–235
interventions and, 245
office location, 55
personalities of, 55
placental stage and, 132–133
practical considerations, 55
prelabor and, 87–88
questions for, 55
recovery and bonding stage, 136
resting phase, 119
role of, 236
transition phase, 112
visiting, 23–24
Castor oil
bowel stimulation with, 215–216
meconium and, 216
Catheter, urinary, 316, 320, 385
Cephalopelvic disproportion (CPD), 287
Cervix. *See also* Dilation stage.
active labor, 102
breech presentation and, 226
early labor and, 92
epidurals and, 321
labor and, 66, 68, 74–75
"lip," 110
prelabor phase, 63, 72–73
prolapsed cord and, 290
resting phase, 117
slow-to-start labor and, 216–217
transition phase and, 109–110
Cesarean births
birth partner and, 347, 353–355
birth plan and, 49
delivery of baby, 349–350
feelings, 355
incision, 348
medical reasons for, 343
nonmedical reasons for, 341–343
pain medications, 347
placenta and, 350
postpartum pain, 385–386
postpartum period, 365
preparations for surgery, 346–348
previous cesarean births and, 345
previous difficult births experiences
with, 231, 233
procedure, 348–349
recovery period, 352

repair procedure, 350–351
support groups, 231
Trial of Labor After Cesarean (TO-
LAC), 356
Vaginal Birth After Cesarean (VBAC),
345, 356–362
Challenges. *See also* Complications
(baby); Complications (mother);
Emergencies.
bed restriction during labor, 224–226
breech presentation, 226–231
descent, encouraging, 223–224
on-the-spot coaching, 204–205
previously difficult birth experiences,
231–233
rapid labor, 208–209, 285–286
self-induction, 212–216
slow progress in active labor, 221–225
slow progress in birthing stage, 221–225
slow-to-start labor, 216–221
Take-Charge routine, 202–207
Chestfeeding
birth partner and, 354, 405
bottle feeding and, 415
colostrum, 378
concerns, 408–411
co-nursing, 414
engorgement, 408
establishment of, 416
first feeding, 375
laid-back position, 375
latch quality, 409–410
milk supply, 406
reasons for, 401–403
resources for, 402–403
schedule, 398
sleep and, 407
sore nipples, 411
starting, 403–404
supplies for, 53
terminology, 400
thrush, 410
24-hour "cure," 412–413
vigorous suckling, 408–409
Chlamydia, 371
Chores, household, 399
Clothes, 33, 34, 52–53
Circumcision, 48, 379–382
Classes
baby care and safety, 51
lesson rehearsals, 32
parent-infant classes, 56
peer support groups, 56
Coaching, on-the-spot, 204–205

Cold, comfort from, 184–185

Colostrum, 298, 378, 408

Combined spinal-epidural, 314, 337

Comfort measures. *See also* Back pain; Pain; Pain medications.

acupressure, 193–194

aromatherapy, 196–197

attention focusing, 158

baths and showers, 176–180

birth ball, 180–183

checklist, 198–199

counterpressure, 194–195

crisscross massage, 188–189

dangle, 175

dangle with partner, 175

directed pushing, 167–168

double hip squeeze, 195

doulas and, 102, 155, 185–186, 199, 200

foot massage, 191–192

hand massage, 190–191

hands-and-knees, 172

hands and knees rocking forward, 176

heat and cold, 184–185

kneeling leaning forward, 172

kneeling lunge, 171

lap squatting, 174

massage, 187–196

movement, 168–176

music, 196

on back with legs drawn up, 175

on-the-spot coaching, 207

open knee–chest, 173

peanut ball, 183–184

position changes, 168–176

pushing techniques, 164–167

relaxation, 153–155, 156–157

rhythmic breathing and moaning, 161–164

rocking chairs, 172

rolling pressure over low back, 196

self-directed pushing, 166

semiprone, 173

semisitting, 171

shoulder massage, 188

side-lying position, 173

sitting leaning forward, 172

sitting on commode, 171

sitting upright, 171

slow dancing, 170

sounds, 196

spontaneous bearing down, 165–166

squatting, 174

standing, 169

standing and leaning, 169

standing lunge, 170, 222

swaying on birth ball, 172

Three Rs, 147–153

Transcutaneous Electrical Nerve Stimulation (TENS), 185–186

visualization, 159–160

walking, 169

Communication

breech presentation and, 228

with caregivers, 234–235

complications with newborns, 298

contact lists, 45

dilation stage, 91–92

with fetus, 44

newborns, 51

pain and, 146

perineal massage, 40

phones, 32

with unborn baby, 44

Complications (baby). *See also* Baby; Challenges; Emergencies.

birth trauma or injury, 300

breathing problems, 299

death, 302–303

fetal distress, 292–295

fetal stage, 290–295

infections, 299–300

jaundice, 301–302

kangaroo care and, 299

legal considerations, 297

low blood sugar, 301

low body temperature, 299

medication effects, 300–301

prematurity, 302

prolapsed cord, 290–292

Complications (mother). *See also* Challenges; Emergencies.

arrest of active labor, 286–289

birth partner and, 271

excessive postpartum bleeding, 295

gestational diabetes mellitus (GDM), 277–280

herpes lesions, 280–281

high blood pressure, 275–277

lacerations, 296–297

placental stage, 295–297

premature labor, 273–275

rapid labor progress, 207–209, 285–286

retained placenta, 295–296

Congenital adrenal hyperplasia (CAH), 379

Congenital hypothyroidism, 379

Contact lists, 45

Contractions

active labor phase, 102
afterpains, 383
attention focusing, 158
Braxton Hicks contractions, 73
dilation stage, 90–91
4–1–1 and 5–1–1 rule, 94
nonprogressive contractions, 72–73
postpartum, 284, 366, 383
prelabor contractions, 72–73, 85–86
timing, 77–80
transition phase, 109
Counterpressure, 194–195
"Count-to-10" fetal movement tracking,
    42–44
Criss-cross massage, 188–189
Crowning and birth phase
    Apgar score, 129
    baby and, 127–128
    birth partner and, 130
    caregivers and, 129
    doulas and, 131
    duration of, 128
    feelings, 128–129
    overview of, 127–128
    summary of, 141

Dancing, 170
Dangle position, 175
Death, 49–50, 302–303
Delayed pushing, 321–322
Descent phase
    birth partner and, 125–126
    caregivers and, 123–124
    doulas and, 126–127
    duration of, 122
    feelings, 122–123, 124–125
    overview of, 120–121
    positions, 122, 124
    pushing, 121–122
    stress hormones, 122
    summary of, 141
Diabetes. See Gestational diabetes
    mellitus (GDM).
Dilation stage. See also Cervix.
    communication with caregiver, 91–92
    contractions, 90–91
    duration of, 91
    light breathing, 163–164
    overview of, 90–91
    pain and, 91, 143, 331
    slow breathing, 162–163
    summary of, 138
Directed pushing, 167–168, 321

Doctors. See Caregivers.
Doulas
    active labor and, 102, 108–109
    arrest of active labor and, 289
    benefits of, 26–27
    birth outcomes and, 27
    breech version and, 230
    comfort measures and, 102, 155,
        185–186, 199, 200
    costs of, 28
    crowning and birth phase, 131
    descent phase, 126–127
    description of, 27
    early labor and, 98–99
    fetal distress and, 295
    gift of, 59
    hypnosis and, 155
    interviewing, 29–31
    lacerations and, 297
    placental stage, 134–135
    popularity of, 21
    postpartum support, 59
    prelabor and, 90
    previously difficult birth experiences
        and, 232
    qualifications of, 27–28
    recovery and bonding stage and, 137
    resting phase, 120
    role of, 18, 21, 25–26
    selection of, 27–28, 29
    Transcutaneous Electrical Nerve Stimu-
        lation (TENS) and, 185–186
    transition phase, 114–116
Dystocia, 286–289

Early labor
    birth partner and, 94–95, 97–99
    cervix and, 92
    doula and, 98–99
    duration of, 92–93
    feelings, 93–94, 96–97
    previous difficult birth experiences and,
        232–233
    trip to birth center, 95–96
    trip to hospital, 95–96
Electronic fetal monitoring (EFM),
    249–252
Emergencies. See also Challenges;
    Complications (baby); Complications
    (mother).
    birth plan and, 48–50
    Cesarean births, 49
    cesarean births and, 344
    emergency deliveries, 209–211

postmaturity syndrome, 64
prolapsed cord, 290–292
rapid labor, 208–209, 285–286
transfer to hospital, 49
Epidurals
administration of, 315–316, 318
birth partner and, 317–323
bladder control, 316
breakthrough pain, 320
combined spinal-epidural, 314
complete dilation, 321–322
delayed pushing, 321–322
directed pushing, 321
distraction from labor and, 319
external breech version and, 229–231
feelings, 318–319
forceps delivery and, 323
other discomforts and, 320
pushing and, 321–322
rectal pain during delivery, 322
requesting, 317
resting and waiting, 320
side effects, 334–335
side effects of, 319–320
vacuum delivery and, 323
vaginal pain during delivery, 322
waiting for, 317–318
Episiotomy, 263–265
Exercises. *See also* Movement (mother);
     Positions (mother).
benefits of, 36–37
pelvic floor (Kegels), 38–39
pelvic rock, 38
squatting, 37
strengthening exercises, 39–40
Eye medications, 371–372

"False" labor. *See* Prelabor.
Feeding. *See* Bottle-feeding; Breastfeed-
     ing; Chestfeeding; Food and meal
     planning; Formula.
Feelings (birth partner)
active labor, 106
crowning and birth phase, 130
descent phase, 124–125
early labor, 96–97
onset of active labor, 101
placental stage, 133
postpartum period, 392, 394
recovery and bonding stage, 136–137
resting phase, 119
transition phase, 112
Vaginal Birth After Cesarean
     (VBAC), 362

Feelings (mother)
active labor, 103–104
arrest of active labor, 288
"baby blues," 391–392
cesarean births, 355
crowning and birth phase, 128–129
descent phase, 122–123
early labor, 93–94
epidurals and, 318–319
excessive bleeding during labor,
     282–283
fetal distress, 294
gestational diabetes mellitus
     (GDM), 279
herpes lesions, 281
high blood pressure, 276–277
lacerations, 296
onset of active labor, 100–101
placental stage, 131–132
postpartum period, 390–392
prelabor, 87
premature labor, 274
previously difficult birth experiences,
     232–233
rapid labor, 208–209
recovery and bonding stage, 136
resting phase, 118
self-assessment, 393–394
transition phase, 110–111
Vaginal Birth After Cesarean (VBAC),
     359–362
Fetal distress, 292–295
Fetal positions. *See also* Baby; Breech
     presentation.
in birthing stage, 115
common, in uterus, 66–67
descent phase, 76–77, 122, 124, 223–224
in dilation stage, 115
early labor, 92–93
encouraging change in, 222–223
epidural side-effects and, 319
occiput anterior (OA), 38, 66–67, 76,
     92, 221
occiput posterior (OP), 66–67, 217, 221
occiput transverse (OT), 66–67, 221
in prelabor, 115
presentation, 66
slow-to-start labor and, 217
tracking, 42–44
Fetus. *See also* Baby.
communicating with, 44
complications with, 290–295
descent of, encouraging, 223–224
descent of, measuring, 76–77

fetal distress, 253, 292–295
head rotation, 76
heart rate, monitoring, 249, 250, 286, 292–293, 359
nonstress tests for, 242
postmature, 64, 66
scalp stimulation test, 253
tracking movements of, 42–44
5-1-1 rule, 94
Food and meal planning, 56–57, 398–399
Foot massage, 191–192
Forceps delivery, 267–268, 323
Formula-feeding
first feeding, 378
supplemental nursing system (SNS), 414
supplies for, 54
4-1-1 rule, 94

Galactosemia, 379
General anesthesia, 324–326, 338
Gestational diabetes mellitus (GDM), 277–280
Gestational hypertension (GH), 275
Glucose tolerance test, 277–278
Gonorrhea, 371
Grandparents, 57, 58, 59, 389
Group B streptococcus, 71, 240–241
"Grunt-pushing," 110

Hand massage, 190–191
Hands-and-knees position, 172
Hearing screening test, 379
Heart rate, fetal, 249, 250, 286, 292–293, 359
Heat, comfort from, 184–185
Heel-stick test, 378
Hemorrhoids, 384, 385
Herpes lesions, 280–281
High blood pressure, 224, 271, 275–277
Home births
cleanup, 388–389
placenta and, 388
settling in for, 95–96
supplies for, 35–36
Homecoming, 387–388
Homocystinuria, 379
Hospital
early labor and, 95
emergency transfer to, 49

length of stay, 387
pre-registering, 25
tour of, 24
trip supplies, 35
Household chores, 399
Hydration, 36, 246–249
Hydrotherapy
active labor and, 178
baby monitoring and, 179
bath vs. shower, 177
infection and, 179
modesty and, 180
overview of, 176–177
pain management with, 177
ruptured membranes and, 179
slow-to-start labor and, 219
timing of, 178
water births and, 180
water temperatures, 178–179, 219
Hypertension, 275, 276
Hyperventilation, 163–164
Hypnosis, 155, 158
Hypoglycemia, 373–374

Induction
acupressure, 214
acupuncture, 214–215
alternatives to, 263
bowel stimulation, 215–216
disadvantages of, 259–260, 261–263
failure of, 258
Group B strep and, 240–241
herpes lesions and, 280
of lactation, 414
medical indications for, 258–259
medications, 257–258
methods, 256–258
nipple stimulation, 213–214
nonmedical indications for, 260
reasons for, 214
self-induction, 212–216
sexual stimulation, 215
walking, 214
Infections
bag of waters and, 71–72
circumcision and, 381
eye medications and, 371–372
newborns and, 299–300
Group B strep, 240
perineal massage and, 40
thrush, 410
Insulin, 278, 279
Internal fetal monitoring, 249–250
Internal rituals, 149

Interventions
 amnioinfusion, 256
 Artificial Rupture of the Membranes
  (AROM), 254–255
 caregivers and, 245
 conditions of use, 245–246
 electronic fetal monitoring (EFM),
  249–252
 episiotomy, 263–265
 forceps delivery, 267–268, 323
 induction, 256–263
 institutional policies and, 245–246
 internal fetal monitoring, 249–250
 intravenous (IV) fluids, 246–249
 portable fetal monitoring (telemetry),
  250, 252
 preferences toward, 246
 questions for, 238
 vacuum extraction, 266–267, 323
Intrauterine pressure catheter, 110, 288
Intravenous (IV) fluids, 246–249

Jaundice, 301–302

Kangaroo care, 299
Kegel exercises, 38–39
Knee–chest position, 173
Kneeling and leaning forward, 172, 223
Kneeling lunge, 171

Labor
 arrested labor, 286–289, 344
 bag of waters, breaking, 71–72
 bed restriction, 224–226
 birth plan options, 47
 cervix and, 74–75
 contraction timing, 77–80
 descent, 77
 duration of, 66–67
 excessive bleeding, 281–283
 gestational diabetes mellitus (GDM)
  and, 279
 herpes lesions and, 281
 high blood pressure, 276, 277
 internal rituals, 149
 observations, 243
 positive signs, 68–69, 70
 possible signs, 67–68, 68–69
 prelabor compared to, 63–64
 prelabor signs, 68, 69
 premature labor, 273–275
 presentation, 66–67, 76
 process of, 63–64

 rapid labor progress, 208–209, 285–286
 rituals, 147–148, 149–151
 signs of, 62–63, 67–70
 supplies for, 33
 unpredictability of, 83
Laboring down. See Delayed pushing.
Lap squatting position, 174
Latent phase. See Early labor.
Light breathing, 163–164, 207
"Lip" of cervix, 110
Local anesthesia, 323–324, 339
Lochia, 283
Low birth weight, 302
Low blood sugar, 301
Low body temperature, 299
Lunges
 kneeling lunge, 171
 standing lunge, 170, 222

Maple syrup urine disease, 379
Massage
 acupressure, 193–194
 basic techniques, 187–188
 "breaking the ice pop" hand
  massage, 190
 crisscross massage, 188–189
 double hip squeeze, 195
 perineal massage, 40–42
 rolling pressure over low back, 196
 three-part foot massage, 191–192
 three-part shoulder massage, 188
Medications. See also Pain medications.
 antibiotics, 240–241, 371
 antinausea, 351
 effect on newborn, 300–301
 eye medications, 371–372
 herpes treatment, 280
 induction medications, 257–258
 post-cesarean births, 351
 questions about, 238, 307
Medium-chain acyl-CoA dehydrogenase
  deficiency (MCAD), 379
Midwives. See Caregivers.
Morphine, 332
Movement (fetus). See Fetal positions.
Movement (mother). See also Exercises;
  Positions (mother).
 abdominal lifting, 220
 birth ball movement, 181
 hands and knees rocking forward, 176
 kneeling lunge, 171
 lunge, 222

rocking in rocking chair, 172
slow dancing, 170
swaying on birth ball, 172
walking, 169, 214, 223
Moxibustion, 227, 228
Music
attention focusing with, 158
breech presentation and, 228
comfort and, 196
communication with, 44

Narcotics
arrest of labor and, 287
birth partner and, 311–312
definition of, 312
overview of, 333
for pain management, 333
regional analgesia and, 312–314
timing of, 331
Natural childbirth, 21, 361
Nipple stimulation
for induction, 213–214
uterine contraction and, 366
Nitrous oxide, 324–325, 334
Nonprogressive contractions, 72–73
Nonstress test, 242–243

Occiput anterior (OA) position, 38,
66–67, 76, 92, 221
Occiput posterior (OP) position, 66–67,
217, 221
Occiput transverse (OT) position, 66–67,
221
On-the-spot coaching, 204–205

Pain. *See also* Back pain; Comfort measures; Pain medications.
active labor phase, 102
afterpains, 383
attention-focusing for, 158
back pain, 194–195
breakthrough pain, 320
causes of, 143–144
counterpressure for back pain, 194–195
dilation stage, 91, 143, 331
hydrotherapy and, 177
managing without medication, 163–164,
305–307
post-cesarean pain, 385–386
suffering compared to, 144–145
Pain medications. *See also* Comfort measures; Medications.

birth partner and, 311–312
cesarean births and, 347, 348
code words for, 330
directives on, 146, 205, 326–327
effect on newborn, 300–301
epidurals, 315–323, 334–335
function of, 309–310
general anesthesia, 324–326, 338
local anesthesia, 323–324, 339
morphine, 332
narcotics, 312, 333
nitrous oxide, 324–325, 334
Pain Medications Preference Scale
(PMPS), 326–327, 328–329
questions about, 238, 307
recommending, 205–206
regional analgesia, 312–315
sedatives, 332, 351
spinal blocks, 315–316, 336–337
systemic drugs, 310–312, 332–333
terminology, 308–309
timing of, 331
tranquilizers, 333
usage preferences, 146
Pain Medications Preference Scale
(PMPS), 326–327, 328–329
Parent-infant classes, 56
Peanut ball, 183–184
Pediatricians. *See* Caregivers.
Pelvic floor (Kegel) exercises, 38–39
Pelvic rock exercise, 38
Perineum
birth plan and, 47
episiotomy, 263–265
local block, 309
massage, 40–42
postpartum care, 365, 384
Phenylketonuria (PKU), 379
Phones, 32, 45
Placental stage
caregivers and, 132–133
cesarean births and, 350
complications, 295–297
doulas and, 134–135
duration of, 131
excessive postpartum bleeding, 295
feelings, 131–132, 133
home birth and, 388
overview of, 131
placental encapsulation, 367–368
retained placenta, 295–296
summary of, 142
Platoon sleeping, 396

Portable fetal monitoring (telemetry), 250, 252

Positions (baby). *See* Fetal positions.

Positions (mother). *See also* Exercises; Movement (mother).
  birth ball positions, 180–182
  birthing beds and, 168
  birth plan and, 47
  breech-tilt, 227–228
  dangle, 175
  dangle with partner, 175
  epidural side-effects and, 319
  hands-and-knees, 172
  kneeling and leaning forward, 172, 223
  laid-back breastfeeding position, 375
  lap squatting, 174
  lying semiprone, 223
  on back with legs drawn up, 175
  open knee–chest, 173
  rocking in rocking chair, 172
  rollover, 319
  semiprone, 173
  semisitting, 171
  side-lying, 173, 222
  sitting leaning forward, 172
  sitting on commode, 171
  sitting upright, 171
  slow dancing, 170
  slow-to-start labor and, 220
  squatting position, 174
  standing, 169, 223
  standing and leaning, 169
  standing lunge, 170, 222

Postmaturity syndrome, 64

Postpartum care (baby). *See also* Baby.
  bathing, 377–378
  blood tests, 372–374
  bowel movements, 377
  circumcision, 379–382
  cleanup, 375
  eye medication, 371–372
  feeding schedule, 398
  first days, 376–382
  first feeding, 375
  first hours, 364–365
  fussiness, 397
  hearing screening test, 379
  homecoming, 387–388
  nose and mouth suctioning, 368
  parent-infant classes, 56
  physical exam and assessment, 376–377
  screening tests, 378–379
  sleep schedule, 398

umbilical cord, 366–367, 369–371, 378
vitamin K, 372
warming unit, 374–375

Postpartum care (mother)
  afterpains, 383
  "baby blues," 391–392
  birth plan and, 48
  bowel movements, 384–385
  cesarean births, 365
  cesarean delivery pain, 385–386
  doulas, 59
  emotional self-assessment, 393–394
  fatigue, 394–395
  feelings, 390–392
  first days, 382–386
  first hours, 364–365
  grandparents and, 57, 58, 59, 389
  homecoming, 387–388
  household chores, 399
  meal preparation, 56–57, 398–399
  offers of assistance, 389–390, 398–399
  perineum care, 365, 384
  parent-infant classes, 56
  placental encapsulation, 367–368
  privacy, 376
  shared responsibilities, 57
  sleep deprivation, 394–395
  supplies for, 34, 56
  urination, 384–385
  uterine care, 383
  uterine contraction, 366
  vaginal discharge, 383
  vital signs, 366

Post-term births, 64, 66

Preeclampsia, 275

Pregnancy
  exercise and, 36–40
  gestational diabetes mellitus (GDM), 278
  high blood pressure and, 275–276
  hydration and, 36

Prelabor
  birth partner and, 88–89
  caregivers and, 87–88
  contractions, 85–86
  doula and, 90
  duration of, 86
  experienced parents and, 86
  feelings, 87
  first-time parents and, 85–86
  labor compared to, 63–64
  nonprogressive contractions, 72–73
  overview of, 85
  signs of, 68, 69

summary of, 138
visualization and, 159–160
Premature births
   birth plan and, 49
   birth weight, 302
   causes of, 64
   complications and, 302
   jaundice and, 301
   rate of, 64
   warming units, 374
Premature labor, 70, 273–275
Pre-registration, 25
Priorities for childbirth, 272–273
Pushing
   avoidance technique, 164–165
   birth partner and, 322
   birth plan and, 47
   delayed pushing, 321–322
   descent phase, 121–122
   directed pushing, 167–168
   epidurals and, 321–322
   "grunt-pushing," 110
   modified directed pushing, 167–168
   resting phase, 118
   self-directed pushing, 166
   spontaneous bearing down, 165–166
   urge to push, 110, 121

Rapid labor, 208–209, 285–286
Recovery and bonding phase
   baby and, 135
   birth partner and, 137
   caregivers and, 136
   doulas and, 137
   duration of, 135
   overview of, 135
   summary of, 142
Regional analgesia, 312–315
Relaxation. See Comfort measures.
Resting phase
   birth partner and, 120
   caregivers and, 119
   doulas and, 120
   duration of, 118
   feelings, 118
   overview of, 117–118
   pushing, 118
Rhythm
   breathing, 204–205
   rhythmic breathing and moaning,
      161–164, 204–205
   ritual and, 148, 152–153
   Take-Charge routine, 203, 204

Rituals
   birth partner and, 149–151
   internal rituals, 149
   interruptions to, 148, 150–151
   labor phase, 147–148, 149–151
   rhythm and, 148, 152–153
   spontaneous rituals, 151–153
Rollover position, 319
Ruptured membranes. See Bag of waters.

Sedatives, 331, 332
Self-directed pushing, 166–167
Self-induction, 212–216
Sexual stimulation, induction and, 215
Shoulder dystocia, 260
Shoulder mini-massage, 188
Siblings, preparing for birth, 44–45
Sickle cell disease, 379
Side-lying position, 173, 222
Sleep
   bed-sharing, 407
   breastfeeding and, 407
   platoon sleeping, 396
   sleep deprivation, 394–395
Slow breathing, 162–163, 204
Slow-to-start labor, 216–221
Sounds
   breech presentation and, 228
   comfort and, 196
   communication with, 44
Spinal blocks
   combined spinal-epidural, 314, 337
   neuraxial analgesics, 309
   overview, 336
   severe bleeding and, 282
   technique for, 315–316
Spontaneous bearing down, 165–166
Squatting position, 37, 174
Standing and leaning position, 169
Standing lunge, 170, 222
Standing position, 169, 223
Stillbirth, 49–50
Strengthening exercises, 39–40
Stress hormones, 111, 122
Supplemental nursing system (SNS), 414
Supplies
   baby equipment, 52
   baby's homecoming, 34
   bedding, 52
   birth center trip, 35
   birth partner, 33–34

breast-feeding, 53
clothing, 52–53
formula-feeding, 54
health supplies, 53
home births, 35–36
hospital trip, 35
labor phase, 33
optional paraphernalia, 54
postpartum period, 34
Support groups, 56
Systemic drugs, 310–312

Take-Charge routine, 202–207
Testing
  Apgar test, 129, 244–245
  biotinidase deficiency, 379
  congenital adrenal hyperplasia
    (CAH), 379
  congenital hypothyroidism, 379
  fetal scalp stimulation test, 253
  gestational diabetes mellitus (GDM)
    screening, 277–278
  galactosemia, 379
  glucose tolerance test, 277–278
  Group B Strep (GBS) screening,
    240–241
  hearing screening test, 379
  heel-stick test, 378
  homocystinuria, 379
  maple syrup urine disease, 379
  medium-chain acyl-CoA dehydrogenase
    deficiency (MCAD), 379
  newborn screening tests, 378–379
  nonstress test, 242
  phenylketonuria (PKU), 379
  postpartum blood tests, 372–374
  questions for, 237
  sickle cell disease, 379
  ultrasonography, 105, 179, 229, 230,
    241–242
Three Rs, 147–153
"3 to 6 phase," 100
Thrush, 410
Tranquilizers, 333
Transcutaneous Electrical Nerve Stimulation (TENS), 185–186
Transition phase
  birth partner and, 113–114
  caregivers and, 112
  cervix and, 109–110

contractions, 109
doulas and, 114–116
duration of, 110
feelings, 110–111
overview of, 109–110
stress hormones and, 111
summary of, 140
urge to push, 110
Trial of Labor After Cesarean
  (TOLAC), 356
24-hour "cure," 412–413

Ultrasonography, 105, 179, 229, 230,
  241–242
Umbilical cord
  blood storage
  cord blood storage, 48, 366–367
  cutting, 133, 367, 369–371
  prolapsed cord, 290–292
  stump care, 378
Urge to push, 121
Urination, 316, 384–385
Uterus. See Contractions.

Vacuum extraction, 266–267, 323
Vaginal Birth After Cesarean (VBAC)
  benefits of, 357
  cesarean births and, 345
  challenge of, 362
  emotional concerns, 359
  fears, 359
  improving chances of, 358–359
  rate of, 345, 357
Verbena oil, for bowel stimulation,
  215–216
Versed (medication), 351
Visualization, 159–160
Vitamin K, 372

Walking
  as comfort measure, 169
  slow labor and, 223
  slow-to-start labor and, 214
Warming units, 374–375
Water births, 180
Water, breaking. See Bag of waters.

Zofran (medication), 351